FUNDAMENTALS AND FRONTIERS OF MEDICAL EDUCATION AND DECISION-MAKING

Fundamentals and Frontiers of Medical Education and Decision-Making brings together international experts to consider the theoretical, practical, and sociocultural foundations of health professions education.

In this volume, the authors review the foundational theories that have informed the early transition to competency-based education. Moving beyond these monolithic models, the authors draw from learning and psychological sciences to provide a means to operationalize competencies. The chapters cover fundamental topics including the transition from novices to experts, the development of psychomotor skills in surgery, the role of emotion and metacognition in decision-making, and how practitioners and laypeople represent and communicate health information. Each section provides chapters that integrate and advance our understanding of health professions education and decision-making.

Grounded in psychological science, this book highlights the fundamental issues faced by healthcare professionals, and the frontiers of learning and decision-making. It is important reading for a wide audience of healthcare professionals, healthcare administrators, as well as researchers in judgment and decision-making.

Jordan Richard Schoenherr is an Assistant Professor in the Department of Psychology, a member of the Applied AI Institute at Concordia University, an Adjunct Research Professor in the Department of Psychology, and a member of the Institute for Data Science at Carleton University, Canada.

Meghan M. McConnell is an Associate Professor in the Department of Innovation in Medical Education, and Department of Anesthesiology and Pain Medicine at the University of Ottawa, Canada.

FUNDAMENTALS AND FRONTIERS OF MEDICAL EDUCATION AND DECISION-MAKING

Educational Theory and Psychological Practice

Edited by Jordan Richard Schoenherr and Meghan M. McConnell

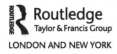

LONDON AND NEW YORK

Designed cover image: Photo by National Cancer Institute; Photo by Robina Weermeijer; Photo by Accuray–all courtesy of Unsplash

First published 2024
by Routledge
4 Park Square, Milton Park, Abingdon, Oxon OX14 4RN

and by Routledge
605 Third Avenue, New York, NY 10158

Routledge is an imprint of the Taylor & Francis Group, an informa business

British Library Cataloguing-in-Publication Data
A catalogue record for this book is available from the British Library

ISBN: 978-1-032-32662-7 (hbk)
ISBN: 978-1-032-32411-1 (pbk)
ISBN: 978-1-003-31609-1 (ebk)

DOI: 10.4324/9781003316091

Typeset in Optima
by Newgen Publishing UK

CONTENTS

ABOUT THE EDITORS

Meghan M. McConnell is an Assistant Professor in the Department of Innovation in Medical Education, and Department of Anesthesiology and Pain Medicine at the University of Ottawa, and is an Assistant Clinical Professor (Adjunct), Psychiatry & Behavioural Neurosciences. She received her doctorate in cognitive psychology from McMaster University and subsequently did two postdoctoral fellowships, the first at the Medical Council of Canada with a focus on psychometrics in high-stakes testing and the second at the University of British Columbia with a concentration in medical education. In 2013, she became an Assistant Professor in the Department of Clinical Epidemiology and Biostatistics at McMaster University. McConnell's research interests lie in three specific areas: (1) emotion research, where she studies the role that emotions and mood play in the training, assessment, and performance of health professionals, (2) educational research, where she studies the cognitive factors modulating learning and knowledge transfer, and (3) assessment research, where she studies the psychometrics of various types of general assessments and the evaluation of skills.

Jordan Richard Schoenherr is an Assistant Professor in the Department of Psychology, is a member of the Applied AI Institute at Concordia University, is an Adjunct Research Professor in the Department of Psychology, and is a member of the Institute for Data Science at Carleton University. Prior to the receipt of his PhD, he began his postdoctoral research in medical education at the University of Ottawa Skills and Simulation Centre. In addition to his academic duties, he has worked for, and consulted with, Health Canada (Office of the Chief Scientist) and the Public Health Agency of Canada (Ombudsman Integrity and Resolution Office) on science policy, science communication, and ethical decision-making. He is the author of the *Ethics of Artificial Intelligence from Popular Science to Cognitive Science* and numerous chapters, proceedings, and peer-reviewed articles that examine applications of decision-making to health, ethics, and cybersecurity. He is currently an Associate Editor for the journal IEEE Transactions on Technology and Society. Dr. Schoenherr's research and writing focuses on the cognitive psychology of learning and metacognition, history and logic of psychometrics, and the sociotechnical systems of higher education.

CONTRIBUTORS

Sandy Abdo is a PhD student in the Faculty of Science at Ontario Tech University, actively contributing as a member of Dr. Bill Kapralos and Dr. Adam Dubrowski's MaxSIMHealth research lab. Her doctoral research focuses on optimizing virtual learning environments, specifically exploring psychomotor-based simulation training for medical professionals. She is particularly passionate about enhancing the customization and personalization of simulation-based training to better meet the needs of individual learners.

Elif Bilgic is an Assistant Professor and Education Scientist in the department, with a cross-appointment at the McMaster Education Research Innovation and Theory (MERIT) program. She received her PhD from McGill University in Surgical Education and completed two postdoctoral fellowships at McGill; one at the Steinberg Centre for Simulation and Interactive Learning, and second at the Simulation, Affect, Innovation, Learning, and Surgery Lab, as a CIHR awarded fellow. Currently, Dr Bilgic's program of research is in the field of performance assessment in the simulation and clinical settings, focusing on technology, innovation, and collaboration, ensuring that trainees are gaining the necessary skills to provide the best patient care possible.

Bapujee Biswabandan is the research program manager at Health Research Services at McMaster University. With an M.Phil in Psychology of Education and a PhD in Education from the Ontario Institute for Studies in Education (OISE) at the University of Toronto, his scholarly work is deeply influenced by Vygotsky's sociocultural theories of learning which emphasize the crucial role of social interaction and cultural context in cognitive development, resonate throughout his research endeavors. His earlier experience includes training community health research workers in Sierra Leone, where he leveraged social frameworks to enhance data collection from local communities. With 15 years of expertise in both qualitative and quantitative research methodologies in low to middle-income countries, he has created various instructional tools, including training modules, infographics, and online teaching modules, all designed to facilitate learning through collaborative and culturally contextual practices. His works in research projects funded by organizations like UNICEF and UNESCO in India, involved leading community researchers in large-scale longitudinal studies, developing training modules for Indigenous teachers, and conducting workshops focused on language education, embodying Vygotsky's principles by integrating social and cultural dimensions into educational practices.

Alice Cavanagh completed concurrent medical and doctoral training at McMaster University in the Michael G. DeGroote School of Medicine and the Health Policy PhD Program. She also holds a Master's in Gender Studies and Feminist Research from McMaster. Alice's doctoral research used qualitative research methodologies to explore how healthcare providers learn to think about intimate partner violence in the course of their professional training. She is presently completing her residency training in family medicine at the University of Toronto.

Teresa Chan is an emergency physician and clinician educator and the founding Dean (School of Medicine) and Vice President (Medical Affairs) at Toronto Metropolitan University. She has previously served as the Director of the McMaster Clinician Educator AFC program and the Competence Committee Chairperson for the Emergency Medicine RCPSC Training Program. She has also been the Assistant Dean of Faculty Development and the Associate Dean of Continuing Professional Development for the Faculty of Health Sciences at McMaster University. She is also currently the national specialty committee chair for the Clinician Educator Area of Focused Competency Diploma program from the Royal College of Physicians and Surgeons of Canada (RCPSC) and holds multiple positions on the editorial boards of new (CanadiEM.org; ALiEM.com) and traditional (*Academic Medicine, JGME, Perspectives on Medical Education, AEM Education & Training* journals) scholarly outlets.

Daisy Minghui Chen is currently a digital pedagogy specialist at McMaster University in the CPD office. She has spent over ten years working collaboratively with teachers and adult learners in higher education, with dedication and commitment to developing learning designs that are pedagogically sound. She is passionate about bringing forward the best learning design practices to facilitate educational professionals, including teachers, instructional designers, and educational technologists to navigate a variety of pedagogies, resources, and tools to design a coherent learning experience for learners in different educational settings. Her pedagogical background includes adult learning theories and strategies, instructional design theories, and assessment and feedback design.

Adam Dubrowski is a Professor and Canadian Research Chair in Health-Care Simulation in the Faculty of Health Sciences, University of Ontario Institute of Technology. He began his research career by studying factors that influence the acquisition of clinical skills, particularly the methods used for optimizing simulation in medical education and training. In this work, he drew on program development and learning theories to evaluate and reshape existing simulation programs, and to develop new ones. As educational technology is constantly evolving, he have his research interests. He now studies the use of disruptive technologies such as virtual learning environments or three-dimensional printing and manufacturing to fill existing gaps in the availability of simulation technology that can help prepare and improve the retention of clinical skills.

Camila López Echagüe is an Assistant Professor at the Science and Development Unit of the Faculty of Science, University of the Republic (Uruguay). She has a degree in Philosophy, a Master's in Social Studies of Science and Technology, and is a PhD student in Logic and Philosophy of Science (University of Salamanca, Spain). Her area of interest is the study of public scientific-technological controversies from an STS approach, as well as the articulation between STS, philosophy, and science education.

Leanne Elliott is a PhD student in the Faculty of Health Sciences at Ontario Tech University. She is a member of Dr. Nick Wattie's Expertise & Skill Acquisition Lab and a recipient of the Vanier Canada Graduate Scholarship. Leanne's research investigates methods for simulation training optimization among medical professionals. She is particularly interested in exploring the effectiveness of the Mastery Learning approach for procedural skill retention and transfer. Leanne is also the owner of LA Power Skating where she directly applies her knowledge of skill acquisition science to her lesson plans and practice designs.

Fiorella Gago is an Assistant Professor at the Medical Psychology Department of the Faculty of Medicine and a researcher at the Science and Development Unit of the Faculty of Science, Universidad de la República (Uruguay). She has a degree in Psychology, a Master's in Public Policy (Universidad Católica del Uruguay), and is a master's student in Biology focusing on Neuroscience (Universidad de la República). Her current interest is the study of science and medical education, specifically on learning outcomes and cognitive processes as well as the evaluation of educational programs and policies.

Stanley J. Hamstra is a Professor and Vice-Chair of Clinical Teaching, Department of Surgery, University of Toronto, a Senior Scientist, Holland Bone and Joint Program, Sunnybrook Research Institute, and Adjunct Professor of Medical Education, Northwestern University, and a Research Consultant for the Accreditation Council for Graduate Medical Education. Hamstra's research addresses the link between graduate medical education and patient outcomes, using large national datasets. Stan continues to work with the ACGME, various medical specialty societies, program director organizations, and specialty certification boards to determine the predictive validity of ACGME milestones for early career performance following graduation. He also works on developing administrative support for educational scholarship and mentorship within academic health settings. Hamstra has had faculty positions at the University of Michigan and the University of Ottawa and continues to work closely with the Royal College of Physicians and Surgeons of Canada and other international accreditation bodies on competency-based medical education. Hamstra holds a PhD in visual neuroscience.

Marila Lázaro is an Adjunct Professor at the Science and Development Unit of the Faculty of Science, University of the Republic (Uruguay). She has a degree and Master's in Biology and a PhD in Philosophy Science Technology Society (University of Basque Country, Spain). Her area of interest is the development and evaluation of collective methods of learning and public deliberation on complex problems and scientific-technological controversies, as well as, in a transversal way, the inclusion of their ethical dimension.

Chel Hee Lee is a senior biostatistician working with the Department of Critical Care Medicine, University of Calgary & Alberta Health Services. He is also an Adjunct Assistant Professor in the Department of Mathematics and Statistics, University of Calgary, and is Co-director of the Data Science Advisory Unit. His research focuses on developing algorithms to quantify the uncertainty associated with clinical reasoning in diagnosis using imprecise probabilities. He has also contributed to the applications of classification and clustering, computational statistics, and Bayesian statistics in health services, metabolomics, and clinical decision systems using advanced statistical models, machine learning algorithms, and artificial intelligence.

Terence P. Ma is Assistant Dean for Assessment and Quality Improvement and Clinical Professor of Biomedical Sciences at the University of Houston Tilman J. Fertitta Family College of Medicine. He has a varied background in health sciences education including being a funded research scientist, faculty member, major course director, Department Chair, Assistant Dean, Associate Dean, and Chief Information Officer. He works in the areas of preclerkship medical education, assessment, program evaluation, accreditation, and technology. His work has focused on educational effectiveness, including the use of competencies. He is an anatomist by training with extensive teaching background in gross anatomy, embryology, and neurosciences. He has been active in developing novel approaches to help students learn anatomy including the use of immersive virtual dissections. The focus of his scholarly work is on the issue of how "we" know that students learned what the faculty said they would teach. Currently, he has been addressing how competency-based medical education can be implemented in preclerkship education and in how the entrustable professional activities resulting in microcredentials can be a model for skills-based learning and hiring. He has been a part of the development of competency standards, learning and employment records (LERs) standard, and health professions education curriculum exchange standards with MedBiquitous and with IEEE representing health sciences education. Additionally, he chairs the Open Competency Network, an international committee focused on competency structures supporting skills-based education and employment in the learner-earner ecosystem.

Julia Micallef is a PhD student in the Faculty of Health Sciences at Ontario Tech University and is a member of the maxSIMhealth lab run by Dr. Adam Dubrowski where she focuses on the designing and testing of simulators for healthcare professionals and trainees. Julia's doctoral work will focus on the development and pre-implementation of the Simulation Technologies, Educational Practices, and Scholarship (STEPS) program – a unique and first-of-its-kind program aiming to train health science students to become simulation assistants.

Dr. Sandra Monteiro is a Faculty of Health Sciences MERIT Scientist appointed to the Department of Medicine. She has a second appointment to the Centre for Simulation Based Learning as the Assistant Director of Simulation Scholarship. Dr. Monteiro is internationally recognized for her research program on clinical reasoning and her expertise in measurement principles and competency assessment. In a prior secondment to Touchstone Institute, (2014–2021), she served as the Director of Research and Analysis, and supported the development of several competency based assessments for various regulated healthcare professions in Canada. At McMaster University, she teaches and supervises students in various graduate programs, including Rehabilitation Sciences, Health Sciences Education and Psychology, Neuroscience and Behaviour. In 2021, she was recognized for her contributions to education and mentorship with a Canadian Association of Medical Education Meridith Marks New Educator Award.

Dr. Matthew Sibbald is an Associate Professor of Medicine, McMaster University and Interventional cardiologist at Hamilton Health Sciences and Niagara Health System. He is a clinician scientist at McMaster Education, Research, Innovation and Theory program with interests in simulation based education, competency based education, clinical reasoning and intravascular imaging. Matt graduated from University of Toronto with an MD in 2004, completing internal medicine and cardiology residencies at University of Toronto. He finished a fellowship in interventional cardiology at University Health Network 2013. He completed a Masters in Health Professions Education in 2011 and PhD in 2013 both from Maastricht University, Netherlands. He is currently director of the Centre for Simulation Based Learning in the Faculty of Health Sciences, cardiology residency program director at McMaster University, and chair-elect of the AFC committee for intervention cardiology at the Royal College of Physicians and Surgeons of Canada.

Mithusa Sivanathan graduated in the Masters of Health Science program at Ontario Tech University, specializing in simulator development methods. She has balanced the rigorous academic journey with a full-time role in the pharmacological industry. Drawing upon practical experience gained from industry, Mithusa bridged the gap between theory and application, ensuring that simulator advancements meet real-world pharmaceutical demands.

Jason Waechter is an intensivist and cardiac anesthesiologist. He has an interest in medical education and is founder of teachingmedicine.com which is a medical education website used at many medical schools in Canada and the United States. He was the Cardiovascular Course Director for 4 years at UBC and currently is very involved with curriculum design and teaching at the University of Calgary. His research interest is competency within medical education.

PREFACE

Personal Paths and Professional Practice

Health professions education is an interdisciplinary field, composed of professionals and practitioners with a variety of skills, expertise, and experience. Here, we provide a few of our personal experiences that led us to study the theoretical and empirical basis of medical decision-making and health professions education.

Like many, my (JRS) interest in the healthcare professions was based on experience. As a child, I was hospitalized with pneumonia for a week – though, it felt like an eternity. The name of the doctor who eventually released me stays with me to this day. The experience instilled respect in me for the medical profession and firmly set their power in our society in my mind. In my teens and twenties, I had undiagnosed sleep apnea. The doctors I would see sporadically at health clinics wrote off my fatigue and erratic sleeping as a function of "growing up" – something that I would overcome at some stage. Who was I to doubt them? As I entered graduate school, I eventually met a nameless clinician at a walk-in clinic who changed all this. He ordered a battery of tests to systematically exclude any possible disorders that might be producing my symptoms. With the diagnosis of sleep apnea and use of continuous positive airway pressure (CPAP), a foggy world became clear again. While I was forever grateful to him for his professionalism and evidence-based approach to medicine, the realization that diagnoses and recommendations – medical decision-making – could be so variable and uncertainty both intrigued and disturbed me.

My entry into, and interest in, health professions education and decision-making were hardly certain. I was merely a health seeker, reliant on the expertise of clinicians. In fact, my mother's reputation as a small-town elementary school teacher made education the last topic of interest to me.

My research focused on judgment, decision-making, reasoning, and learning through controlled experimentation. I drank the academic Kool-Aid and avoided applied questions other than to "pay the bills" while I worked in a science policy office (the Office of the Chief Scientist) at Health Canada. I'd even discounted an offer from a clinician at a sleep clinic I'd attended to examine the effect of apnea on attention. However, social networks have a way of influencing you that is not always immediately visible.

My cousin and his partner were both in healthcare (a nurse and doctor, respectively), and he'd always insisted that what I worked on was directly applicable to medical education. Eventually, I relented. He introduced me to the head of the ICU at a hospital in Ottawa. He (Dr. Pierre Cardinal) was a humble man with no sign of pretense. In addition to my surprise at his command of cognitive psychology, he also introduced me to new applied perspectives that I hadn't encountered during my degree.

Before I had completed my PhD, he urged me to talk to the medical director of the University of Ottawa Skills and Simulation Centre (uOSSC). During the first 30 minutes of that conversation, neither he nor I seemed to speak the same language. The conversation was fizzling. In retrospect, we had very different priorities that came from our respective professional backgrounds. While I had worked for and with Canada's federal health organizations (Health Canada, Public Agency of Canada), I examined science policy and medical research, not practice. The terminology I used for decision-making would have been well known to cognitive scientists, but is undoubtedly esoteric outside my field. Eventually, I uttered something about "diagnostic evidence". That keyword unlocked our conversation. After speaking to the research director (Dr. Stanley Hamstra), I was offered a position. He was perceptual psychologist and was interested in medical education as a social and philosophical system. I would later learn that he was one of a small cohort that had made the transition from perceptual and cognitive psychology to health professions education.

When I first stepped into the simulation center, I wore a three-piece suit. I watched the learners and educators interact, trying to understand how the learner–educator dyads worked. It was a place filled with research opportunities with diverse task and eager students (Figure 0.1). Almost immediately, a problem emerged: the learners often wanted to socialize with me. For young medical students, opportunities for training and learning were also opportunities for developing their social network and advancing their careers. Students weren't just interested in obtaining and demonstrating their competence; they wanted to integrate themselves into the social network of medicine. They were perhaps too concerned about "networking" with me. Within a few days, I adopted a more casual look: a collared shirt and blue jeans. The learners and most clinical educators began to ignore me. My

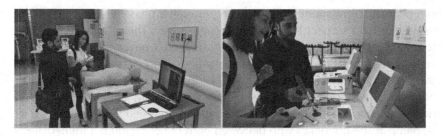

FIGURE 0.1 Simulation tasks performed at the simulation center as demonstrated by research assistants. Tasks include an ultrasound task with prefabricated mannequin (left) and laparoscopic trainers requiring the use of an endoscope and movement of rings between pegs (right).

observations now continued unnoticed, with one nurse educator remarking after my introduction "Oh, *you* don't look like a doctor!".

In another session, we used a laparoscopic cholecystectomy ("lap choly") trainer which had been developed by an interprofessional team: an experimental psychologist, a clinician, an engineer, and likely many technicians who constantly made contributions that often went unseen and unacknowledged. This task required that the learner would have to separate the gallbladder from the liver of a porcine specimen that was obtained from a local abattoir – pig gallbladders aren't in high demand in the culinary world.

When running the training activity, clinical educators would ask the odd student about their thoughts: Did this session help you? Did you have fun? Do you feel like you can perform this procedure better? Based on the social dynamic I'd observed previously, there was considerable pressure for socially desirable responses. The learners invariably said that it was a great experience, that they learned a lot, and that they felt more confident in performing the procedure. It wasn't clear to me that this kind of informal debriefing would provide the kind of feedback that would help shape the development of a task. It also raised doubts in me about the belief that high-fidelity simulations did much more than increase learner confidence (Schoenherr & Hamstra, 2024; Schoenherr et al., 2024) and impressed upon me the need for translational research in medical education (Schoenherr, 2024; Schoenherr & Hamstra, 2024).

My [MMM] interest in health professions education started with my mother. I grew up on the west coast of Canada in a small town of about 50,000 people, where my mum was a family physician. To say that my mum was highly regarded in our community is an understatement. As a child, anywhere we went, people would stop and talk to my mum for what seemed like forever in my young mind. As a teenager, I can remember several occasions where people stopped me as I walked down the street to say they recognized me from pictures in my mum's office (I went through a phase where I had bright purple hair, so I suspect I was easily recognizable). They would always tell me what a wonderful doctor my mum was, and I never quite knew what to say during these interactions. These dealings didn't stop after my mother moved away from the west coast. In my late 20s, I moved to Vancouver while completing my postdoctoral fellowship at the University of British Columbia, and the receptionist at my new dentist's office mentioned that I had the same last name as the physician who delivered both of her children. I immediately knew it was my mother. I'll always remember the smile on the receptionist's face as she gushed over how wonderful my mum had been to her and her children, and how much she missed my mother now that she had moved her practice to another province.

The reason my mother had such a powerful impact on her patients' lives is clear to me now, although I certainly didn't understand it when I was younger. She was invested emotionally in her patients. She cared for them deeply. She knew that people came to her in times of distress, and she wanted to help. But the compassion she had for her patients came with a cost, one that her patients did not see. I cannot count the number of times I found my mum crying silently for reasons she could not and would not share.

When I was about ten years old, I remember my mum picking me up from one of my extra-curricular activities. I was annoyed because she was late, which was a common occurrence. But my annoyance quickly subsided when I realized she had been crying. A patient of hers had died after a long battle with breast cancer; she was my mother's age and left behind two young daughters. The only reason I knew why my mum was upset was because I went to school with this woman's daughters and had found out earlier that day that their mother had passed away. Mum would never talk about her patients, as she took patient confidentiality very seriously. This meant mum was never able to share her pain with those close to her.

When I was in high school, another one of mum's patients, "Sandra", gave birth to little girl with hypoplastic heart syndrome, where half of her heart had not fully formed. Her baby would die at home just a few days later. The only reason I know about this story is because Sandra wrote a memoir about her life and described in detail how impactful my mother was during this difficult experience. Upon taking her baby girl home, my mum came to their house to explain to Sandra and her husband what to expect. She reminded them to take pictures of their baby girl, something that Sandra thought was futile at the time, but afterward, she was so grateful to have those photographs. Mum told them that when their baby passed away, they should call her and not 911, as the paramedics would only try to resuscitate the baby, and that would be of no benefit. When the baby died at 3:00 in the morning, my mother came over right away and sat with Sandra until the morning came. Mum called the funeral home for the family and only left because she needed to go to work. Sandra describes the day of the funeral, sitting in the front pew with her husband and young son, staring at a picture of her baby girl, a picture that she wasn't certain she would have taken had my mother not made that recommendation. My mum was late in arriving to the funeral, but Sandra insisted that the pastor wait until my mother arrived and asked mum to sit with her and her family. Again, I only know the details of this story because of Sandra's memoir. Sandra reached out to me as an adult and sent me a copy of her book, because she wanted me to know the impact my mother had on her life.

These two experiences are the few that I know the details about, because mum would never share the details of her work. She couldn't due to patient confidentiality, but even if she could, she wouldn't, as my mum was a deeply private person. I can only image what other stories my mother could tell. To say these experiences took an emotional toll on my mother is an understatement, to say the least. As a young child, I learned early on to give mum space when she came home. I was an incredibly energetic child, and every ounce of me would want to jump on my mother the moment she came through the door, to tell her about my adventures in excruciating detail. But mum simply didn't have to the emotional bandwidth to deal with my brothers and I after a long day at work. She needed time to decompress from her workday before she could deal with us. Many times, mum had to cancel plans with my brothers and me. Or she was late to pick me up. Or she was too tired to play. And for good reason – there was someone who was sick and in pain and my mum could help. But my young mind couldn't understand this. She was doing good in the world, but I was upset at her for it. I regret those feelings, but I was a child that didn't understand her perspective.

Many healthcare professionals – and their children – likely relate to this account. This portrayal of my mum does not imply that she was anything but a loving, wonderful mother. But the fact of the matter was that she – like many in healthcare – simply didn't have much emotional energy left for her family. If she could go back in time to start her medical practice over again, I have no doubt she would have done things differently. But she was never taught how to deal with the emotional aspects of medicine. She was from the generation of "detached concern", where the goal was to distance yourself from your patients and be an objective, cool-headed clinician. She was told to simply "find a closet to cry in" to deal with the emotional complexities embedded throughout in medical training and practice. Clearly, my mother didn't excel at emotional detachment from her patients, partly because she never fully agreed with that approach to doctor–patient interactions, but also because my mum was compassionate to a fault when she saw someone in distress. In a fashion typical for her, my mother has had to process a lot of guilt over her decision to spend her emotional energy on her patients rather than her children. And I am happy to say that she now has a phenomenal relationship with her children, and she is one of the strongest, most amazing people I know.

As a child, I was often asked whether I was going to be a doctor like my mum. Without hesitation, I would answer the question with an emphatic "No". I had witnessed firsthand the impact of being a doctor had on my mum's emotional well-being, and I had no desire to put myself through that. And while I didn't follow in my mum's footsteps, she undoubtedly impacted my career trajectory. I became fascinated by the emotional experiences of healthcare professionals, and how these emotions impacted all facets of their practice. I went on to get my PhD in cognitive psychology, where I studied the impact of emotions on cognitive processes in controlled, experimental settings. And while this research fascinated me, I wanted to move beyond the laboratory setting and examine how my dissertation research transferred to the real world. This led me to complete a postdoctoral fellowship with Dr. Kevin Eva, a world-renowned researcher in health professions education and clinical decision-making.

Kevin encouraged me to explore how emotions influenced clinical training and practice. I spent the first year of my fellowship talking to every doctor I could about how emotions impacted their practice. Funnily enough, the majority of them denied that emotions impacted their clinical performance. Like my mother, most of them were from the generation of "detached concern" – you were not supposed to show emotions, let alone them influence you. But when I asked physicians to talk to me about their emotional experiences during training and practice, the stories were rich and detailed. Most were negative. But all were clearly impactful. And so I started my career in health professions education.

Our book examines how healthcare professionals learn and make decisions. Many of the contributors here are, or have, conducted research in the psychological science. In fact, this volume is the result of the first editor (JRS) being asked to contribute an edited volume on medical decision-making to a series on perception and decision-making. When he began to solicit interest in the project from the co-editor (MMM) and colleagues, it became clear that there was ample quality content, but not all of it fit into the mold of *learning* and *decision-making*. Many of the proposals considered how the antecedent processes of learning are related to the conceptual foundations of learning (e.g., what are competencies in the healthcare professions), psychometrics issues (e.g., what is construct validity), and operationalizing these concerns (e.g., entrustable professional activities). Still more considered issues related to putting the empirical evidence into practice by examining how educational innovations and medical education programs were implemented at an institutional and national level (e.g., translational research, program evaluation, and medical pluralism).

The core of this book stems from cognitive psychology. Both editors (JRS and MMM) have backgrounds in cognitive psychology as do most of the contributors to this volume. Arguably, they share the same histories of starting in a highly theoretical field where precision is key to adapting and applying their knowledge to the fast and furious practices of the healthcare professions. Meeting at a conference, once JRS discovered the right "Meghan" he'd heard so much about; they kept in correspondence over the years. The COVID-19 pandemic and a mutated book proposal finally provided the opportunity for collaboration.

While directed toward academics, the book's intended audience is diverse. When assembling this volume, we wanted a book that could speak to fundamental issues faced by healthcare professionals and the frontiers of learning and decision-making yet remain accessible to a wide audience of healthcare professionals. Each section seeks to provide a basic background – outlining and defining basic terms and issues – while providing other chapters meant to integrate and advance our understanding of health professions education and decision-making. While no volume can capture all issues relevant to these domains, the book offers a representative – and diverse – sample. Many chapters that explored innovation, implementation, and medical pluralism in health professions education and healthcare delivery would come to form the core of a second volume (Schoenherr, 2024).

References

Schoenherr, J. R. (2024). *Fundamentals and frontiers in medical education and decision-making: Innovation, implementation, and translational research*. Routledge.

Schoenherr, J. R., & Hamstra, S. J. (2024). Validity in health professions education: From assessment instruments to program innovation and evaluation. In Schoenherr, J. R. & McConnell, M. (eds.), Fundamentals and Frontiers in Medical Education: Educational Theory and Psychological Practice. Routledge.

SECTION 1

Conceptual Issues

1

HUMAN-CENTERED DESIGN IN HEALTH PROFESSIONS EDUCATION

Informing Competency-Based Education with Psychological Science

Jordan Richard Schoenherr and Meghan M. McConnell

The healthcare professions occupy a central role in human societies. At their best, they preserve health and ameliorate illness, contributing to the physical and psychological well-being of communities and society. Beyond fundamental concerns of health and well-being, the healthcare professions are granted special access to financial, social, and material resources (Freidson, 1970; Starr, 1981; Sturdy & Cooter, 1998; Turner, 1995). The unique status granted to the health professions in contemporary society comes with the responsibility to deliver effective care, administer resources appropriately, and advocate for the health of their patients and communities (Board, 1999; Plochg et al., 2009; Rocks et al., 2020; Sturmberg et al., 2012). As we move into an era informed by 'big data' analytics and artificial intelligence (AI), concerns remain about candidate selection, the adequacy of a curriculum in identifying when learners' reach milestones, and how the outcomes of health professions education relate to patient care (Chahine et al., 2018; Mansouri & Lockyear, 2007; Patel et al., 2009; Patterson et al., 2016).

Undergirding all issues in health professions education is the need to identify competencies to develop effective assessment and educational interventions, that are informed by learners' abilities and constraints. Human-centered approaches to learning engineering present an effective means to achieve this, by balancing the needs of the learner with performance criteria and milestones developed around essential knowledge and skills (Thai et al., 2022; Schoenherr et al., 2023; Zoltowksi et al., 2012). By taking into consideration learners' affective, cognitive, and social responses, we can gain a better understanding of the factors that facilitate and interfere with the acquisition of knowledge and skills that define competencies in healthcare.

DOI: 10.4324/9781003316091-2

Adapting research from psychological sciences presents a valuable resource for educators and administrators.

Translating research findings from scientific studies to inform health professions education is not an easy task. Research in psychological science is directed toward generalizable knowledge about mental representations, mental processes, and their relationship to neuroanatomy and neurophysiology. In contrast, research in health professions education is directed toward applied questions such as identifying and delineating necessary competencies, milestones and entrustable professional activities (EPAs), evaluating the impact of training on the standard-of-care, and using human resources and learners' time efficiently.[1] As translational research, health professions education must adapt findings from controlled experimental studies to the human-centered clinical context and adapt findings from clinical settings to large-scale educational and healthcare delivery programs, with recognizable gaps in those programs informing what kind of bench science and clinical research should be conducted (Figure 1.1). In this volume, we focus on the relationship between basic educational theory and models and evidence derived from psychological science. A subsequent volume considers translational research and the problems of implementation in greater depth (Schoenherr, 2024a).

Medical Decision-Making as Core Competency. Decision-making is at the core of the healthcare professions. It requires that healthcare professionals accumulate evidence to inform their judgments and choose from among the available treatment options, while seeking closure to provide timely recommendations to patients, colleagues, and policymakers. This is not a solitary task. Healthcare professionals must work in teams, communicating and coordinating their activities in large social networks (Tasselli, 2015).

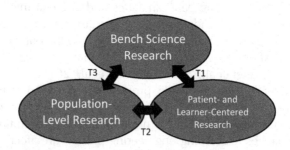

FIGURE 1.1 Typology of translational research practices in health professions education. T_1 research translates evidence from bench science research to patient-or learned centered research settings. T_2 research translates evidence from patient-or learned centered research to population-level research. T_3 translates population-level research to bench science research. Adapted from Rubio et al. (2010) and Schoenherr (2024).

Despite the common goal of providing the best care, each member of a healthcare team will have different knowledge and skills that must be brought together to achieve collective competence, such that the whole proves to be equal to, or more effective than, the sum of its member's competency (Schoenherr & Mahias-Ito, 2024). Psychological science provides a firm theoretical and empirical foundation that can help operationalize critical features of competencies and adapt to a human-centered approach to health professions education.

Competencies represent often complementary or overlapping sets of skills and knowledge (Batalden et al., 2002; Frank et al., 2010). Rather than being defined objectively, competencies are created by organizations that seek to represent and standardize the healthcare professions to provide an adequate standard-of-care (Boyd et al., 2018; Hawkins et al., 2015; Whitehead et al., 2011; Whitehead et al., 2015). These organizations can be regional, national, or international, varying in their degree of authority to monitor and regulate educational institutions (e.g., accreditation) or provide advice to healthcare professionals (e.g., Bedoll et al., 2021; van Zanten et al., 2008; Schoenherr & Beaudoin, 2024).

With the demands of the healthcare, it is unsurprising that health professions education is an interdisciplinary field focused on applied research (Gwee et al., 2013; O'Sullivan et al., 2010; Teodorczuk et al., 2017). Ideally, it combines educational research, anthropology and sociology, psychological science, as well as the innovation and implementation sciences. Rather than respecting disciplinary silos, broad questions and approaches must be adopted to provide educators with evidence-based practices that can be implemented within an institutional context (Schoenherr & Hamstra, 2024).

Despite claims of interdisciplinarity, health professions education typically draws from applied health and health professions education research literatures (Albert et al., 2020). Efforts to implement competency-based approach in education have historically met with difficulty due to failures to adequately identify and operationalize competencies (Morcke et al., 2013). This, the first of a two-volume series, is an attempt to integrate educational theory with the learning and psychological sciences (Volume I) with social, cultural, and innovation theory (Volume II).

No single work can capture the complexity of health professions education; however, critical features and insights can be highlighted to bridge these gaps. This volume addresses two themes in health professions education, each defining a different level of analysis. Section 1 considers how we formulate the problem of health professions education. The shift to competency-based education models requires the identification of skills and knowledge that are both individually necessary and jointly sufficient to ensure that healthcare professionals engage in effective practice. It considers the nature of competency, its operationalization and measurement, and the role of technology in health professions education and medical decision-making during implementation.

Beyond educational philosophies, frameworks, and principles, the development of effective curricula requires specific theories to assess competency development in learners. Effective learning engineering (e.g., educational interventions and assessment instruments) requires understanding the process of learning and how knowledge is represented and changed over time. Section 2 examines how to operationalize competencies using research in psychological science and health professions education. Rather than viewing competencies as abstract ideas, they must be grounded in the mental representations and processes that are used in practice. This section examines the nature of expertise in the healthcare professions, the process of psychomotor skill development, the role of affect and emotion in decision-making, and how the representations of health and illnesses can improve health communication in healthcare teams and social networks. In the remainder of this introductory chapter, we provide a basic overview of these themes.

1.1 From Apprenticeships to Competency-Based Education in the Health Professions

All human societies have developed their own indigenous approaches to healthcare (e.g., Chan, 2024; Venosa et al., 2024; Schoenherr, 2024; Schoenherr & Beaudoin, 2024). Humans are driven to find causal explanations within nature, to differentiate the 'normal' from 'abnormal'. Healers can be found in all societies. Traditionally, this knowledge was passed down in an idiosyncratic manner from mentor to mentee, defining an apprenticeship model. As institutionalized medicine emerged as a dominant social institution, establishing standards became paramount to reinforce a common professional identity and ensure consistency in practice (Freidson, 1970; Starr, 1982; Schoenherr & Beaudoin, 2024; Sturdy & Cooter, 1998; Turner, 1995).

Professional education and professionalization are not new concerns. In varied forms, the imperial examination system (Kējǔ) evolved in China for over a millennium which attempted to standardize education for entry into the civil service (Elman, 2000; Hu, 1984; Lai, 1970; Liu, 2018). Test-takers were rank-ordered based on their knowledge of classic texts on associated reasoning, moral norms, and conventions, permitting the selection of the most competent individuals. This approach to assessment had wide regional influence, with variants adopted in Korea, Japan, Vietnam (Kang, 1974; Ko, 2017; Liu, 2007) and possibly Western education traditions (Chang, 1942; Deng, 1943). Health professions education emerged as a parallel social system, based on an apprenticeship model (Deng, 1990; Schoenherr & Beaudoin, 2024). While more unsystematic and comparatively recent, a similar evolution is observed in the Western tradition of health professions education, initially defined by a division between academic doctors and surgeons representing a distinction between theory and practice (Custers & ten Cate, 2018; Starr, 1982).

In the history of the healthcare professions in Europe (e.g., Granshaw & Porter, 1989) and North America (e.g., Starr, 1982), historical trends in disciplinary specialization increased the importance of the hospital as a locus of education. Early efforts resulted in the introduction of standards and a centralized approach for the accreditation of universities as teaching institutions (e.g., Beck, 2004; Duffy, 2011; Flexner, 1910/2002), a process defined by the negotiation of roles, increased social stratification, and established physicians in a position of dominance relative to other professions (e.g., Coburn, 1988; Coburn et al., 1983; Freidson, 1970; Sinclair, 1997; Starr, 1981; Strauss et al., 1963; Turner, 1995). However, these standards were necessarily general. In the learning context, medical experts were deemed to have specialized knowledge of their profession, and this was reasoned to be adequate for teaching. For instance, the idea of 'see one, do one, teach one' often attributed to William Stewart Halstead reflects a training method wherein the learner observes a clinician perform a task and then practices on patients until they are proficient.

Retrospectively, this approach to education has come to be known as the 'apprenticeship model' (e.g., Rodriguez-Paz et al., 2009; Vozenilek et al., 2004) or 'time-based' approach to health professions education (e.g., Frank et al., 2010; Mazmanian & Davis, 2012; Shah, 2016). It is the focus on the development of practical knowledge that is often contrasted with a scientific approach to evidence-based decision-making (Marckmann, 2001). While occurring in unique settings (e.g., academic hospitals, clinics), apprenticeships are a common feature of healer training across cultures (e.g., Hsu, 1999; Walsh, 1994; for East Asian examples, see Schoenherr & Beaudoin, 202; for discussion of European guilds, see Ackernecht, 1984; Himmelmann, 2007). Table 1.1 presents a generalized list of features of this educational model.

The apprenticeship model can be conceived of as a folk theory of expertise defined by a simple continuum based on the similarity of a learner to an 'expert' prototype by educators. With sufficient attention and time, learners could acquire the necessary knowledge and practical skills through observation, emulation, and conformity through clerkships/apprenticeships. Medical errors could be understood as deviations from the methods of the clinician providing the instruction (Bosk, 1979; Lester & Tritter, 2001; Sinclair, 1997).[2] Moreover, the recognition that multiple approaches to treatment were permissible emphasized the autonomy of practice of an individual clinician, as well as the importance of the preceptor–learner relationship. In later stages of this paradigm, greater emphasis was placed on summative testing to assess

TABLE 1.1 Description of Approaches to Healthcare Professions Education

Traditional Approaches	Competency-Based Approaches
Expertise is based on specialized knowledge that produces intuitions.	Expertise is based on specific, identifiable competencies in relevant domains.
Expert-based knowledge transfer through learner conformity and teacher authority.	Competency-based knowledge transfer through validated learning and assessment methods.
With sufficient time and attention, learners will acquire expert knowledge.	Learning is dependent on the nature of the tasks used to train and available assessment instruments.
Unmediated assessment wherein only experts are qualified to determine whether novices have achieved an adequate level of performance.	Mediated assessment wherein specialized tools must be tested and have sufficient evidence to support their validity.
Training conduct by healthcare professionals.	Training conduct by education and healthcare experts.
Idiosyncratic.	Standardized.
Standardized tests determine entry into expert-level training.	Quantifiable outcomes based on assessment instruments. Qualitative assessments.
Expert intuitions determine expertise of learners.	Diverse quantity and quality of evidence demonstrating a pattern of expertise.

learners' medical expertise. However, with ill-defined knowledge and skills, idiosyncratic apprentice-teacher relationships, and variability in the kinds of cases that a learner is exposed to during the period of an apprenticeship, such approaches to training will produce inconsistent learner outcomes. Consequently, these traditional methods of education have been framed using the 'tea steeping' metaphor.

More recently, effort have been made to formalize this process. The goal of the 'cognitive apprenticeship' is to make the often implicit (tacit) knowledge of experts explicit to facilitate communicate with leaners. Learning is framed as a guided experience to develop both cognitive and metacognitive abilities (Collins et al., 1998). This is achieved through modelling expertise-in-use, coaching and social scaffolding, exploration of the problem space, and articulation and reflection that motivate explicit and controlled use of knowledge and skills (for discussions in medical education, see Stalmeijer et al., 2010; Stalmeijer et al., 2013; for reviews, see Lyons et al., 2017). Crucially, this approach leaves the specific competencies as well as the methods of assessment underspecified.

Relative to these traditional education approaches, competency-based medical education (CBME) is considered a 'paradigm shift'. CBME requires that expertise in the healthcare professions can be divided into specific *competencies* such as those defined by the Accreditation Council for Graduate Medical Education (ACGME) in the United States and the World Health Organization (WHO) or *roles* such as those defined by the Royal College of Physicians and Surgeons of Canada (RCPSC), which can be further subdivided into skills that can be assessed with appropriate tools. However, the extent to which competency-based approaches reflect a true paradigm defined by theory, methods, and data and whether a paradigm shift has occurred remains to be seen. By translating and adopting the theory, methods, and findings of psychological science, a more compelling argument can be made for a coherent evidence-based educational paradigm.

Competency-Based Education in the Healthcare Professions. Within recent decades, educators have recognized the need to identify specific skills and knowledge required for clinical practice, as well as ways to assess and document the progression of such skills and knowledge throughout training. In the United States and Canada, the ACGME and RCPSC have developed related frameworks that define the general competencies and roles, respectively, that learners should demonstrate. More recently, the World Health Organization has released its own competency-based framework that attempts to generalize this to all health professionals (WHO, 2022). Despite differences in terminology, the competency-based approaches share many features. Arguably, the competencies and roles related to medical expertise/ knowledge, communication, systems-based approaches and collaboration, and professionalism are inseparable. However, depending on the role that healthcare professionals occupy, they will likely have need for different competency profiles (Schoenherr, 2020).

Dissimilarities in these frameworks must not be deemphasized. For instance, the competency-based approaches of the ACGME and WHO stress *individual characteristics*, whereas the role-based approach of the RCPSC refers to skills that are defined relative to a healthcare professional's *relationships* with those around them. The ACGME guidelines are also directed toward residents, whereas the RCPSC guidelines refer to physicians and, despite the organizations' name, do not explicitly refer to surgeons. However, this difference is likely attributable to the ACGME framework being based on the development of milestones for residency. In comparison to the approaches adopted by the ACGME and RCPS, the WHO framework is more closely aligned with ACGME. Moreover, this model assumes that competencies are defined by behaviors with *competence* reflecting a 'holistic measure of performance' (WHO, 2022, p. 10). Table 1.2 presents the competencies, roles, and their definitions across the three frameworks.

As is clear from Table 1.2, there are numerous similarities among the frameworks. At a general level, competency-based approaches emphasize the importance of operationalization, the need to translate an abstract concept (e.g., communicator) into more specific behaviors. However, this is not always achieved. As Monteiro and McConnell (2024) recently demonstrated in a 12-station objective structured clinical examination (OSCE) that assessed the same ten competencies at each station, ratings of different competencies were strongly correlated within training station, whereas weaker correlations were observed for the same competency assessed at the same station. Such studies suggest that competencies are often not adequately delineated.

One common means to operationalize competencies is the concept of an entrustable professional activity (EPA), which reflects the belief that a learner has achieved a professional milestone that is essential for independent practice (e.g., Ma, 2024).[3] This requires the development of effective assessment instruments to determine whether learners have sufficiently attained specific knowledge or skills within a particular domain or task. Entrustment scales have been developed in many clinical settings to measure the actual practice of learners (Dubois et al., 2021; George et al., 2014; Halman et al., 2018; Mink et al., 2018; Rekman et al., 2016; Warm et al., 2014; Warm et al., 2016; Weller et al., 2014; Weller et al., 2017). Despite these advances, we must also note that competencies and milestones reflect *minimal* criteria rather than a standard of excellence, with competencies defined along continua (Blömeke et al., 2015).

A major restriction of the multiple definitions of competency, including that of the WHO, is that they focus on an individual and neglects the social networks that define healthcare delivery. Consequently, we must also consider *collective competency*, the extent to which a group of individuals can effectively perform a task (Lingard, 2012). While this term itself is abstract, it can be operationalized in terms of communication skills at an individual level and transactive memory on a group-level (Schoenherr & Mahias-Ito, 2024; Schoenherr & Le-Bouar, 2024). Transactive memory represents the extent to which a defined group of individuals can collectively perform a task effectively, based on their mutual awareness of the competencies of other team members (Hollingshead, 1998; Lewis & Herndon, 2011; Peltokorpi, 2008; Wegner, 1987). Thus, collective competence is evidenced by effective gathering and sharing of information, coordination, and delegation of activities in the delivery of healthcare. New methods of assessment are required to capture improvements in knowledge and skills (Lockyear et al., 2017).

TABLE 1.2 ACGME, RCPSC, and World Health Organization (WHO) Competencies

ACGME (Competencies)	RCPSC (Roles)	WHO (Competency Domains)
Medical Knowledge Residents must be able to demonstrate knowledge about established and evolving biomedical, clinical, and cognate (e.g., epidemiological and social-behavioral) sciences and the application of this knowledge to patient care.	**Medical Expert** As medical experts, physicians integrate all of the CanMEDS Roles, applying medical knowledge, clinical skills, and professional values in their provision of high-quality and safe patient-centered care. Medical expert is the central physician role in the CanMEDS framework and defines the physician's clinical scope of practice.	**Decision-Making (2)** Competencies related to the approach to decision-making.
Professional Residents must be able to demonstrate a commitment to carrying out professional responsibilities, adherence to ethical principles, and sensitivity to a diverse patient population.	**Professional** As professionals, physicians are committed to the health and well-being of individual patients and society through ethical practice, high personal standards of behavior, accountability to the profession and society, physician-led regulation, and maintenance of personal health.	**Evidence-Informed Practice (5)** Competencies related to the generation of evidence and information and their integration into practice.
Interpersonal and Communication Skills Residents must be able to demonstrate interpersonal and communication skills that result in effective information exchange and teaming with patients, patients' families, and professional associates.	**Communicator** As communicators, physicians form relationships with patients and their families* that facilitate the gathering and sharing of essential information for effective healthcare.	**Communication (3)** Competencies related to effective communication.
Systems-Based Practices Residents must be able to demonstrate an awareness of and responsiveness to the larger context and system of healthcare and the ability to effectively call on system resources to provide care that is of optimal value.	**Collaborator** As collaborators, physicians work effectively with other healthcare professionals to provide safe, high-quality, patient-centered care.	**Collaboration (4)** Competencies related to the practice philosophy of teamwork.

(Continued)

TABLE 1.2 (Continued)

ACGME (Competencies)	RCPSC (Roles)	WHO (Competency Domains)
Patient Care and Procedural Skills Residents must be able to provide patient care that is compassionate, appropriate, and effective for the treatment of health problems and the promotion of health.	**Leader** As leaders, physicians engage with others to contribute to a vision of a high-quality healthcare system and take responsibility for the delivery of excellent patient care through their activities as clinicians, administrators, scholars, or teachers.	**Personal Conduct (6)** Competencies related to self-governed behaviors.
Practice-Based Learning and Improvement Residents must be able to investigate and evaluate their patient care practices, appraise and assimilate scientific evidence, and improve their patient care practices.	**Health Advocate** As health advocates, physicians contribute their expertise and influence as they work with communities or patient populations to improve health. They work with those they serve to determine and understand needs, speak on behalf of others when required, and support the mobilization of resources to effect change.	**People-Centeredness (1)** Competencies related to the provision of health services that incorporate perspectives of individuals, caregivers, families, and communities as participants in and beneficiaries of health systems.
	Scholar As scholars, physicians demonstrate a lifelong commitment to excellence in practice through continuous learning and by teaching others, evaluating evidence, and contributing to scholarship.	

Note: WHO Competencies are numbered in order listed in WHO (2022).

Despite the claims of a paradigm shift, the CBME approach is neither the dominant nor the sole educational paradigm used in the health professions. Many challenges are evidenced in terms of how to operationalize and implement competency frameworks (Epstein & Hundert, 2002; van Der Vleuten & Schuwirth, 2005; Wass et al., 2001). Healthcare professionals, educators, and administrators cannot simply replace one learning paradigm for another, i.e., the problem of de-implementation (Prasad & Ioannidis, 2014; Prusaczyk et al., 2020; Schoenherr, 2024b; van Bodegom-Vos et al., 2017). The clear benefit of CBME is that by making knowledge and skills concrete and measurable, they can be used as a common standard for educators. Yet, many logistical issues remain in terms of developing and delivering assessment opportunities for learners who are accurate, reliable, and providing sufficient feedback while avoiding assessment fatigue. Moreover, while the prospective benefits of learning analytics are appealing, simply having data is insufficient to assessment competence (Bilgic et al., 2024). Data must be labeled, cleaned, and issues arising from missing data must be addressed prior to analysis, regardless of whether educators are considering single experiments, programs, and large data sets (McConnell et al., 2016; Schoenherr & Michael, 2024). Indeed, overreliance on quantification has led to criticism of psychometrics as an effective approach to assessment clinical competence (Hodges, 2013; cf. Schoenherr & Hamstra, 2016), extending to concerns in the development and use of AI (e.g., Chellen et al., 2019; Cirrillo et al., 2020; Kim et al., 2023; Schoenherr, 2022a).

In psychological science, the abstract abilities, knowledge, attitudes, emotions, and motivations are referred to as *construct*. Stakeholders in health professions education must ensure that they understand the constructs that define a competency, how they have been operationalized, the context in which data has been collected, and how it is used to inform the development of educational activities, as well as curriculum and program development (Ma, 2024; Schoenherr, 2024b; Schoenherr & Hamstra, 2024). For instance, while a task might work in a teaching hospital in one country, it might be less effective in other settings due to differences in educator familiarity with pedagogical technique, material and financial resources, or conventions, roles, and norms within a community (Schoenherr, 2024d; Schoenherr & Beaudoin, 2024).

Frameworks for Competency Assessment. Any successful attempt to shift to a CBME program requires identifying education and assessment principles. Yet, frameworks are highly conceptual, developed by consensus and interpersonal agreement within a community of practitioners or institutional committees. They need not adequately specify the features of skills and knowledge to a sufficient degree to *operationalize* specific competencies to allow for observation or measurement. Even if informed by popular educational frameworks, there is no guarantee that a task adequately assesses competence. Instead, a need remains to make direct and explicit links with psychological sciences to create a successful human-centered approach to learning engineering.

Perhaps the most prominent model within health professions education is Bloom's taxonomy (Anderson & Kratwohl, 2001; Bloom et al., 1956; Kratwohl, 2002; for further discussion, see Ma, 2024). Rather than focusing on the development of affective (McConnell, 2024) or psychomotor skills (Abdo et al., 2024), Bloom's taxonomy considers the development of *general* cognitive processes from those which are comparatively concrete and simple to those which are abstract and complex: knowledge acquisition, comprehension, application, analysis, synthesis, and evaluation.

Despite the intuitive simplicity of Bloom's taxonomy, cognitive science defines expertise in terms of the interaction between decision-making systems and knowledge structures. Along these lines, Kratwohl (2002) refined Bloom's taxonomy by distinguishing between two facets[4] of cognition: mental processes and mental representations.[5] Table 1.3 provides a summary of these dimensions. However, much like Bloom's original taxonomy, the underlying cognitive domains are not specified and do not necessarily correspond to processes distinguished in cognitive science, reflecting a similar approach as apprenticeship. The specifics of sensory modalities, working memory, attentional networks, and problem-solving are not directly addressed in a manner that would help inform educators and learning engineers to design

TABLE 1.3 Krathwohl's Modified Learning Taxonomy

Cognitive Representations	*Cognitive Prcocesses*
Factual Knowledge: The basic elements that learners must know to be acquainted with a discipline or solve problems in it.	**Remember**: Retrieving relevant knowledge from long-term memory.
	Understand: Determining the meaning of instructional messages, including oral, written, and graphic communication.
Conceptual Knowledge: The interrelationships among the basic elements within a larger structure that enable them to function together.	**Apply**: Carrying out or using a procedure in a situation.
Procedural Knowledge: How to do something; methods of inquiry, and criteria for using skills, algorithms, techniques, and methods.	**Analyze**: Breaking material into its constituent parts and detecting how the parts relate to one another and to an overall structure or purpose.
	Evaluate: Making judgments based on criteria and standards.
Metacognitive Knowledge: Knowledge of cognition in general as well as awareness and knowledge of one's own cognition.	**Create**: Putting elements together to form a novel, coherent whole or make an original product.

or assess educational interventions. As we discuss below, this is especially concerning given that these systems interact to determine information gathering, diagnosis, treatment recommendations, and interpersonal communication.

An alternative model of skill acquisition in health professions education was developed by Dreyfus and Dreyfus (1980). Learners are assumed to pass through five stages of skill development: novice, competence, proficiency, expertise, and mastery. As learners progress through these stages, recollection, recognition, decision-making processes, and awareness are defined by fundamental shifts in performance. The novice skill-level is defined by abilities that are not adapted to specific situations, and problems are decomposed and analytic decision-making processes dominate with self-observation and feedback driving skill development. By the time a learner has reached the mastery level, his performance is defined by contextual-bound recollection, wholistic pattern recognition, intuitive decision-making, and low levels of monitoring. Despite failing to address specific interactions between systems, this model does capture robust patterns of skill development. Research in psychomotor skills (Abdo et al., 2024) and diagnostic reasoning (Schmidt et al., 1990) qualify these findings, demonstrating the process of automaticity and how experts must assess trade-offs between speed and accuracy while avoiding being misled by overconfidence (Schoenherr et al., 2024).

Finally, Miller (1990) has developed another influential framework that considers the development of clinical competence, skills, and performance. Defined by a pyramidal structure, *knowledge* provides the foundation that can be assessed using standardized testing to determine how much a learner knows. Building on this foundation, *competence* assumes that the learner knows how to apply this knowledge. Assessment of this level requires examining reasoning skills, information search, synthesis, and implementation. Miller notes that traditional examinations can address these skills, while leaving open the question of whether competencies can be applied in realistic settings. He refers to this next level as *performance*, whereby learners demonstrate that they can behaviors in an appropriate manner when presented with a specific scenario. Here, specific skills and competencies can be assessed in whole or part by using simulation studies that vary in their degree of perceived realism ('fidelity'). The final level of assessment concerns whether the learner independently engages in behaviors that are appropriate to the task, i.e., professional activities (Ma, 2024; WHO, 2022). Here, the healthcare professional must be observed in the real world. Despite the ubiquitous use of Miller's pyramid, like other learning frameworks, it has been criticized on the grounds that it also lacks specificity (Kahlke et al., 2020; Witheridge et al., 2019) and is not aligned with contemporary empirical studies.

The emphasis placed on performance assessment has led to an increased need to include simulation in health professions education. Here, educators often assume that high-fidelity simulation (e.g., realistic mannequins, mock-up operating rooms, virtual reality) are ideal means to providing learners with a realistic training experience that will produce transferrable knowledge and skills. While technology can enhance learning outcomes (Cook et al., 2011), critical theoretical reviews (Dieckmann et al., 2007; Hamstra et al., 2014; Norman et al., 2012; Schoenherr & Hamstra, 2017) and empirical studies (Liu et al., 2013; Massoth et al., 2019; Matsumoto et al., 2002; de Giovanni et al., 2009; Sidhu et a., 2007) have repeatedly reinforce that 'fidelity' is not a meaningful criterion to evaluate learning interventions and assessment instruments. This insight is also critical in that simulation might be disproportionately expensive, making such instructional interventions inaccessible to countries and healthcare institutions that have comparatively limited funds (Schoenherr, 2024b). Moreover, questions remain concerning the extent to which skills learned in simulations are in fact transferable to practice (Grierson, 2014). Instead, learning engineers, educators, and program administrators must question whether their approach to assessment and training is *valid* based on theoretical and empirical information from the learning and psychological sciences (Messick, 1995).

Even if an educational activity or assessment instrument is adequately designed, it must be compatible with learning objectives while also fitting into a programmatic context. In this volume, Schoenherr and Hamstra (2024) review the concept of construct validity and contrast it with implementation validity. Construct validity requires that evidence is accumulated about learner performance from an educational intervention or assessment instrument and that this evidence is used in a validity argument to demonstrate that instructional designers have adequately sampled tasks from a target domain (e.g., neonatology would include reasoning, empathy, and communication skills; ultrasound diagnostics would include psychomotor skills, reasoning, visualization capabilities). However, these educational activities must be embedded within a curriculum, thereby requiring that educational program developers critically evaluate whether a task occupies a distinct niche relative to other educational interventions and assessments within a program and that they can be sustained with appropriate human, financial, and material resources.

By identifying tasks with construct validity that can be administered in a principled and consistent manner within a program, educational institutions are then able to employ sophisticated learner analytics. Beyond accurately and adequately capturing learner performance, learning analytics also requires critical reflection on how data are presented in the form of visualization, as visualizations and graphical perception can affect interpretation and perceived accuracy (e.g., Schoenherr & Davies, 2009). In the health professions, learning analytics can consider educational and clinical outcomes, how performance changes during training, transition to practice, and practice on multiple levels (e.g., macro, meso, or micro; Hall et al., 2021). In this volume, Bilgic et al. (2024) review and provide recommendations as to how learning analytics can be applied in admissions, undergraduate health professions education, postgraduate health professions education, continuing professional development, and health systems. As health professions education begins to adopt new learning technologies, learning analytics provide an indispensable set of techniques to help shape and maintain quality education programs. They are not a panacea, as the validity of the data collection, processing, and presentation must be considered.

Paralleling advancements in learning analytics, learning engineering has advanced considerably within recent decades, largely driven by a variety of approaches collectively referred to as artificial intelligence (AI). Beyond relatively common techniques such as virtual reality training (Barteit et al., 2021; Baniasadi et al., 2020; Pottle, 2019), adaptive instructional systems (AIS) and intelligent tutoring systems (ITS) can tailor instruction to the learner, realizing the notion of social scaffolding[6] (Schoenherr, 2020). However, the accuracy and validity of these methods remains an open question (Schoenherr & Michael, 2024). For instance, recent interest in generative AI such as large language models (LLM; e.g., ChatGPT) has been tempered with realizations that while replicating the content and structure of human performance, many of the products are inaccurate. Illustrating this, Kim et al. (2023) presented vignettes to ChatGPT-4 and Bard that controlled for differences in the standard-of-care based on race/ethnicity, gender, and socioeconomic status. They found discrepancies both between the recommendations of the two chatbots and between the clinicians and chatbots' recommendations based on race and gender. These observations also introduce many ethical questions in terms of when, where, and who uses AI-based learning technologies as well as who benefits from their use (Schoenherr et al., 2023). It remains clear then that the frontiers of health professions education must be informed by fundamental theories and issues of psychometrics and psychological science.

We must also consider how health professionals adopt AI in their practice as it will also affect patients. How health information seekers gather and use information raises important questions that must be addressed by the healthcare professions such as how to address disinformation and competing recommendations. More training and education need to consider how health information seekers in the clinic and the public understand disease. In addition to understanding the mental models of disease and illness maintained by health information seekers (Schoenherr & Le-Bouar, 2024), healthcare professionals must understand how medical beliefs are shaped by cultural traditions (Schoenherr, 2024b; Schoenherr & Beaudoin, 2024) and novel technologies (Schoenherr, 2022a, 2022b; Schoenherr et al., 2023).

1.2 Learning and Decision-Making in the Health Professions

To operationalize competencies in human-centered design, educators must be able to identify the mental representations and processes that constitute a given competency or EPA. Decision-making in the healthcare professions requires the integration of multiple sources and types of information including understanding probability, assessing the accuracy and reliability of information, using multivariate information, engaging in differential diagnosis, communicating this information to other healthcare professionals and patients, and using information acquired from others to adjust their own diagnoses, recommendations, and the clinical and social environment.

Psychological science emerged as a discipline focused on learning and decision-making, with some of the earliest experiments identifying stages of mental processing (Donders, 1868), the operations of memory systems (Ebbinghaus, 1885), and distinguishing conscious from unconscious knowledge (Pierce & Jastrow, 1884). Fundamental features include attention and working memory limitations (Cowan, 2001; Miyake & Shah, 1999), distinct attention functions including capture, task-switching, and regulation (Fan et al., 2002), and increased automaticity in practice that results from extensive training over time (Schneider & Shiffrin, 1977; Logan, 1988) leading to the rapid use of available and recognizable patterns (Gigerenzer & Goldstein, 2011; Klein, 1993). Expertise isn't simply about responding quickly. Contemporary models of learning and decision-making assume that multiple processes contribute to our behavior (Evans & Stanovich, 2013; Kahneman & Klein, 2009), with each system competing for activation during response selection (e.g., Ashby et al., 1998; Logan, 1988). An effective human-centered approach to learning engineering in health professions education requires taking these cognitive processes and responses into account.

A broad distinction can be made between fast, automatic processes ('Type 1') and slow, deliberate processes ('Type 2'; Figure 1.2). Research suggests that, when presented with a novel task, learners rely on effortful learning processes defined by testing simple hypotheses, e.g., 'Is cancer associated with alcohol consumption?', 'Is the intestinal cramping experienced by the patient a result of polyps blocking a portion of their bowel?'. In parallel, associative learning mechanisms accumulate traces that are integrated into more complex rules based on feedback, e.g., experience clinical intuitions that merely suggest the patient is 'sick', a perceived mismatch, or leaps of abductive reasoning (O'Neill et al., 2021; Vanstone et al., 2019).

The two kinds of cognitive processes are neuroanatomically distinct and susceptible to different kinds of task-based interference: Type 1 processes are affected by feedback delays, whereas Type 2 processes are affected by the availability of attention and working memory capacity of the learner (Ashby

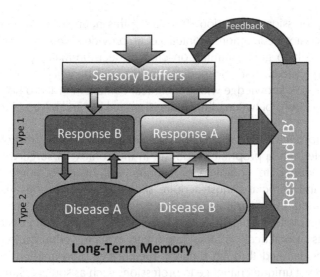

FIGURE 1.2   Model of learning and decision-making. A stimulus (patient, diagnostic test, illness narrative, health message, etc.) is presented to the learner, clinician, or health information seeker. Sensory information is processed, activating information in long-term memory with a subset of information kept active in working memory. In experts, attention is drawn to diagnostically relevant features due to chronically accessible representations in long-term memory, leading to more efficient exchanges of information in working memory. Once enough evidence is accumulated based on accuracy or speed criterion, the decision-maker responds. The response solicits feedback from the environment and the decision-maker processes it implicitly and/or explicitly.

& Valentin, 2017). Health professions education must account for how these systems cooperate and compete during learning and healthcare delivery.

Expertise Development. Medical expertise tends to be defined as a form of *pattern recognition*. Whether in terms of proprioceptive information gathered during a physical examination, assessing the size and shape of subdermal tissue, or the assessment of results from blood work or cardiac monitoring, learners must organize evidence into mental representations. Pattern recognition is determined by the learner's ability to encode, store, and retrieve information effectively and efficiently. This reflects a process of automaticity (Ashby et al., 1998; Logan, 1988). Automaticity reflects a major facet of expertise, one that is often taken to be the defining feature. In this volume, Monteiro et al. (2024) examine the transition from medical student (novice) to experienced clinician (expert). Building on neuroscientific research, they argue that models of experience-dependent learning and neuroplasticity that characterize early childhood development can also be applied to adults learning a new skill in health professions education. Translating this neuroscientific evidence to health professions education, Monteiro et al. provide several 'decision-tuning strategies' to help guide training on clinical decision-making. For instance, novice learners (e.g., first-year medical students) will benefit from instructor-led framing of book knowledge within a clinical context in order to help learners make connections between clinical decision-making and basic science.

Psychomotor Skills. Once a pattern has been identified, healthcare professionals need to select an appropriate response. In the context of surgery, the motor program required to complete procedures will be exceedingly complex. Surgeons and clinicians must acquire skills that involve both visuospatial reasoning and the coordination of sensorimotor systems, e.g., physician examination methods such as auscultation, palpitation, and percussion. While many areas of practices are associated with explicit, verbalizable processes that can be learned through didactic methods, motor, implicit, nonverbal skills present a unique challenge to professions such as surgery. Surgical skills require a high degree of technical proficiency, integrating sensorimotor skills to perform complicated surgical procedures. For instance, minimally invasive surgical (MIS) techniques such as laparoscopy require surgeons to indirectly monitor the anatomy and physiology of patients, while using visual and proprioceptive feedback to cut, cauterize, and suture. The learner is faced with a dynamic system that they must master which cannot necessarily be captured in declarative knowledge transmitted through didactic lectures.

The earliest models of psychology suggested that more complex task represents a combination of simpler tasks (Donders, 1868; Sanders, 1980). Using this logic, to acquire complex clinical skills, tasks can be analyzed, and the individual elements can be presented to learners (e.g., verbal protocol analysis; Hoffman et al., 2009; Korovin et al., 2020; cf. Hamm, 2004). Over time, the elements of a task become associated and activate seamlessly from start to completion, i.e., automaticity. This has been a persistent focus in psychomotor skill acquisition (e.g., Fitts & Posner, 1967) and its application to surgical skill development (Kopta, 1971; Resnick & McRae, 2006[7]). As in other technical skills (Wulf & Shea, 2002[7]), surgical skills require considering situational dynamics that include both the task demands and environmental constraints.

In this volume, Abdo et al. (2024) examine models of technical skill development in simulation-based health professions education. While focusing on psychomotor skill development, they highlight key features of learning in the context that are applicable to all areas of health professions education, such as maintaining learner motivation, providing effective feedback and observation, including variability in training, and ensuring distribution of practice (rather than mass practice). These proposals are also supported by studies of learning, problem-solving, and sleep which demonstrate that unfilled intervals (e.g., sleep) can improve motor skill performance acquisition and problem-solving, referred to as *offline memory reprocessing* (Walker & Stickgold, 2004; Stickgold, 2005).

Affect and Emotion. Healthcare is a challenging environment, defined by noise, incomplete information, and changing contexts. Healthcare professionals must ultimately engage in effortful *reasoning* that allows them to interpolate missing information, extrapolate as-yet available information, and identify vulnerabilities and biases in the decision-making process. Beyond these concerns, we must also recognize that clinical cognition is rarely 'cold'. The knowledge and experiences of illness are often associated with strong affective and emotional responses. Healthcare professionals will also experience stress in delivering healthcare in time-limited environments (e.g., Intensive Care Unit, Emergency Room) and empathize with patients and family members. Despite the emotive nature of clinical practice, the impact of emotions on clinical decision-making is still in its infancy. However, cognitive psychologists have a long history of examining the impact of emotions on a variety of cognitive processes involved in clinical decision-making, such as attention, memory, judgment, decision-making, and reasoning. In this volume, McConnell (2024) summarizes cognitive psychology research documenting how emotions influence what people pay attention to, what they remember, and how they make decisions and reason about the world around them. Building on this research, McConnell then makes several recommendations for how clinicians and educators can incorporate emotions into their clinical training and practice.

Metacognition and Reflective Practices. Competencies reflect a combination of verbal and nonverbal knowledge and skills. The presence of affective and psychomotor skills that are largely impenetrable to conscious reflection and those associated with effortful learning of novices and explicit reasoning point to the need to coordinate multiple learning and decision-making systems. Despite the potential need to rely on clinical intuition in critical care situations where time and information are limited (Schmidt et al., 1990), extensive research has demonstrated that deliberate accumulation and weighing of evidence is superior approach (Ægisdóttir et al., 2006; Grove et al., 2000). Indeed, studies have indicated that medical errors are attributable to the ineffective information gathering (e.g., patient history, laboratory results) or cognitive reasoning biases (Graber et al., 2005; Zwann et al., 2012). Moreover, learning outcomes are also improved when explicit deliberation is required (e.g., MaGaghie et al., 2011). To ensure that they know when to stop and think (Moulton et al., 2010a, 2010b), healthcare professionals must acquire metacognitive skills to effectively monitor their performance and regulate their behavior. This requires the adoption of strategies to understand when there are vulnerable decision points in the process of healthcare delivery (e.g., Croskerry, 2009; Croskerry & Norman, 2008; Norman, 2009; Norman & Eva, 2010).

Verbal reports have proven to be a fruitful means to gain insight into the nature of expertise (e.g., Ericsson & Simon, 1980; Klein, 1993; for a review, see Ericsson, 2006), allowing the learners to reflect on how they learn and decide. As Gago et al. (2024) demonstrates, written reports (learning logs) suggest that learners have varying degrees of insight into their emotional responses and personal biases when considering ethical challenges that are present in biomedical sciences. The ability to observe changes (e.g., features/dimensions and complexity) and motivations for engaging with ethical dilemmas. Conforming to the human-centered design approach, such methods also provide opportunities to gain insight into how learners understand the curriculum and to use this as feedback to improve the delivery of assessment and educational interventions.

While qualitative methods can be used to understand the learners' experiences of reflection, operationalization of competency-based approaches clearly favors the use of quantitative methods (Nisbett & Wilson, 1977). In this volume, Schoenherr et al. (2024) consider conjoint measures to assess the development of expertise and self-assessment of performance. Rather than limiting expertise to an exclusive focus on automatic pattern recognition and response, they note that healthcare professionals must consider trade-offs between the speed of their response and the accuracy of their diagnostic and treatment recommendations. According to their account, expertise should be judged in terms of an absence of a speed-accuracy trade-of (Schoenherr, 2020). However, identifying the key decision-points in a diagnostic or surgical procedure that require slowing – or stopping – requires that healthcare professions engage in performance monitoring. In concluding their chapter, they consider measure of confidence calibration of both the accuracy and subjective confidence of learners when performing a task. They note that experience is inversely related to overconfidence bias.

1.3 Summary: Health Professions Education as Translational Research

The future of learning engineering in health professions education must be built on a foundation of human-centered design. Novel educational paradigms and technologies appear to hold promise for health professions education. CBME represents a progressive step away from apprenticeship models. When informed by the learning and cognitive sciences, CBME can promote greater validity in educational activities and assessment instruments used in the healthcare professions. As the evidence accumulated from educational activities increases in its validity, we will undoubtedly see improved patient outcomes.

The lessons of the learning and psychological sciences can also be used to inform the development of novel learning technologies. Technologies such as AI systems (AIS and ITS) present a promising means to provide learners with supplementary feedback, interoperable credential wallets that allow learners to obtain validated continuing professional development credits, and big data analytics potential can be used to identify areas of the health professions curriculum that require improvement (Chahine et al., 2018; Chan et al., 2019; Masters, 2019; Paranjape et al., 2019; Schoenherr et al., 2023). However, calls to 'move from an information age to [an] age of artificial intelligence' are premature if the data used to train AI for education (Wartman & Combs, 2018; Brigic et al., 2024) or to supplement human decision-making have been developed on erroneous assumptions about learning and decision-making (Schoenherr, 2022a; Schoenherr & Michael, 2024). Moreover, the feedback provided to learners and inferences made about them can potentially be even more harmful due if their operations are neither explainable nor contestable by learners or educators. Similar criticism can be raised about CBME training more generally when they are not girded by strong theoretical models and empirical evidence.

In this volume, we demonstrate that the gap between underspecified models of competence development and the demands of CBME can be addressed by turning to the learning and psychological sciences (Kahlke et al., 2020; Regher & Norman, 1996). As a translational research program, we hope to refocus health professions education to draw more extensively from fundamental decision-making research to clarify the nature of competencies while highlighting unexplored areas in the learning and cognitive sciences that merit further exploration.

We do not suggest this is more than a preliminary step. As a translational research program, health professions education requires that educators and psychological scientists can translate the knowledge of bench science (T_1) to training groups of learners in clinical settings (T_2) and inform program evaluation and development (T_3; see Figure 1.1; e.g., McGaghie, 2010; Schoenherr, 2024c). As previous studies have demonstrated, challenges in implementing CBME educational intervention such as simulation-based training and assessment (e.g., 'high' fidelity simulations and OSCEs) or problem-based learning (PBL) are at least partially attributable to failing to understand the social and cognitive processes associated with learning and implementation issues that arise due to institutional and sociocultural factors (Amoako-Sakyi & Amonoo-Kuofi, 2015; Hamstra et al., 2014; Hamstra & Schoenherr, 2017; Kwan, 2019; Lim, 2012; Monteiro & McConnell, 2023; Norman et al., 2012; Park et al., 2015). To retain focus, issues of cultural traditions (Schoenherr & Beaudoin, 2024), social inequalities in health professions and healthcare delivery (Khan, 2024), social instability due to conflict, and issues of regional diversity (e.g., Oluwabunmi et al., 2024; Venosa et al., 2024) and the need to indigenize healthcare (Chan, 2024; Schoenherr, 2024d) are largely left for a subsequent volume (Schoenherr, 2024a).

By reviewing issues associated with defining competencies, measurement, and learning and decision response processes, we hope to highlight theories of learning that can be used to inform the development of more effective competency-based curriculum and healthcare delivery. Here, we simply hope to demonstrate how a human-centered approach to learning engineering in the healthcare professions must address the affective, cognitive, and social processes associated with the learning environment.

Notes

1 As evidence of this, the review of Messick's (1995) validity framework conducted by Cook et al. (2013) excluded generalizability as a source of evidence. While this might be a deliberate exclusion (e.g., Schoenherr & Hamstra, 2016), it minimally highlights the applied focus of the research.
2 This is also found in the history of science where 'involuntary constant differences' in response time (bias) were attributed to failing to adhere to a 'right method' of observation (Canales, 2010; Schoenherr, 2016).
3 The WHO (2022) defines 'practice activities' as "[a] core function of health practice comprising a group of related tasks. Practice activities are time limited, trainable and, through the performance of tasks, measurable. Individuals may be certified to perform practice activities" (p. 10).
4 Referred to as dimensions in the original paper.
5 Kratwohl (2002) referred to these as the 'structure of knowledge' and the 'structure of cognitive processes', respectively.
6 Based on the work of Lev Vygotsky, social scaffolding reflects the activities performed by a teacher or peer who facilitates learning. Like physical scaffolding, they are eventually removed allowing the learner to perform the activities on their own. Social scaffolding can be partially understood in terms of a joint attention process (Schoenherr & Mahias-Ito, 2024).
7 Illustrating the issues of health professions education as translational research, Kopta (1971) redefined stages of the Fitts and Posner (1967) model when adapting it to surgery. Namely, although Fitts and Posner originally emphasized the development of associations between motor programs in their intermediate stage (they referred to the intermediate stage as associative, emphasizing stimulus-response association that define the gradual onset of automaticity in now what is defined as Type 1 processes), Kopta (1971) suggested that integration of information include declarative medical knowledge also occurs here. Thus, Kopta fundamentally changed the model which has been adopted in surgical skills training.

References

Abdo, S., Elliot, L., Micallef, J., Sivanathan, M., & Dubrowski, A. (2024). Optimizing psychomotor skills acquisition in healthcare simulation through knowledge mobilization. In Schoenherr, J. R. & McConnell, M. M. (eds.) *Fundamentals and*

Frontiers in Health professions education and Decision-Making: Educational Theory and Psychological Practice. Routledge.

Ackerknecht, E. H. (1984). From barber-surgeon to modern doctor. *Bulletin of the History of Medicine*, 58(4), 545–553.

Ægisdóttir, S., White, M. J., Spengler, P. M., Maugherman, A. S., Anderson, L. A., Cook, R. S., ... & Rush, J. D. (2006). The meta-analysis of clinical judgment project: Fifty-six years of accumulated research on clinical versus statistical prediction. *The Counseling Psychologist*, 34(3), 341–382.

Albert, M., Rowland, P., Friesen, F., & Laberge, S. (2020). Interdisciplinarity in health professions education research: Myth and reality. *Advances in Health Sciences Education*, 25, 1243–1253.

Amoako-Sakyi, D., & Amonoo-Kuofi, H. (2015). Problem-based learning in resource-poor settings: Lessons from a medical school in Ghana. *BMC Health Professions Education*, 15, 1–8.

Anderson, L.W., & Kratwohl (Eds.). (2001). *A Taxonomy for Learning, Teaching, and Assessing: A Revision of Bloom's Taxonomy of Educational Objectives.* Longman.

Ashby, F. G., Alfonso-Reese, L. A., Turken, A. U., & Waldron, E. M. (1998). A neuropsychological theory of multiple systems in category learning. *Psychological Review*, 105(3), 442–481.

Ashby, F. G., & Valentin, V. V. (2017). Multiple systems of perceptual category learning: Theory and cognitive tests. In *Handbook of Categorization in Cognitive Science* (pp. 157–188). Elsevier.

Baniasadi, T., Ayyoubzadeh, S.M. and Mohammadzadeh, N. (2020). Challenges and practical considerations in applying virtual reality in medical education and treatment. *Oman Medical Journal*, 35(3), p.e125.

Batalden, P., Leach, D., Swing, S., Dreyfus, H., & Dreyfus, S. (2002). General competencies and accreditation in graduate health professions education. *Health Affairs*, 21(5), 103–111.

Beck, A. H. (2004). The Flexner report and the standardization of American health professions education. *Journal of the American Medical Association*, 291(17), 2139–2140.

Bedoll, D., van Zanten, M., & McKinley, D. (2021). Global trends in health professions education accreditation. *Human Resources for Health*, 19(1), 1–15.

Bilgic, E., Chen, D. M., and Chan, T. (2024). Implementation of learning analytics in medical education: Practical considerations. In Schoenherr, J. R. & McConnell, M. M. (eds.) *Fundamentals and Frontiers in Health professions education and Decision-Making: Educational Theory and Psychological Practice.* Routledge.

Blömeke, S., Gustafsson, J. E., & Shavelson, R. J. (2015). Beyond dichotomies: Competence viewed as a continuum. *Zeitschrift für Psychologie*, 223(1), 3.

Bloom, B.S. (Ed.), Engelhart, M. D., Furst, E. J., Hill, W. H., & Kratwohl, D. R. (1956). *Taxonomy of Educational Objectives: The Classification of Educational Goals. Handbook 1: Cognitive Domain.* David McKay.

Board, S. (1999). Medical professionalism in society. *The New England Journal of Medicine*, 341, 1612–1616.

Bosk, C. (1979). *Forgive and Remember: Managing Medical Failure.* University of Chicago Press.

Boyd, V. A., Whitehead, C. R., Thille, P., Ginsburg, S., Brydges, R., & Kuper, A. (2018). Competency-based health professions education: The discourse of infallibility. *Health Professions Education*, 52(1), 45–57.

Canales, J. (2010). *A Tenth of a Second: A History*. University of Chicago Press.

Chahine, S., Kulasegaram, K. M., Wright, S., Monteiro, S., Grierson, L. E., Barber, C., ... & Touchie, C. (2018). A call to investigate the relationship between education and health outcomes using big data. *Academic Medicine*, 93(6), 829–832.

Challen, R., Denny, J., Pitt, M., Gompels, L., Edwards, T., & Tsaneva-Atanasova, K. (2019). Artificial intelligence, bias and clinical safety. *BMJ Quality & Safety*, 28(3), 231–237.

Chan, K. S., & Zary, N. (2019). Applications and challenges of implementing artificial intelligence in health professions education: Integrative review. *JMIR Health Professions Education*, 5(1), e13930.

Chang, Y. Z. (1942). China and English civil service reform. *The American Historical Review*, 47(3), 539–544.

Cirillo, D., Catuara-Solarz, S., Morey, C., Guney, E., Subirats, L., Mellino, S., ... & Mavridis, N. (2020). Sex and gender differences and biases in artificial intelligence for biomedicine and healthcare. *NPJ Digital Medicine*, 3(1), 81.

Coburn, D. (1988). Canadian medicine: Dominance or proletarianization? *The Milbank Quarterly*, 66(2), 92–116.

Coburn, D., Torrance, G. M., & Kaufert, J. M. (1983). Medical dominance in Canada in historical perspective: The rise and fall of medicine? *International Journal of Health Services*, 13(3), 407–432.

Collins, A., Brown, J. S., Newman, S. E. (1989). Cognitive apprenticeship: Teaching the crafts of reading, writing, and mathematics. In Resnick, L.B. (ed.) *Knowing, Learning, and Instruction: Essays in Honor of Robert Glaser* (pp. 453–494). Lawrence Erlbaum.

Cook, D. A., Brydges, R., Zendejas, B., Hamstra, S. J., & Hatala, R. (2013). Technology-enhanced simulation to assess health professionals: A systematic review of validity evidence, research methods, and reporting quality. *Academic Medicine*, 88(6), 872–883.

Cook, D. A., Hatala, R., Brydges, R., Zendejas, B., Szostek, J. H., Wang, A. T., ... & Hamstra, S. J. (2011). Technology-enhanced simulation for health professions education: A systematic review and meta-analysis. *Journal of the American Medical Association*, 306(9), 978–988.

Cowan, N. (2001). The magical number 4 in short-term memory: A reconsideration of mental storage capacity. *Behavioral and Brain Sciences*, 24, 87–185.

Croskerry, P. (2009). Clinical cognition and diagnostic error: Applications of a dual process model of reasoning. *Advances in Health Sciences Education*, 14, 27–35.

Croskerry, P., & Norman, G. (2008). Overconfidence in clinical decision making. *The American Journal of Medicine*, 121(5), S24–S29.

Custers, E. J., & ten Cate, O. (2018). The history of health professions education in Europe and the United States, with respect to time and proficiency. *Academic Medicine*, 93(3), S49–S54.

de Giovanni, D., Roberts, T., & Norman, G. (2009). Relative effectiveness of high- versus low-fidelity simulation in learning heart sounds. *Medical Education*, 43(7), 661–668.

Deng, Y. (1990). Development of health professions education in China. *Academic Medicine*, 65(8), 512–514.

Deng, S.-Y. (1943). Chinese influence on the Western examination system *Harvard Journal of Asiatic Studies*, 7, 267–312.

Dieckmann, P., Gaba, D., & Rall, M. (2007). Deepening the theoretical foundations of patient simulation as social practice. *Simulation in Healthcare, 2*, 183–193.

Donders, F. C. (1868). *Die Schnelligkeit Psychischer Processe: Erster Artikel. Archiv für Anatomie, Physiologie und Wissenschaftliche Medicin*, 657–681.

Dreyfus, S. E. & Dreyfus, H. L. (1980). A five-stage model of the mental activities involved in directed skill acquisition. *Operation Research Center Report* (pp. 80–82). University of California.

Dubois, D. G., Lingley, A. J., Ghatalia, J., & McConnell, M. M. (2021). Validity of entrustment scales within anesthesiology residency training Validité des échelles de confiance dans le cadre de la résidence en anesthésiologie. *Canadian Journal of Anesthesia /Journal canadien d'anesthésie, 68*, 53–63.

Duffy, T. P. (2011). The Flexner report—100 years later. *The Yale Journal of Biology and Medicine, 84*(3), 269.

Ebbinghaus, H. (1885). *Über das Gedächtnis: Untersuchungen zur Experimentellen Psychologie*. Duncker & Humblot.

Elman, B. A. (1991). Political, social, and cultural reproduction via civil service examinations in late imperial China. *The Journal of Asian Studies, 50*(1), 7–28.

Elman, B. A. (2000). *A Cultural History of Civil Examinations in Late Imperial China*. University of California Press.

Elman, B. A. (2013). *Civil Examinations and Meritocracy in Late Imperial China*. Harvard University Press.

Epstein, R. M., & Hundert, E. M. (2002). Defining and assessing professional competence. *Journal of the American Medical Association, 287*(2), 226–235.

Ericsson, K. A. (2006). Protocol analysis and expert thought: Concurrent verbalizations of thinking during experts' performance on representative tasks. In Ericsson, A., Hoffman, R. R., Kozbelt, A., & Williams, A. M. (eds.) *The Cambridge Handbook of Expertise and Expert Performance* (pp. 223–241). Cambridge University Press.

Ericsson, K. A., & Simon, H. A. (1980). Verbal reports as data. *Psychological Review, 87*(3), 215.

Evans, J. S. B., & Stanovich, K. E. (2013). Dual-process theories of higher cognition: Advancing the debate. *Perspectives on Psychological Science, 8*(3), 223–241.

Fan, J., McCandliss, B. D., Sommer, T., Raz, A., & Posner, M. I. (2002). Testing the efficiency and independence of attentional networks. *Journal of Cognitive Neuroscience, 14*(3), 340–347.

Fitts, P. M., & Posner, M. I. (1967). *Human Performance*. Belmont: Brooks/Cole Pub. Co.

Flexner, A. (1910/2002). Health professions education in the United States and Canada. *Bulletin of the World Health Organization, 80*, 594–602.

Frank, J. R., Snell, L. S., Cate, O. T., Holmboe, E. S., Carraccio, C., Swing, S. R., ... & Harris, K. A. (2010). Competency-based health professions education: Theory to practice. *Medical Teacher, 32*(8), 638–645.

Freidson, E. (1970). *Professional Dominance: The Social Structure of Medical Care*. Transaction Publishers.

Frohlich, K. L., Ross, N., & Richmond, C. (2006). Health disparities in Canada today: Some evidence and a theoretical framework. *Health Policy, 79*(2–3), 132–143.

Gago, F., Echagüe, C. L., & Lázaro, M. (2024). Reflection as a core skill in bioethics education: Application to the scientific and healthcare professions.

In Schoenherr, J. R. & McConnell, M. M. (Eds.), *Fundamentals and Frontiers in Medical Education and Decision-Making: Educational Theory and Psychological Practice*. Routledge.

Gallagher, J. (2019, January). Indigenous approaches to health and wellness leadership: A BC First Nations perspective. *Healthcare Management Forum*, 32(1), 5–10. SAGE Publications.

George, B. C., Teitelbaum, E. N., Meyerson, S. L., et al. (2014). Reliability, validity, and feasibility of the Zwisch scale for the assessment of intraoperative performance. *Journal of Surgical Education*, 71, e90–e96.

Gigerenzer, G., & Goldstein, D. G. (2011). The recognition heuristic: A decade of research. *Judgment and Decision Making*, 6(1), 100–121.

Graber, M. L., Franklin, N., & Gordon, R. (2005). Diagnostic error in internal medicine. *Archives of Internal Medicine*, 165(13), 1493–1499.

Granshaw, L., & Porter, R. (1989). *The Hospital in History*. Routledge.

Grierson, L. E. (2014). Information processing, specificity of practice, and the transfer of learning: Considerations for reconsidering fidelity. *Advances in Health Sciences Education*, 19, 281–289.

Grove, W. M., Zald, D. H., Lebow, B. S., Snitz, B. E., & Nelson, C. (2000). Clinical versus mechanical prediction: A meta-analysis. *Psychological Assessment*, 12(1), 19.

Gwee, M. C. E., Samarasekera, D. D., & Chong, Y. (2013). APMEC 2014: Optimising collaboration in health professions education: Building bridges connecting minds. *Health Professions Education*, 47(s2), iii–iv.

Hall, A. K., Schumacher, D. J., Thoma, B., Caretta-Weyer, H., Kinnear, B., Gruppen, L., Cooke, L. J., Frank, J. R., Van Melle, E. & ICBME Collaborators (2021). Outcomes of competency-based medical education: A taxonomy for shared language. *Medical Teacher*, 43(7), 788–793.

Halman, S., Rekman, J., Wood, T., et al. (2018). Avoid reinventing the wheel: Implementation of the Ottawa Clinic Assessment Tool (OCAT) in internal medicine. *BMC Medical Education*. https://doi.org/10.1186/s12909-018-1327-7

Hamm, R. M. (2004). Theory about heuristic strategies based on verbal protocol analysis: The emperor needs a shave. *Medical Decision Making*, 24(6), 681–686.

Hamstra, S. J., Brydges, R., Hatala, R., Zendejas, B., & Cook, D. A. (2014). Reconsidering fidelity in simulation-based training. *Academic Medicine*, 89(3), 387–392.

Hawkins, R. E., Welcher, C. M., Holmboe, E. S., Kirk, L. M., Norcini, J. J., Simons, K. B., & Skochelak, S. E. (2015). Implementation of competency-based health professions education: Are we addressing the concerns and challenges? *Health Professions Education*, 49(11), 1086–1102.

Himmelmann, L. (2007). From barber to surgeon-the process of professionalization. *Svensk Medicinhistorisk Tidskrift*, 11(1), 69–87.

Hodges, B. (2013). Assessment in the post-psychometric era: Learning to love the subjective and collective. *Medical Teacher*, 35, 564–568.

Hoffman, K. A., Aitken, L. M., & Duffield, C. (2009). A comparison of novice and expert nurses' cue collection during clinical decision-making: Verbal protocol analysis. *International Journal of Nursing Studies*, 46(10), 1335–1344.

Hollingshead, A. B. (1998). Communication, learning, and retrieval in transactive memory systems. *Journal of Experimental Social Psychology*, 34(5), 423–442.

Hsu, E. (1999). *The Transmission of Chinese Medicine*. Cambridge University Press.

Hu, C. T. (1984). The historical background: Examinations and controls in pre-modern China. *Comparative Education*, 20(1), 7–26.

Kahlke, R. M., McConnell, M. M., Wisener, K. M., & Eva, K. W. (2020). The disconnect between knowing and doing in health professions education and practice. *Advances in Health Sciences Education*, 25, 227–240.

Kahneman, D., & Klein, G. (2009). Conditions for intuitive expertise: a failure to disagree. *American Psychologist*, 64(6), 515.

Kang, H. W. (1974). Institutional borrowing: The case of the Chinese civil service examination system in early *Koryŏ*. *The Journal of Asian Studies*, 34(1), 109–125.

Khan, K. (2024). Inequality and social mobility in the medical professions in India: Career availability and vulnerabilities. In Schoenherr, J. R. & McConnell, M. M. (eds.), *Fundamentals and Frontiers in Health professions education and Decision-Making: Educational Theory and Psychological Practice*. Routledge.

Kim, J., Cai, Z. R., Chen, M. L., Simard, J. F., & Linos, E. (2023). Assessing Biases in Medical Decisions via Clinician and AI Chatbot Responses to Patient Vignettes. *JAMA Network Open*, 6(10), e2338050–e2338050.

Kim, M., Sohn, H., Choi, S., & Kim, S. (2023). Requirements for Trustworthy Artificial Intelligence and its Application in Healthcare. *Healthcare Informatics Research*, 29(4), 315.

Klein, G. A. (1993). A recognition-primed decision (RPD) model of rapid decision making. *Decision Making in Action: Models and Methods*, 5(4), 138–147.

Ko, K. H. (2017). A brief history of imperial examination and its influences. *Culture and Society*, 54, 272–278.

Kopta, J. A. (1971). The development of motor skills in orthopaedic education. *Clinical Orthopaedics and Related Research (1976-2007)*, 75, 80–85.

Korovin, L. N., Farrell, T. M., Hsu, C. H., White, M., & Ghaderi, I. (2020). Surgeons' expertise during critical event in laparoscopic cholecystectomy: An expert-novice comparison using protocol analysis. *The American Journal of Surgery*, 219(2), 340–345.

Kratwohl, D. R. (2002). A revision of Bloom's taxonomy: An overview. *Theory into Practice*, 41(4), 212–218.

Krupinski, E. A., Tillack, A. A., Richter, L., et al. (2006). Eye-movement study and human performance using telepathology virtual slides: Implications for health professions education and differences with experience. *Human Pathology*, 37, 1543–1556.

Kwan, C. Y. (2019). A thorny path: The developmental course of problem-based learning for health sciences education in Asia. *Advances in Health Sciences Education*, 24(5), 893–901.

Lai, C. T. (1970). *A Scholar in Imperial China*. Kelly & Walsh.

Lester, H., & Tritter, J. Q. (2001). Medical error: A discussion of the medical construction of error and suggestions for reforms of health professions education to decrease error. *Health Professions Education*, 35(9), 855–861.

Lewis, K., & Herndon, B. (2011). Transactive memory systems: Current issues and future research directions. *Organization Science*, 22(5), 1254–1265.

Lim, W. K. (2012). Dysfunctional problem-based learning curricula: Resolving the problem. *BMC Health Professions Education*, 12(1), 1–7.

Lingard, L. (2012). Rethinking competence in the context of teamwork. In Hodges, B. L. & Lingard, L (eds.), *The Question of Competence: Reconsidering Health Professions Education in the Twenty-First Century*, (pp. 42–69). Cornwell University Press.

Liu, H. (2007). Influence of China's imperial examinations on Japan, Korea and Vietnam. *Frontiers of History in China*, 2(4), 493–512.

Liu, H. (2018). *The Examination Culture on Imperial China*. Paths International.

Liu, Y., Glass, N. L., Glover, C. D., Power, R. W., & Watcha, M. F. (2013). Comparison of the development of performance skills in Ultrasound-guided regional anesthesia simulations with different phantom models. *Simulation in Healthcare*, 8, 368–375.

Lockyear, J., Carraccio, C., Chan, M. K., Hart, D., Smee, S., Touchie, C., … & ICBME Collaborators. (2017). Core principles of assessment in competency-based health professions education. *Medical Teacher*, 39(6), 609–616.

Logan, G. D. (1988). Toward an instance theory of automatization. *Psychological Review*, 95(4), 492.

Lyons, K., McLaughlin, J. E., Khanova, J., & Roth, M. T. (2017). Cognitive apprenticeship in health sciences education: A qualitative review. *Advances in Health Sciences Education*, 22, 723–739.

Ma, T. (2024). Considerations for implementation of a competency-based education program for preclerkship courses. In Schoenherr, J. R. & McConnell, M. M. (eds.), *Fundamentals and Frontiers in Health professions education and Decision-Making: Educational Theory and Psychological Practice*. Routledge.

Mansouri, M., & Lockyer, J. (2007). A meta-analysis of continuing medical education effectiveness. *Journal of Continuing Education in the Health Professions*, 27(1), 6–15.

Marckmann, G. (2001). Teaching science vs. the apprentice model – Do we really have the choice? *Medicine, Health Care and Philosophy*, 4, 85–89.

Massoth, C., Röder, H., Ohlenburg, H., Hessler, M., Zarbock, A., Pöpping, D. M., & Wenk, M. (2019). High-fidelity is not superior to low-fidelity simulation but leads to overconfidence in medical students. *BMC Health Professions Education*, 19(1), 1–8.

Masters, K. (2019). Artificial intelligence in health professions education. *Medical Teacher*, 41(9), 976–980.

Matsumoto, E. D., Hamstra, S. J., Radomski, S. B., & Cusimano, M. D. (2002). The effect of bench model fidelity on endourological skills: A randomized controlled study. *The Journal of Urology*, 167(3), 1243–1247.

McConnell, M. (2023). Emotions and clinical decision-making. In Schoenherr, J. R. & McConnell, M. (eds.), *Fundamentals and Frontiers of Health professions education and Decision-Making: Educational Theory and Psychological Practice*. Routledge.

McConnell, M., & Eva, K. W. (2022). Emotions and learning: Cognitive theoretical and methodological approaches to studying the influence of emotions on learning. In Cleland, J. & Durning, S. J. (eds.), *Researching Health Professions Education, Second Edition*, (pp. 279–290). Wiley.

McConnell, M., Monteiro, S., Pottruff, M. M., Neville, A., Norman, G. R., Eva, K. W., & Kulasegaram, K. (2016). The impact of emotion on learners' application of basic science principles to novel problems. *Academic Medicine*, 91(11), S58–S63.

McConnell, M., Sherbino, J., & Chan, T. M. (2016). Mind the gap: The prospects of missing data. *Journal of Graduate Health Professions Education*, 8(5), 708–712.

McGaghie, W. C. (2010). Health professions education research as translational science. *Science Translational Medicine*, 2(19), 1–3.

McGaghie, W. C., Issenberg, S. B., Cohen, E. R., Barsuk, J. H., & Wayne, D. B. (2011). Does simulation-based health professions education with deliberate practice yield better results than traditional clinical education? A meta-analytic comparative review of the evidence. *Academic Medicine*, 86(6), 706–711.

Meier, K. M. & Blair, M. R. (2013). Waiting and weighting: Information sampling is a balance between efficiency and error-reduction. *Cognition*, 126, 319–325.

Messick, S. (1995). Validity of psychological assessment: Validation of inferences from persons' responses and performances as scientific inquiry into score meaning. *American Psychologist*, 50(9), 741.

Miller, G. E. (1990). The assessment of clinical skills/competence/performance. *Academic Medicine*, 65(9), S63–S67.

Mink, R. B., Schwartz, A., Herman, B. E., et al. (2018). Validity of level of supervision scales for assessing pediatric fellows on the common pediatric subspecialty entrustable professional activities. *Academic Medicine*, 93, 283–291.

Miyake, A., & Shah, P. (1999). *Models of Working Memory*. Cambridge University Press.

Monteiro, S., Cavanaugh, A., Biswabandan, B., & Sibbald, M. (2024). Separating the noise from the signal: The role of familiarity and pattern recognition in the development of clinical expertise. In Schoenherr, J. R. & McConnell, M. (eds.), *Fundamentals and Frontiers of Health professions education and Decision-Making: Educational Theory and Psychological Practice*. Routledge.

Monteiro, S., & McConnell, M. M. (2023). Evaluating the construct validity of competencies: A retrospective analysis. *Medical Science Educator*, 33(3), 729–736.

Morcke, A. M., Dornan, T., & Eika, B. (2013). Outcome (competency) based education: An exploration of its origins, theoretical basis, and empirical evidence. *Advances in Health Sciences Education*, 18, 851–863.

Moulton, C. A., Regehr, G., Lingard, L., Merritt, C., & MacRae, H. (2010a). 'Slowing down when you should': Initiators and influences of the transition from the routine to the effortful. *Journal of Gastrointestinal Surgery*, 14, 1019–1026.

Moulton, C. A., Regehr, G., Lingard, L., Merritt, C., & MacRae, H. (2010b). Operating from the other side of the table: Control dynamics and the surgeon educator. *Journal of the American College of Surgeons*, 210(1), 79–86.

Nisbett, R. E., & Wilson, T. D. (1977). Telling more than we can know: Verbal reports on mental processes. *Psychological Review*, 84(3), 231.

Norman, G. (2009). Dual processing and diagnostic errors. *Advances in Health Sciences Education*, 14, 37–49.

Norman, G., Dore, K., & Grierson, L. (2012). The minimal relationship between simulation fidelity and transfer of learning. *Medical Education*, 46(7), 636–647.

Norman, G. R., & Eva, K. W. (2010). Diagnostic error and clinical reasoning. *Health Professions Education*, 44(1), 94–100.

Oluwabunmi O.-O., E., Adisa, A. O., Olopade, F. E., Lawal1, T. A., Hammad, N., Iputo, J. E., & Scott-Emuakpor, A. B. (2024). Medical education in Sub-Saharan Africa. *Fundamentals and Frontiers in Medical Education and Decision-Making: Innovation, Implementation, and Translational Research*. Routledge.

O'Neill, L. B., Bhansali, P., Bost, J. E., Chamberlain, J. M., & Ottolini, M. C. (2021). "Sick or not sick?" A mixed methods study evaluating the rapid determination of illness severity in a pediatric emergency department. *Diagnosis*, 9(2), 207–215.

O'Sullivan, P. S., Stoddard, H. A., & Kalishman, S. (2010). Collaborative research in health professions education: A discussion of theory and practice. *Health Professions Education*, 44(12), 1175–1184.

Paranjape, K., Schinkel, M., Panday, R. N., Car, J., & Nanayakkara, P. (2019). Introducing artificial intelligence training in health professions education. *JMIR Health Professions Education*, 5(2), e16048.

Park, W. B., Kang, S. H., Myung, S. J., & Lee, Y. S. (2015). Does objective structured clinical examinations score reflect the clinical reasoning ability of medical students? *The American Journal of the Medical Sciences*, 350(1), 64–67.

Patel, V. L., Yoskowitz, N. A., & Arocha, J. F. (2009). Towards effective evaluation and reform in medical education: A cognitive and learning sciences perspective. *Advances in Health Sciences Education*, 14, 791–812.

Patterson, F., Knight, A., Dowell, J., Nicholson, S., Cousans, F., & Cleland, J. (2016). How effective are selection methods in medical education? A systematic review. *Medical Education*, 50(1), 36–60.

Peltokorpi, V. (2008). Transactive memory systems. *Review of General Psychology*, 12(4), 378–394.

Pierce, C. S., & Jastrow, J. (1884). On small differences in sensation. *Memoirs of the National Academy of Science*, 3, 75–83.

Plochg, T., Klazinga, N. S., & Starfield, B. (2009). Transforming medical professionalism to fit changing health needs. *BMC Medicine*, 7, 1–7.

Pottle, J., 2019. Virtual reality and the transformation of medical education. *Future Healthcare Journal*, 6(3), 181.

Prasad, V., & Ioannidis, J. P. (2014). Evidence-based de-implementation for contradicted, unproven, and aspiring healthcare practices. *Implementation Science*, 9, 1–5.

Prusaczyk, B., Swindle, T., & Curran, G. (2020). Defining and conceptualizing outcomes for de-implementation: Key distinctions from implementation outcomes. *Implementation Science Communications*, 1, 1–10.

Regehr, G., & Norman, G. R. (1996). Issues in cognitive psychology: Implications for professional education. *Academic Medicine*, 71(9), 988–1001.

Rekman, J., Hamstra, S. J., Dudek, N., et al. (2016). A new instrument for assessing resident competence in surgical clinic: The Ottawa Clinic Assessment Tool. *Journal of Surgical Education*, 73, 575–582.

Reznick, R. K., & MacRae, H. (2006). Teaching surgical skills—Changes in the wind. *New England Journal of Medicine*, 355(25), 2664–2669.

Rocks, S., Berntson, D., Gil-Salmerón, A., Kadu, M., Ehrenberg, N., Stein, V., & Tsiachristas, A. (2020). Cost and effects of integrated care: A systematic literature review and meta-analysis. *The European Journal of Health Economics*, 21, 1211–1221.

Rodriguez-Paz, J. M., Kennedy, M., Salas, E., Wu, A. W., Sexton, J. B., Hunt, E. A., & Pronovost, P. J. (2009). Beyond "see one, do one, teach one": Toward a different training paradigm. *Postgraduate Medical Journal*, 85(1003), 244–249.

Rubio, D. M., Schoenbaum, E. E., Lee, L. S., Schteingart, D. E., Marantz, P. R., Anderson, K. E., … & Esposito, K. (2010). Defining translational research: Implications for training. *Academic Medicine*, 85(3), 470.

Sanders, A. F. (1980). 20 stage analysis of reaction processes. *Advances in Psychology*, 1, 331–354. North-Holland.

Schatz, S., Thai, K. P., Criag, S. D., Schoenherr, J. R., Lis, J., & Kolodner, J. (2022). Human-centered design tools. In *Learning Engineering Toolkit* (pp. 279–301). Routledge.

Schmidt, H. G., Norman, G. R., & Boshuizen, H. P. (1990). A cognitive perspective on medical expertise: theory and implication. *Academic Medicine*, 65(10), 611–21.

Schneider, W., & Shiffrin, R. M. (1977). Controlled and automatic human information processing: I. Detection, search, and attention. *Psychological Review*, 84(1), 1.

Schoenherr, J. R. (2017). Prestige technology in the evolution and social organization of early psychological science. *Theory & Psychology*, 27(1), 6–33.

Schoenherr, J. R. (2020). Adapting the zone of proximal development to the wicked environments of professional practice. In *Adaptive Instructional Systems: Second International Conference, AIS 2020*, July 19–24, 2020 (pp. 394–410). Springer International Publishing.

Schoenherr, J. R. (2022a). *Ethical Artificial Intelligence from Popular to Cognitive Science*. Taylor & Francis.

Schoenherr, J. R. (2022b). Folkmedical technologies and the sociotechnical systems of healthcare. *IEEE Technology and Society Magazine*, 41(3), 38–49.

Schoenherr, J. R. (2024a). Innovation and implementation in health professions education and healthcare delivery. In Schoenherr, J. R. (ed.), *Fundamentals and Frontiers in Medical Education and Decision-Making: Innovation, Implementation, and Translational Research*. Routledge.

Schoenherr, J. R., Mahias-Ito, Y., & Li, X.Y. (2024). Collective competence and social learning in the health professions: learning, thinking, and deciding in groups. In Schoenherr, J. R. (ed.), *Fundamentals and Frontiers in Medical Education and Decision-Making: Innovation, Implementation, and Translational Research*. Routledge.

Schoenherr, J. R. (2024b). The development and dynamics of Mayan healthcare systems: A socioecological approach. In Schoenherr, J. R. (ed.), *Fundamentals and Frontiers in Medical Education and Decision-Making: Innovation, Implementation, and Translational Research*. Routledge.

Schoenherr, J. R. (2024c). The translational research process. In Eltorai, A. E. M., et al. (eds.), *Translational Neurosurgery*. Elsevier.

Schoenherr, J. R., Abbas, R., Michael, K., Rivas, P., & Anderson, T. D. (2023). Designing AI using a human-centered approach: Explainability and accuracy toward trustworthiness. *IEEE Transactions on Technology and Society*, 4(1), 9–23.

Schoenherr, J. R. & Beaudoin, J. (2024). Medical pluralism in East Asian medical education: The evolving landscape of health professions education in East Asia. In Schoenherr, J. R. (ed.), *Fundamentals and Frontiers in Medical Education and Decision-Making: Innovation, Implementation, and Translational Research*. Routledge.

Schoenherr, J. R., Chiou, E., and Goldshtein, M. (2023). Building trust with the ethical affordances of education technologies: A sociotechnical systems perspective, In *Putting AI in the Critical Loop* (pp. 127–165). Elsevier.

Schoenherr, J. R., & Davies, J. (2009). Aesthetics and accuracy in graphical representations of science. *Proceedings of the 12th International Conference on Scientometrics and Infometric*, Rio de Janiero, Brazil.

Schoenherr, J. R., & Hamstra, S. J. (2016). Psychometrics and its discontents: An historical perspective on the discourse of the measurement tradition. *Advances in Health Sciences Education*, 21, 719–729.

Schoenherr, J. R., & Hamstra, S. J. (2017). Beyond fidelity: Deconstructing the seductive simplicity of fidelity in simulator-based education in the health care professions. *Simulation in Healthcare*, 12(2), 117–123.

Schoenherr, J. R., & Hamstra, S. J. (2024). Validity in health professions education: From assessment instruments to program innovation and evaluation. In

Schoenherr, J. R. & McConnell, M. (eds.), *Fundamentals and Frontiers in Medical Education: Educational Theory and Psychological Practice*. Routledge.

Schoenherr, J. R. & Le-Bouar, C. (2024). Representing and communicating health information: Fundamentals of persuasive health communication. In Schoenherr, J. R. & McConnell, M. (eds.), *Fundamentals and Frontiers in Medical Education: Educational Theory and Psychological Practice*. Routledge.

Schoenherr, J. R., & Michael, K. (2024). AI-based technologies in the healthcare ecosystem: Applications in medical education and decision-making. In Schoenherr, J. R. (ed.), *Fundamentals and Frontiers in Medical Education and Decision-Making: Innovation, Implementation, and Translational Research*. Routledge.

Schoenherr, J. R., Waechter, J., Lee, C. H. (2024). Quantifying expertise in the healthcare professions: cognitive efficiency and metacognitive calibration. In Schoenherr, J. R. & McConnell, M. (eds.), *Fundamentals and Frontiers in Medical Education: Educational Theory and Psychological Practice*. Routledge.

Shah, N., Desai, C., Jorwekar, G., Badyal, D., & Singh, T. (2016). Competency-based medical education: An overview and application in pharmacology. *Indian Journal of Pharmacology*, 48(Suppl 1), S5.

Sidhu, R. S., Park, J., Brydges, R., MacRae, H. M., and Dubrowski, A., (2007). Laboratory-based vascular anastomosis training: A randomised controlled trial evaluating the effects of bench model fidelity and level of training on skill acquisition. *Journal of Vascular Surgery*, 45, 343–349.

Sinclair, S. (1997). *Making Doctors: An Institutional Apprenticeship*. Routledge.

Spilg, E., Siebert, S., & Martin. G. (2012). A social learning perspective on the development of doctors in the UK National Health Service. *Social Science & Medicine*, 75, 1617–1612.

Stalmeijer, R. E., Dolmans, D. H., Wolfhagen, I. H., Muijtjens, A. M., & Scherpbier, A. J. (2010). The Maastricht Clinical Teaching Questionnaire (MCTQ) as a valid and reliable instrument for the evaluation of clinical teachers. *Academic Medicine*, 85(11), 1732–1738.

Stalmeijer, R. E., Dolmans, D. H., Snellen-Balendong, H. A., van Santen-Hoeufft, M., Wolfhagen, I. H., & Scherpbier, A. J. (2013). Clinical teaching based on principles of cognitive apprenticeship: views of experienced clinical teachers. *Academic Medicine*, 88(6), 861–865.

Stanovich, K. E. (2018). Miserliness in human cognition: The interaction of detection, override and mindware. *Thinking & Reasoning*, 24(4), 423–444.

Starr, P. (1981). *The Social Transformation of American Medicine: The Rise of a Sovereign Profession and the Making of a Vast Industry*. Hachette UK.

Starr, P. (1982). *The Social Transformation Of American Medicine*. Basic Books, Inc.

Stickgold, R. (2005). Sleep-dependent memory consolidation. *Nature*, 437(7063), 1272–1278.

Strauss, A., Schatzman, L., Ehrlich, D., Bucher, R., & Sabshin, M. (1963). The hospital and its negotiated order. In Freidson, E. (ed.), *The Hospital in Modern Society* (pp. 147–169). Free Press.

Sturdy, S., & Cooter, R. (1998). Science, scientific management, and the transformation of medicine in Britain c. 1870–1950. *History of Science*, 36(4), 421–466.

Sturmberg, J. P., O'Halloran, D. M., & Martin, C. M. (2012). Understanding health system reform – A complex adaptive systems perspective. *Journal of Evaluation in Clinical Practice*, 18(1), 202–208.

Tasselli, S. (2015). Social networks and inter-professional knowledge transfer: The case of healthcare professionals. *Organization Studies*, 36(7), 841–872.

Teodorczuk, A., Yardley, S., Patel, R., Rogers, G. D., Billett, S., Worley, P., Hirsh, D., & Illing, J. (2017). Health professions education research should extend further into clinical practice. *Health Professions Education*, 51(11), 1092–1100.

Thai, K. P., Craig, S. D., Goodell, J., Lis, J., Schoenherr, J. R., & Kolodner, J. (2022). Learning engineering is human-centered. In *Learning Engineering Toolkit* (pp. 83–123). Routledge.

Turner, B. S. (1987/1995). *Medical Power and Social Knowledge*, Second edition. Sage Publications.

van Bodegom-Vos, L., Davidoff, F., & Marang-Van De Mheen, P. J. (2017). Implementation and de-implementation: Two sides of the same coin?. *BMJ Quality & Safety*, 26(6), 495–501.

van der Vleuten, C. P., & Schuwirth, L. W. (2005). Assessing professional competence: From methods to programmes. *Health Professions Education*, 39(3), 309–317.

Vanstone, M., Monteiro, S., Colvin, E., Norman, G., Sherbino, J., Sibbald, M., ... & Peters, A. (2019). Experienced physician descriptions of intuition in clinical reasoning: A typology. *Diagnosis*, 6(3), 259–268.

van Zanten, M., Norcini, J. J., Boulet, J. R., & Simon, F. (2008). Overview of accreditation of undergraduate health professions education programmes worldwide. *Health Professions Education*, 42(9), 930–937.

Venosa, A. R., Baroneza, J. E., & Fernandes, R. A. F. (2024). Medical education in Brazil: A history of an evolving pluralistic healthcare system. In Schoenherr, J. R. (ed.), *Fundamentals and Frontiers in Medical Education and Decision-Making: Innovation, Implementation, and Translational Research*. Routledge.

Vozenilek, J., Huff, J. S., Reznek, M., & Gordon, J. A. (2004). See one, do one, teach one: advanced technology in medical education. *Academic Emergency Medicine*, 11(11), 1149–1154.

Walker, M. P., & Stickgold, R. (2004). Sleep-dependent learning and memory consolidation. *Neuron*, 44(1), 121–133.

Walsh, R. (1994). The making of a shaman: Calling, training, and culmination. *Journal of Humanistic Psychology*, 34(3), 7–30.

Warm, E. J., Held, J. D., Hellmann, M., et al. (2016). Entrusting observable practice activities and milestones over the 36 months of an internal medicine residency. *Academic Medicine*, 91, 1398–1405.

Warm, E. J., Mathis, B. R., Held, J. D., et al. (2014). Entrustment and mapping of observable practice activities for resident assessment. *Journal of General Internal Medicine*, 29, 1177–1182.

Wartman, S. A., & Combs, C. D. (2018). Health professions education must move from the information age to the age of artificial intelligence. *Academic Medicine*, 93(8), 1107–1109.

Wass, V., van der Vleuten, C., Shatzer, J., & Jones, R. (2001). Assessment of clinical competence. *The Lancet*, 357(9260), 945–949.

Wegner, D. M. (1987). Transactive memory: A contemporary analysis of the group mind. In Mullen B. & Goethals G. R. (eds.), *Theories of Group Behavior* (pp. 185–208). Springer-Verlag.

Weller, J. M., Castanelli, D. J., Chen, Y., & Jolly, B. (2017). Making robust assessments of specialist trainees' workplace performance. *British Journal of Anesthesiology*, 118, 207–214.

Weller, J. M., Misur, M., Nicolson, S., et al. (2014). Can I leave the theatre? A key to more reliable workplace-based assessment. *British Journal of Anesthesiology*, 112, 1083–1091.

Whitehead, C. R., Austin, Z., & Hodges, B. D. (2011). Flower power: the armoured expert in the CanMEDS competency framework? *Advances in Health Sciences Education*, 16, 681–694.

Whitehead, C. R., Kuper, A., Hodges, B., & Ellaway, R. (2015). Conceptual and practical challenges in the assessment of physician competencies. *Medical Teacher*, 37(3), 245–251.

Witheridge, A., Ferns, G., & Scott-Smith, W. (2019). Revisiting Miller's pyramid in health professions education: The gap between traditional assessment and diagnostic reasoning. *International Journal of Health Professions Education*, 10, 191.

WHO (2022). *Global Competency and Outcomes Framework for Universal Health Coverage*. World Health Organization.

Wu, H., & Cheng, P. (2000). A comparison of ancient and modern methods of education in traditional Chinese medicine [Chinese]. *Shanghai Journal of Traditional Chinese Medicine*, 12, 10–13.

Wulf, G., & Shea, C. H. (2002). Principles derived from the study of simple skills do not generalize to complex skill learning. *Psychonomic Bulletin & Review*, 9(2), 185–211.

Zoltowski, C. B., Oakes, W. C., & Cardella, M. E. (2012). Students' ways of experiencing human-centered design. *Journal of Engineering Education*, 101(1), 28–59.

Zwaan, L., Thijs, A., Wagner, C., van der Wal, G., & Timmermans, D. R. (2012). Relating faults in diagnostic reasoning with diagnostic errors and patient harm. *Academic Medicine*, 87(2), 149–156.

2

CONSIDERATIONS FOR IMPLEMENTATION OF A COMPETENCY-BASED EDUCATION PROGRAM FOR PRECLERKSHIP COURSES

Terence P. Ma

2.1 Theoretical Considerations

In North America, Flexner (1910) proposed a system wherein a learner would first earn a baccalaureate degree and then attend medical school. In medical school (undergraduate medical education, UME), learners would start with two years of foundational sciences followed by two years of clinical training. This is the model used in the USA and Canada (Nara et al., 2011; Wijnen-Meijer et al., 2013). The past 30 years have been defined by an ongoing review of how the Flexnerian model can evolve to meet the needs of learners and educators as they strive to produce optimal outcomes for patients (Blumenthal, 2002; Committee on the Health Professions Education Summit, 2003; Cooke et al., 2006; HHMI and AAMC, 2009; Cooke et al., 2010). To address this change in focus, many medical educators are advocating an outcomes-based (Harden et al., 1999a) or competency-based medical education (CBME) approach (Frank et al., 2010b). This approach has been adopted worldwide (Olapade-Olaopa et al., 2024; Schoenherr and Beaudoin, 2024; Venosa et al., 2024; Wijnen-Meijer et al., 2013; Weggemans et al., 2017). The goal of this approach is to be patient-focused and learner-centered (Frenk et al., 2010; Schumacher et al., 2024).

2.1.1 Competency-Based Medical Education (CBME)

Outcomes-based medical education defines learning "by what [students] can demonstrate they have learned" (McNeir, 1993, pg. 2). In this approach, "The educational outcomes are clearly specified and decisions about the content and how it is organised, the educational strategies, the teaching methods,

DOI: 10.4324/9781003316091-3

the assessment procedures and the educational environment are made in the context of the stated learning outcomes" (Harden et al., 1999a, pg. 8). The focus is on what learners can demonstrate at the end of their training. Thus, it is necessary to identify the knowledge, skills, and abilities that our graduates should have and then determine the pathways which lead to those results (Harden et al., 1999a). Outcomes-based education in health sciences has become synonymous with CBME (Morcke et al., 2013; Harden and Laidlaw 2021).

CBME was first promoted by McGaghie et al. (1978). It has become the dominant approach for medical education (Harden et al., 1999b; Tamblyn, 1999; Carraccio et al., 2002; Cooke et al., 2010; Frank et al., 2010b; Frenk et al., 2010; Harris et al., 2010; Carraccio and Englander, 2013; Englander et al., 2017; Van Melle et al., 2019; Hamza et al., 2023). In this model, competencies are "The abilities of a person to integrate knowledge, skills, and attitudes in their performance of tasks in a given context. Competencies are durable, trainable and, through the expression of behaviors, measurable" (World Health Organization, 2022). Thus, competencies are the attributes that an individual attains (ten Cate et al., 2015; Ma and ten Cate, 2023). Table 2.1 lists the definitions that are used in this chapter (World Health Organization, 2022).

The core components of a CBME program include (Van Melle et al., 2019) the following: (1) *outcome competencies* – the final expected outcome is clearly articulated; (2) *sequenced progressively* – competencies and developmental markers are sequenced; (3) *tailored learning experiences* – experiences facilitate the acquisition of competencies; (4) *competency-focused instruction* – teaching promotes acquisition of competencies; and

TABLE 2.1 Definitions Used

Competencies	The abilities of a person to integrate knowledge, skills, and attitudes in their performance of tasks in a given context. Competencies are durable, trainable, and, through the expression of behaviors, measurable.
Competence	The state of proficiency of a person to perform the required practice activities to the defined standard. This incorporates having the requisite competencies to do this in a given context. Competence is multidimensional and dynamic. It changes with time, experience, and setting.
Competent	Descriptive of a person who has the ability to perform the designated practice activities to the defined standard. This equates to having the requisite competencies.
Domain	A broad, distinguishable area of content; domains, in aggregate, constitute a general descriptive framework. Based on Englander et al. (2013).

(5) *programmatic assessment* – assessments support and document the development of competencies. The rationales that underlie CBME are (Frank et al., 2010b) as follows: (1) to focus on outcomes to be accountable that medical graduates are competent in all domains; (2) to emphasize the abilities and attitudes to be acquired by the trainee and not just knowledge; (3) to de-emphasize time-based training so that the learner actually achieves the desired outcomes; and (4) to promote learner-centeredness to ensure the learner is engaged in the process. The World Health Organization (2022) summarized that CBME is an "approach to preparing [health workers] for practice that is fundamentally oriented to outcome abilities and organized according to competencies. It de-emphasizes time-based training and facilitates greater accountability, flexibility and learner-centeredness." The emphasis of this approach is on "what sort of doctor will be produced–rather than on the educational process" (Harden et al., 1999a, pg. 7).

Competencies are contextual (Frank et al., 2010a; World Health Organization, 2022). A competency can have different thresholds for competence in different contexts (Smith et al., 2007). For example, in the competencies on diversity, equity, and inclusion (Association of American Medical Colleges [AAMC], 2022), the Association of American Medical Colleges (AAMC) describes competencies along a "learning continuum": *Entering residency* (New to the journey), *Entering practice* (Advancing along journey), *Faculty Physician Teaching and Leading* (Continuing the journey). For each stage along that continuum, there is a different expectation for competence.

The educational paradigm needs to shift from focusing on educational activities as a means to teach objectives and move to tailoring experiences to facilitate the gaining of competence (Van Melle et al., 2019; Schoenherr, Mahias-Ito, & Li, 2024). It is, essentially, "a highly individualized learning process rather than the traditional, one-size-fits-all curriculum" (Frenk et al., 2010, pg. 1943). At the GME level, fully competency-based training programs have had numerous successes internationally (Caccia et al., 2015; Schultz and Griffiths, 2016; Nousiainen et al., 2018; Sherbino et al., 2020). The USA also has competency-based GME programs (Eno et al., 2020), although graduation from these training programs is not competency based (Carraccio et al., 2023).

2.1.2 Foundational Educational Approaches

2.1.2.1 Learning Outcomes

Learning objectives define the end results of educational experiences (Bloom et al., 1956; Harden et al., 1999a; Anderson et al., 2001; Harden, 2002; Harden, 2007). Anderson et al. (2001) separated them into *Global Objectives* (vision) that reflect institutional learning objectives (ILOs), *Educational*

Objectives (curricular design) that reflect course-level objectives, and *Instructional Objectives* (educational activities) that reflect session-level objectives.

In medical education, Harden defined learning outcomes as "broad statements of what is achieved and assessed at the end of a course of study" (Harden, 2002, pg. 151). Harden's description of learning outcomes fits with the concept of ILOs. He further distinguishes between learning outcomes, which are more general, and "learning or instructional objectives," which are highly specified, and thus align with instructional objectives. For the purposes of this chapter, learning outcomes are global objectives and learning objectives define the learning to occur within an educational experience such as a session or course.

2.1.2.2   Bloom's Taxonomy

The predominant approach to addressing educational outcomes is embodied in the work of Bloom and colleagues (Bloom et al., 1956; Krathwohl et al., 1956; Anderson et al., 2001; Krathwohl, 2002). While Bloom described three educational domains, cognitive (knowledge), psychomotor (skills), and affective (attitudes) (Bloom et al., 1956; Krathwohl et al., 1956), foundational science education has focused primarily using on the knowledge domain (Chatterjee and Corral, 2017). Knowledge is a series of progressive steps that progress from factual knowledge to conceptual knowledge to procedural knowledge to metacognitive knowledge (Anderson et al., 2001). However, having knowledge does not imply that the learner can use that knowledge effectively. Thus, Bloom's taxonomy (Bloom et al., 1956; Anderson et al., 2001) focuses on cognitive processing of the knowledge as essential for meaningful learning. Students should develop the ability to use knowledge in a progressively complex manner and progress from Remember to Understand to Apply to Analyze to Evaluate to Create (see Table 2.2). As the learner ascends the cognitive learning scale, we presume the learner retains and is able to use earlier levels of knowledge and cognitive processing (Forehand, 2010).

The purposes of the higher orders of metacognitive processing (specifically, evaluate and create) (Table 2.2, Two rightmost columns) are probably inappropriate for preclerkship medical students as they are not being trained to be an expert in scientific disciplines or medicine. Therefore, there are four levels of cognitive processing that could be appropriate for medical students. Further, based on the educational and experiential level of preclerkship students, they are most likely limited to the first two levels of cognitive processing (Table 2.2, Two leftmost columns), Remember and Understand. Application and Analysis (Table 2.2, Two middle columns) is most appropriate to clinical education experiences.

TABLE 2.2 Bloom's Taxonomy Levels as Revised by Anderson et al.

Remember	Understand	Apply	Analyze	Evaluate	Create
Recognizing (identify)	Interpreting (clarify, paraphrase, represent, translate)	Executing (carry out)	Differentiating (discriminate, distinguish, focus, select)	Checking (coordinate, detect, monitor, test)	Generating (hypothesize)
Recalling (retrieve)	Exemplifying (illustrate, instantiate)	Implementing (use)	Organizing (find coherence, integrate, outline, parse, structure)	Critiquing (judge)	Planning (design)
	Classifying (categorize, subsume)		Attributing (Deconstruct)		Producing (construct)
	Summarizing (abstract, generalize)				
	Inferring (conclude, extrapolate, interpolate, predict)				
	Comparing (contrast, map, match)				
	Explaining (construct models)				

Source: Table modified from Anderson et al. (2001, pp. 67–68).

The verb form is used to guide assessment of what the learner does with the learning (Anderson et al., 2001; Krathwohl, 2002). They guide learners regarding the expected outcome (Chatterjee and Corral, 2017).

Regretfully, there is not much consistency in the construction of the lists of verbs available for instruction (Stanny, 2016; Newton et al., 2020; Larsen et al., 2022). Each UME program ought to utilize a single verb list across its courses and clerkships to ensure consistency.

2.1.2.3   Fink's Taxonomy of Significant Learning

Fink (2003) proposed a "Taxonomy of Significant Learning" as a successor to Bloom's taxonomy and suggested that it should consist of (1) foundational knowledge, (2) application learning, (3) integration, (4) the human dimension – caring, and (5) learning how to learn. This taxonomy appears to have limited adoption within medical education (Branzetti et al., 2019). In this approach, the first three dimensions are consistent with elements of Bloom's knowledge domain and are also consistent with competencies of medical practitioners (Edgar et al., 2020).

The idea that there should be learning devoted to the human dimension is consistent with much of what we want our learners to develop (Branch, 2000; MacLeod, 2011). Further, the Fink concept that we should be teaching learners how to learn is not emphasized in any other educational framework. Yet, it should be an essential element in medical education (Mayer, 2010; Branzetti et al., 2019).

2.1.2.4   Miller's Pyramid

Miller (1990) proposed a framework for assessing physicians (see Figure 2.1). In his pyramid, the lowest level, Knows, is that trainees need to know what is required to carry out professional functions. This is applicable to preclerkship education. At the next level, Knows How, learners need to demonstrate competence, which Miller defines as "the quality of being functionally adequate, or of having sufficient knowledge, judgement, skill, or strength for a particular duty" (Miller, 1990, pg. S63). This is the skill of acquiring "information from a variety of human and laboratory sources, to analyze and interpret these data, and finally to translate such findings into a rational diagnostic or management plan" (Miller, 1990, pg. S63). While some of this is applicable to clinical preclerkship education, the development of management plans is usually beyond the scope of foundational sciences education. At the next higher level, trainees need to "Show How" they can perform the professional task. Finally, in the final level of the triangle, Does, when the physician is no longer a trainee and is functioning independently. Recently, ten Cate and others (2021) have proposed extending the pyramid

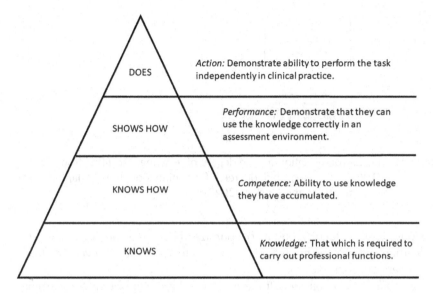

FIGURE 2.1 Miller's pyramid. Modified from Miller (1990).

to a fifth level, entrustment. Miller's Pyramid recognizes knowledge, including foundational sciences, as the basis for clinical medicine at its foundational level.

2.1.2.5 Mastery Learning

Bloom (1968, 1971) proposed an approach to education called "Mastery Learning," which was derived from the work of Carroll (1963, 1971). Carroll proposed that aptitude, or ability to achieve, is not a function of ability to learn but is a function of how much time the learner needs. Thus, the degree of learning is defined by a ratio between "time spent" and "time needed" (see Figure 2.2a). He further argued that "time spent" and "time needed" can be subdivided into component parts (see Figure 2.2b).

Consequently, the degree of learning by an individual student is based on the optimization of these component parts (Carroll, 1963; Block et al., 1971; Bloom, 1971; Guskey, 2023):

1. *Learner perseverance*: This is the amount of time that the learner is willing to spend in learning actively. If a learner is not willing to spend adequate time, they will not attain mastery. However, perseverance "is not fixed; it can be increased by increasing the frequency of reward and the evidence of learning success. Furthermore, the need for perseverance can be decreased by high quality instruction" (Bloom, 1971, pg. 54).

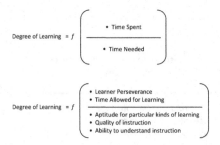

FIGURE 2.2 (a) Carroll equation for the degree of learning. Modified from Carroll (1963). (b) Expanded degree of learning equation. Adapted from Bloom (1971) and Guskey (2023).

Consequently, faculty ought to optimize the quality of instruction and learners ought to be motivated by rewards to stimulate perseverance (e.g., success on assessments).

2. *Time allowed for learning*: If there is a fixed amount of time for learning, it will either be too much or too little for some students. "The learning time needed will be affected by his aptitudes, his ability to understand instruction, and the quality of instruction he receives in class and outside of class" (Bloom, 1971, pg. 55). Thus, a curriculum ought to have flexibility in the timing for how a learner achieves the expected outcomes.

3. *Aptitude for particular kinds learning*: Different students have different aptitudes for different subjects. Bloom argued that "it is highly probable that more effective learning conditions can reduce the amount of time to learn a subject to mastery for all students and especially for the students with lower aptitudes" (Bloom, 1968, pg. 4). Thus, a learner can attain mastery in some subjects faster than in others. In a group of learners, different learners will learn with different aptitudes for different subjects; thus, an educational curriculum optimized for outcomes must take different aptitudes into consideration.

4. *Quality of instruction*: The concept is based on the idea that different students learn differently (Hernández-Torrano et al., 2017). While the general presumption is that there is a standard way to teach, the assumption used in mastery learning is "that individual students may need very different types of instruction" (Bloom, 1971, pg. 52). Carroll (1963) suggests that it is the degree, presentation, explanation, and ordering of the elements of the learning task that are optimized for the learner. Thus, a curriculum should have options that enable learners to learn according to their learning strategies.

5. *Ability to understand instruction*: Bloom defines this variable as "the ability of the learner to understand the nature of the task he is to learn and the procedures he is to follow in the learning of the task" (Bloom,

1968, pg. 5). This variable addresses the instructional ability of the faculty member and the resources provided to the learner.

Additionally, Bloom (1971) introduced the ideas of (1) the frequent use of formative assessments (Scriven, 1967) to guide student progress and provide feedback and (2) the use of alternative learning resources to provide "corrective activities" for the student to guide them toward success once formative assessments diagnose deficiencies in the student's learning. Bloom observed that teaching should occur sequentially. That is, the curriculum is sequenced from Block 1, to Block 2, to some Block x, which represents the end of the instruction (Bloom, 1971; Guskey, 2023). Each sequential block builds upon the prior knowledge and requires the ability to use that knowledge.

Figure 2.3 summarizes Bloom's model for mastery learning. A learner goes through the content of Block 1 and then takes a formative exam. If they pass the formative exam, they then receive some enhancement materials on that content before moving onto Block 2. If a learner fails the formative exam, they receive feedback and corrective activities. If they pass the subsequent formative exam, they progress to Block 2. If they fail, they receive additional feedback and more corrective activities. In this iterative manner, a learner can attain mastery of the material (Guskey, 2023).

Mastery learning is recognized as a foundational concept for CBME (Bordage, 2009; Van Melle et al., 2019). This approach has been proposed for clinical training (McGaghie, 2015) and adopted in simulation training (Cook et al., 2013; McGaghie et al., 2014; Griswold-Theodorson et al., 2015; Reed et al., 2016; Soetikno et al., 2020), ultrasound training (Jensen et al., 2018; Østergaard et al., 2019; Hagopian, 2020). This approach has also been used in preclerkship education (Colbert-Getz et al., 2023).

In McGaghie's (2015) formulation, mastery learning has at least seven features:

(1) baseline or diagnostic testing, (2) clear learning objectives sequenced as units usually in increasing difficulty, (3) engagement in educational activities focused on reaching the objectives, (4) a set of minimum passing standard for each educational unit, (5) formative testing to gauge unit completion at a preset minimum passing standard for mastery, (6) advancement to the next educational unit given measured achievement at a preset minimum passing standard for mastery, and (7) continued practice or study on an educational unit until the mastery standard is reached.

(McGaghie, 2015, pg. 1439)

While McGaghie focused on clinical education, these features can be applied to preclerkship education.

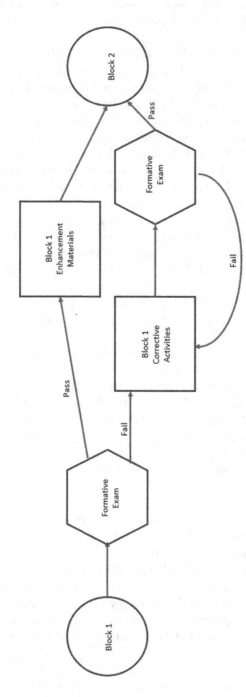

FIGURE 2.3 Bloom's mastery learning model. After time is provided to learn material from Block 1, the learner takes a formative exam. If they pass the formative exam, they move onto doing some enhancement content to reinforce Block 1 content. After experiencing that learning, they will move onto Block 2. If they fail the formative exam, they are provided with supplemental materials optimized to their learning. Subsequently, they take another formative exam. If they fail, they repeat the cycle with additional supplemental materials. If they pass, then they move onto Block 2. Modified from Guskey (2023).

2.1.2.6 *Master Adaptive Learning*

The Master Adaptive Learning approach (Schumacher et al., 2013; Cutrer et al., 2017; Cutrer et al., 2019) is founded on self-determined theory (Deci and Ryan, 2012) and self-directed learning (Knowles, 1975) or self-regulated learning (White et al., 2013). Three broad principles underlie this approach:

> (1) While learners must take responsibility for their learning, they must also seek external information to guide their efforts and calibrate their self-assessments; (2) While teachers must allow learners to assume responsibility for their learning, they must provide the role modeling, support, and feedback necessary to guide learning and assessment; and (3) While the learning environment impacts learners and teachers through defining the culture and context in which professional formation occurs, learners and teachers must attend to the reciprocal impact they have on the learning environment so as to ensure they are also creating a meaningful learning environment for others.
>
> *(Schumacher et al., 2013, pg. 1640)*

In combination with Deming's quality assurance PDCA (plan-do-check-act) cycle (Moen and Norman, 2006), Cutrer et al. (2017) proposed that the master adaptive learner would use four general phases to learn:

1. *Planning.* In this phase, learners would identify a gap, select an opportunity to learn, and search for resources for learning.
2. *Learning.* In this phase, the learners internalize the new material.
3. *Assessing.* In this phase, the learners try out the new materials.
4. *Adjusting.* In this phase, the learners incorporate their learning into daily routines.

While the adaptive master learning process was developed for clinical education, it can be adapted to preclerkship education (Cutrer et al., 2021). The key element of this educational approach is to enhance the environment for student learning. It promotes learner identification of knowledge gaps and how to fill them. The most essential element in this approach is the continued educational cycle that master adaptive learners go through to refine and improve their learning and understanding. This element is consistent with CBME.

2.1.2.7 *Forgetting Curve*

Retention of content decreases over time. This is described by Ebbinghaus' forgetting curve (Murre and Dros, 2015; Rivera-Lares et al., 2022). Ebbinghaus demonstrated that a learner will initially forget at an exponential rate and then come to some lower level in retention, typically around 20% of the content within a month (Swart and Venter, 2018). This forgetting has been demonstrated in medical education (Custers, 2010; Custers and ten Cate, 2011; Pusic et al., 2012; Weggemans et al., 2017; Kooloos et al., 2020). Custers and ten Cate (2011) showed that unrehearsed (not used or not repeated) basic science information was retained relatively well (up to 50%) in a select sample of medical students and physicians for up to two years and then started to decline. However, retention of rehearsed information (information that was reviewed and/or repeated) was significantly improved over time.

Consistent with CBME, as learners progress in a medical education program, effort must be made to ensure retention of content from prior learning and minimize forgetting. This is accomplished through intentional reintroduction – spaced repetition – of the material (Swart and Venter, 2018; Wollstein and Jabbour, 2022).

2.1.2.8 Entrustable Professional Activities

Entrustable Professional Activities (EPAs) have gained significant currency in the medical education landscape (Ma and ten Cate, 2023). EPAs are units of professional practice that a clinician needs to perform on a regular basis (ten Cate, 2005, 2019a). While competencies and skills are possessed by individuals, EPAs refer to work that must be done by healthcare professionals (ten Cate et al., 2015; ten Cate and Taylor, 2021; ten Cate and Schumacher, 2022). This approach has been implemented extensively around the world in medicine (Pangaro and ten Cate, 2013; Carraccio et al., 2017; O'Dowd et al., 2019; Edgar et al., 2020; Harris et al., 2020; de Graaf et al., 2021; Karpinski and Frank, 2021; Watson et al., 2021; Mueller et al., 2022; Nousiainen et al., 2022; Yap et al., 2023), pharmacy (Haines et al., 2017; Haines et al., 2018; Abeyaratne and Galbraith, 2023), nursing (Alexander et al., 2022; Corrigan et al., 2022; Spies and Feutz, 2023), physician assistant studies (Mulder et al., 2010; Acker et al., 2021), dentistry (Arunachalam et al., 2022; Cully et al., 2023; Ehlinger et al., 2023), and dietetics (Bramley et al., 2021; Bramley et al., 2023).

EPAs were developed for the UME level in the USA (AAMC, 2014; American Association of Colleges of Osteopathic Medicine, 2016) and Canada (The AFMC EPA Working Group, 2019). The focus of much research has been on the AAMC Core EPAs for Entering Residency in the USA (Meyer et al., 2019). However, this UME effort has had mixed success (Amiel et al., 2022; Harvey et al., 2023) and did not focus on preclerkship education. There have been attempts to develop EPAs for preclerkship learners (Chen et al., 2016).

However, ten Cate (2022) has recently suggested that the EPA approach is most appropriate for GME.

The general EPA approach (ten Cate, 2005, 2019b) – start by observing, progress to doing under tight supervision, then progress to doing under light supervision, then progress to being trusted to do the activity without supervision – is consistent with the mastery learning approach of moving along a sequential learning curve with increasing complexity and mastery. A key concept is whether an individual is ready to perform an activity with a specific level of trust: entrustability (ten Cate et al., 2016; Ma and ten Cate, 2023). This specific concept could be included in a CBME-based approach to preclerkship education through activities that start with supervised guidance leading toward the ability of the learner to perform the activities with minimal supervision.

2.1.3 Educational Expectations

In USA medical school accreditation standards, educational institutions must develop and demonstrate program outcomes (Commission on Osteopathic College Accreditation, 2023; Liaison Committee on Medical Education, 2023). These outcomes have been often linked to the Physician Competency Reference Set (Englander et al., 2013), the AAMC Core EPAs for Entering Residency (AAMC, 2014), the Osteopathic Core Competencies (American Association of Colleges of Osteopathic Medicine, 2012), and/or the Accreditation Council for GME's (ACGME's) core competencies (Swing, 2007).

To ascertain educational activities, such as lectures, labs, and small groups, are related to ILOs, session learning objectives are mapped to ILOs, often through course/clerkship learning objectives (Harden, 2001). The assumption is that graduates will meet the session learning objectives, and thus, by completing the courses and clerkships which have those learning objectives, the learner has achieved the ILOs. The validity of this assertion, however, is dependent on how the learning objectives are written, assessed, and documented at the course level (Schoenherr & Hamstra, 2024). Further, this follows a feed-forward curriculum design whereby the educational objectives in the sessions define those in the course which then define the educational outcomes.

In a CBME model, however, the converse approach is taken. The outcomes, what a graduate can demonstrate, are initially designed. Figure 2.4a shows the typical USA medical education model. Figure 2.4b shows the process for developing educational outcomes in the CBME model. The institution defines what the graduate should be able to demonstrate through its Mission and ILOs. In each of the prior curriculum stages, the learner is prepared so that they can be successful at the next stage of training. Hence, the goal of the

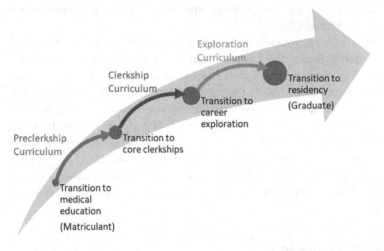

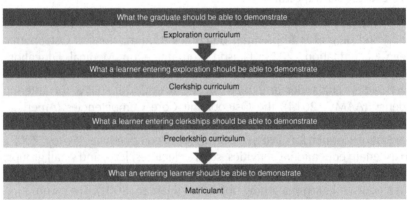

FIGURE 2.4   (a) The typical educational pathway for a US medical student. There is a transition from premedical to medical education when they become matriculants. There is a second transition from the preclerkship curriculum to the core clerkships. A third transition occurs when they transition into a curriculum focused on career exploration in electives and advanced clerkships. Lastly, as a graduate, they transition to residency. (b) Backwards curriculum design in medical education. The Exploration Curriculum should refine the trainee so that they represent what the institution has decided a graduate should be able to demonstrate program outcomes. The Clerkship Curriculum prepares a trainee to be able to demonstrate the knowledge, skills, and attitudes necessary to be successful in the Exploration Curriculum. The Preclerkship Curriculum prepares learners to be successful in the Clerkship Curriculum. There should also be a baseline which outlines what an entering learner should be able to demonstrate as a matriculant to medical school.

preclerkship curriculum is to prepare learners for their core clerkships; it is not to prepare learners for clinical practice.

Matriculants to medical school may have experienced courses with similar titles at different institutions. However, just because the titles are similar does not mean they have been exposed to the same content or have the same level of proficiency in the subject. Further, some students may not have had equivalent courses at all. Thus, consistent with McGaghie's (2015) first feature in clinical mastery learning, it is incumbent upon the institution to assess the matriculants and then ensure they have the same educational foundation so that they can be successful in the curriculum.

2.2 Implementation Strategies

2.2.1 Learning Objectives and Competency Objectives

2.2.1.1 What Are Learning Objectives?

Learning objectives, or session objectives, are specific, measurable outcomes due to an educational activity (Bloom et al., 1956; Anderson et al., 2001; Thomas, 2016; Chatterjee and Corral, 2017; Ryan et al., 2022). They typically comprise five elements (Thomas, 2016): (1) who is to accomplish the objective, (2) what they will be able to accomplish, (3) the criteria that they must accomplish, (4) of what action (e.g., demonstration of knowledge, skills, attitudes, abilities (KSAs)), and (5) by when. A learning objective expresses a target of an educational activity as defined by an action verb (Anderson et al., 2001; Thomas, 2016; Chatterjee and Corral, 2017), which allows measurement of the criteria required to meet the objective. Consequently, a learning objective defines the measurable end goal of a learning experience. Learning objectives are independent of educational progression; they specify what a learner should be able to achieve at the end of an educational activity. The results of learning objectives are binary: did the learner achieve the objective or not.

2.2.1.2 Achievement of Competence

In CBME, we measure whether a learner has achieved competence along learning curves (ten Cate et al., 2010; Pusic et al., 2011; Pusic et al., 2015). Thus, competence is a performance threshold within a continuum and is not an endpoint. The medical education community has adopted the Dreyfus and Dreyfus (1986) model of skills acquisition to categorize the learning curve (Batalden et al., 2002; Carraccio et al., 2008). Figure 2.5 shows a plot for progression to competence using the Dreyfus and Dreyfus (1986) model. A learner starts as a "Novice" (Level 1), progresses to "Advanced Beginner"

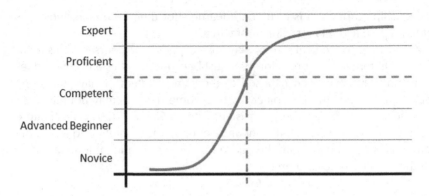

FIGURE 2.5 The Dreyfus and Dreyfus (1986) model. It is based on a learning curve and progresses from novice (follows the rules) to advanced beginner (all rules have equal importance) to competent (some perception of the relativity of rules and actions) to proficient (ability to prioritize actions) to expert (transcends rules and actions to act as necessary).

(Level 2), then to "Competent" (Level 3), "Proficient" (Level 4), and then "Expert" (Level 5). The threshold dotted line between Competent and Proficient indicates that the learner has achieved a predetermined, required level of proficiency for that competency within a specific context (e.g., level of training). The learner can continue development along the continuum of a competency after attaining competence. In a different context (e.g., a higher level of training), the required level of proficiency may be much higher and have additional components. Furthermore, the speed by which a learner gains or loses competence varies (ten Cate et al., 2010; Colbert-Getz and Shea, 2021).

Competence is the achievement of a standard of performance. It is evidence-based. The methodology by which the standard of performance is set is an important topic of discussion (Cusimano, 1996; Nabishah et al., 2011; Barsuk et al., 2018) that is beyond the scope here. This chapter will focus on the assessments necessary to determine the level of competence a learner demonstrates in the cognitive domain. As competence is achievement of a predetermined standard, the assessment of competence is criterion referenced and not norm referenced (Pereira et al., 2018). Competence is not a minimum pass level, but the level of achievement required to meet the competency within a context.

2.2.1.3 What Are Competency Objectives?

Competency objectives are specific measurable expressions of achievement required to meet standards of performance within specific contexts. The assertion of competence is that a learner has achieved a predetermined threshold for a competency objective. These are granular expressions of expected proficiency at a specific level of training. A competency objective is similar to a learning objective, excepting that it defines a threshold for competence and is not session dependent.

Features of competency objectives are that they are (1) observable and/or measurable, (2) designed for the specific context of the learner, (3) independent of specific learning activities, (4) have a pre-determined required level of proficiency, and (5) must be demonstrated prior to progression.

2.2.1.3.1 Observable and/or measurable

Ideally, acquisition of competence is documented along a learning curve that is aligned to a learning achievement scale. Thus, when writing a competency objective, an appropriate verb must be used to enable the observation and/ or measurement of the progression toward and beyond the competence threshold.

2.2.1.3.2 Designed for the specific context of the learner

The institution (or faculty member) must establish the educational context for the learner. Contexts could be "preclerkship," "clerkship," "transition to residency," "transition to unsupervised practice," and "leading/teaching as clinicians." Another set of contexts could be "first block," "second block," etc. A competency objective would have different expectations for each context. The threshold for competence in the early part of the preclerkship phase would require less proficiency than at the end of the clerkship phase. For example, in the first semester of medical school, a learner may meet a competency objective if they can distinguish different heart sounds; in the core clerkships, they may need to provide an appropriate, reasoned, diagnosis based on the heart sounds; and in the exploration phase of the curriculum, they may need to provide an appropriate treatment plan for the patient. Thus, competency objectives define the progression of the learner from matriculant to graduate for an institutional competency.

Ideally, ILOs would be consistent with an accepted national/international standard for medical education competencies (Rubin and Franchi-Christopher, 2002; Simpson et al., 2002; Frank and Danoff, 2007). There is currently no single medical education framework in the USA at the time of this writing. Institutions should align to these external standards. Individual institutions can define their own institutional contexts and competencies for their unique programs. However, aligning institutional competencies with national frameworks enables third parties to understand the curriculum and learner competencies at the institution.

2.2.1.3.3 Independent of specific learning activities

A foundational tenet of CBME is that learners can use a variety of learning experiences to gain competence. Educational activities are designed to enhance the progress of students in gaining competence (Van Melle et al., 2019). Attending a learning activity does not mean that the learner has or will achieve competence because of that activity. The learner may already have gained competence before the activity; the learner may need additional time and effort to gain competence after the activity. Thus, gaining competence is not the end goal of a learning experience, rather the learning experience provides opportunities for the learner to develop their competence.

2.2.1.3.4 Have a predetermined level of proficiency

Much has been written about learner assessment in competency programs (Shumway and Harden, 2003; Harden, 2007; Frank et al., 2010b; Harris et al., 2010; Holmboe et al., 2010; Pangaro and ten Cate, 2013; Van Melle et al., 2019; Colbert-Getz and Shea, 2021). It is not the purpose of this chapter to establish the method for setting the threshold for competence (Cusimano, 1996; Nabishah et al., 2011; Yudkowsky et al., 2015; Lok et al., 2016; Barsuk et al., 2018; Pereira et al., 2018). However, the institution or faculty member should pre-determine a specific level of proficiency for each competency objective. Thus, it is possible to collect evidence of achievement to demonstrate proficiency within the defined context.

2.2.1.3.5 Must be demonstrated prior to progression

As competency objectives define the proficiency of a learner in a progression toward a competency, a learner should demonstrate that they have achieved a level of proficiency prior to moving onto the next level of proficiency. The AAMC notes that "building competence … is a journey and not a destination" (AAMC, 2022). This concept of having sequenced competency objectives with increasing difficulty, set passing standards, formative assessments, and advancement to the next context based on achievement is consistent with mastery learning (McGaghie, 2015; Barsuk et al., 2018; Van Melle et al., 2019).

2.2.2 Assessment for Competence

"A competency-based approach to medical education relies on continuous, comprehensive, and elaborate assessment and feedback systems" (Holmboe et al., 2010, pg. 676). Data can be collected for a single competency or a competency and associated subcompetencies. Evidence should demonstrate progression along a learning curve and retention over time. Thus, assessment for competence should not be a single snapshot of the learner's performance. Further, the data collected should be valid and reliable (Iliya, 2014; Kibble, 2017). In practice, this usually means multiple formative assessments over time that examine the level of performance for each competency objective or combinations of competency objectives.

2.2.2.1 Summative Assessments vs Formative Assessments

Summative assessments are "usually applied at the end of a period of instruction to measure the outcome of student learning" (Kibble, 2017, pg. 110) and produce a singular snapshot of a learner's performance. Similar high-stakes exams include the licensure exams (e.g., USMLE and COMLEX). There is a place for summative exams in educational programs, especially if there is a need to rank order the learners (Bloom, 1971), track learner outcomes to inform the next instructor (Iliya, 2014), or assess program outcomes at a particular point in time (Iliya, 2014; Heeneman et al., 2015). In a pass/fail curriculum, especially one which constantly assesses for competence, whether summative examinations are always necessary is an open question.

Bloom introduced the use of "formative assessments" as "brief diagnostic-progress tests to determine which of the unit's tasks the student has or has not mastered and what he must do to complete his unit learning" (Bloom, 1971, pg. 58). The definition of formative assessments has evolved. Assessment is formative

> to the extent that evidence about student achievement is elicited, interpreted and used by teachers, learners, or their peers, to make decisions about the next steps in instruction that are likely to be better, or better founded, than the decisions they would have taken in the absence of the evidence what was elicited.
>
> *(Black and Wiliam, 2009, pg. 6)*

The purposes of formative assessments are as follows:

> 1. clarifying, sharing, and understanding learning intentions and criteria for success; 2. engineering effective classroom discussions, questions, and tasks that elicit evidence of learning; 3. providing feedback that moves learners forward; 4. activating students as instructional resources for one another; and 5. activating students as the owners of their own learning.
>
> *(Wiliam, 2010, pg. 31)*

"Assessment for learning" is a term that was introduced to advance the definition of a "formative assessment" (Wiliam, 2010). However,

> Assessment for learning is any assessment for which the first priority in its design and practice is to serve the purpose of promoting students' learning. It thus differs from assessment designed primarily to serve the purposes of accountability, or of ranking, or of certifying competence. An assessment activity can help learning if it provides information that teachers and their students can use as feedback in assessing themselves and one another and in modifying the teaching and learning activities in which they are engaged. Such assessment becomes "formative assessment" when the evidence is actually used to adapt the teaching work to meet learning needs.
>
> *(Black et al., 2004, pg. 10)*

Assessments in a CBME program modify teaching and learning activities as well as to certify competence. Therefore, the term "formative assessment" is most appropriate for CBME.

2.2.2.2 Criterion- vs. Norm-Referenced Assessments

For both summative and formative assessments, a question revolves around what constitutes "passing." There are two basic methods to determine passing. One is "criterion-referenced" and the other is "norm-referenced." A "criterion-referenced" assessment is one in which "each student is judged against predetermined absolute standards or criteria without regard to other students" (Lok et al., 2016). Passing is meeting the criteria. In norm referencing, students are compared and ranked to each other along a Gaussian curve which enables a rank order of students compared to their peers (Turnbull, 1989). Using the Gaussian curve, one then assigns specific percentages of the class to specific "grades," regardless of whether the class had a high performance or a low performance (Lok et al., 2016). Score normalization techniques, such as using *z-scores* (Winters, 2002), are common in norm-referenced examinations. Passing is usually set at some arbitrary "grade" based on the distribution of scores.

The majority (129 of 155 of USA MD schools in 2021–2022) have moved to a pass/fail grading system (AAMC, 2023) for the preclerkship curriculum. This type of curriculum is successful for student well-being (Robbins et al., 2008; Bloodgood et al., 2009; Reed et al., 2011; Spring et al., 2011). It would be reasonable to assert that for these pass/fail schools, which theoretically do not rank order their students, a criterion-based assessment system would be adequate. All these schools need to demonstrate is that the learner has met the outcomes required (i.e., achieved the competencies). However, there are many challenges to this approach (Pereira et al., 2018; Ryan et al., 2023) which focus on how grading has been traditionally done, reporting of student performance to residency program directors, and other similar factors.

2.2.2.3 Learning Achievement Scale

There is no significant guidance on how learners gain competence in preclerkship education. I have developed a learning achievement scale based on the Dreyfus and Dreyfus (1986) model to aid curriculum development in preclerkship education. This scale is based on learning curves (Pusic et al., 2015) wherein the levels of proficiency are as follows: Level 1 – Identify; Level 2 – Assemble; Level 3 – Utilize; Level 4 – Elaborate; and Level 5 – Assimilate. Figure 2.6 shows graphically the learning curve and Table 2.3 provides the definition for each level. A faculty member could articulate which level demonstrates competence within an educational context.

The following is an example of using this scale in a gross anatomy course to determine competence within different contexts of learning. The curriculum has an initial introductory block at the start of the academic year and then subsequent systems-based blocks for the remainder of the preclerkship curriculum. The example competency objective is "Discuss coronary circulation." Early in the introductory block, learners must meet the "Identify" level by naming the various vessels of the heart and where they were located on the heart. Later in that block, learners must meet the "Assemble" level where they could name the origins and relationships of the vessels (e.g., what vessel is a branch of what other vessel; what vessel drains into what vessel; how to determine if the heart is right or left dominant). In the cardiovascular (systems based) block, learners were expected to utilize their knowledge. For

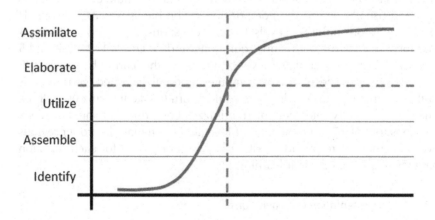

FIGURE 2.6 A learning achievement scale for preclerkship CBME based on Dreyfus and Dreyfus (1986).

TABLE 2.3 Learning Achievement Scale

Level	Explanation
Assimilate (Level 5)	Learners can *assimilate* the elements of the competency with other competencies or subcompetencies to address a challenge.
Elaborate (Level 4)	Learners can *elaborate* on the elements of the competency to address a challenge (knowledge, skill, or attitude).
Utilize (Level 3)	Learners can *utilize* the elements of the competency.
Assemble (Level 2)	Learners can *assemble* the elements of the competency together.
Identify (Level 1)	Learners can *identify* the elements of that comprise the competency.

example, if a portion of the heart is ischemic, the learner can explain what vessel might be occluded. Conversely, if a blockage of a vessel (e.g., in an imaging study) was presented to the learner, they need to name the areas of the heart that would be hypoxic.

As the learner gained clinical information during the unit, they were to elaborate what the appropriate treatment might be (e.g., angioplasty of a specific vessel when given an area of the heart that is hypoxic). As they approached the end of their preclerkship education, the learners should be able to assimilate from a different domain of information (e.g., the most appropriate vessels from outside the domain of the heart to use in a coronary artery bypass graft [CABG] procedure).

Learners need to have frequent feedback on their performance as they progress along the learning achievement scale. Thus, in this example, there were question banks for each achievement level (a minimum of 30 questions each and usually more). The composition of the banks was as follows: (1) Level 1 questions only; (2) Levels 1 and 2 questions; (3) Levels 1, 2, and 3 questions; (4) Levels 1, 2, 3, and 4 questions; and (5) Levels 1, 2, 3, 4, and 5 questions. To move to a higher level of questions, the learner had to pass (9 out of 10) the prior level. As the computer randomly selected the questions for these formative quizzes, learners could return to take the quiz up to three times before faculty intervention. The quizzes comprised a minimum of six questions (out of 10) from the highest level and the remainder from previous levels. Learners were provided with a keyword or phrase for each question that they missed to cue their learning.

2.2.2.4 Implementation Considerations

There is an assumption that it is essential that learners retain the information that they have learned in their foundational sciences curriculum into their clinical years (Flexner, 1910; Cooke et al., 2010). However, the educational process by which the basic sciences and clinical sciences are integrated has been the subject of extensive discussion (Harden, 2000; Pawlina, 2009; Bandiera et al., 2013; Kulasegaram et al., 2013; Dominguez and Zumwalt, 2020; Wijnen-Meijer et al., 2020; Khalil et al., 2021). Fundamentally, learners need to retain information from their foundational sciences studies as they progress into the clinical sciences.

As retention of basic sciences content is subject to the Ebbinhaus' forgetting curve (Custers, 2010; Custers and ten Cate, 2011), we should include a form of spaced repetition (Deng et al., 2015; Yeh and Park, 2015; Kang, 2016; Jape et al., 2022; Marinelli et al., 2022) to enhance retention. We can achieve this goal through the repetition of prior material in formative quizzes.

2.2.2.5 Progression in Learning

Establishing a progression in the training is key to CBME (Frank et al., 2010a; Frank et al., 2010b; Van Melle et al., 2019; World Health Organization, 2022). We accomplished this, in part, by increasing complexity of the learning achievement as the learner progressed. At the same time, the learner receives feedback on their deficits. This process guided their use of supplemental materials to address their deficits.

2.2.3 Time in CBME Preclerkship Education

By aiming at the acquisition of competence, time is less of a focus (Kogan et al., 2018). The focus should be on the progression toward acquisition of competence and not how long it takes to achieve competence. There are structural barriers currently in place for a fully time-variable competency educational program (Kogan et al., 2018; ten Cate et al., 2018; Carraccio et al., 2023). However, there are methods to move toward CBME within those structural barriers. For example, during a time-delimited unit for learning (e.g., a semester, block), it is possible to allow learners to achieve competencies at their own rate. Progression to the next unit of training would be dependent on whether they achieved the required competency objectives before the end of the current unit of learning. Learners can be provided with multiple opportunities (e.g., formative assessments) to help them determine their level of achievement. These opportunities would also provide faculty with information on learner progress so that individualized interventions can take place.

In every unit of training, a learner would have all the required competencies to move to the next unit presented to them on the first day of classes. They will progress at their own pace during that unit. As there are multiple competencies, they might complete some competencies quickly and other competencies at a slower pace. Faculty responsibilities are to (1) design learning experiences that supplement the learning taking place, (2) provide guidance to the learner when they experience difficulty in a specific competency, (3) curate and provide alternative learning resources to enable better learning, and (4) determine when to intervene with an individual student. Thus, it is possible to determine progression toward competence through multiple formative assessments which document and provide feedback to the learner and inform faculty of the learner's progress. A learner would be able to progress to the next unit of training after reaching the predetermined level of competence for all the competencies in that unit of training. A program such as this could meet the precepts of a CBME program without the structural changes to a more traditional time-dependent educational program. Figure 2.7 illustrates how this process would progress.

Two common challenges are (1) time dependency and (2) individualization. Both three- and four-year medical education programs leading to the MD degree in the USA must meet the accreditation standard of providing at least 130 weeks of instruction (Liaison Committee on Medical Education, 2023). Further, many medical schools allow learners to extend their time to six or more years after matriculation. Thus, time allocation within a medical education program to meet competencies requires management, not a change to accreditation standards (Stamy et al., 2018).

Individualized learner programs are not new (Markee, 1968), especially for remediation (Guevara et al., 2011). However, the concept of CBME requires a more comprehensive approach to individualized education (Irby et al., 2010; ten Cate, 2017; Schwinn et al., 2019; Gifford et al., 2021; Triola and Burk-Rafel, 2023). Individual educational plans are one approach to individualized learning and are used in pediatrics (Li and Burke, 2010; Tewksbury et al., 2018). However, providing options for multiple learning and instructional resources could also be effective. This effort could be assisted through the use of artificial intelligence (Holmes et al., 2023).

2.3 Educational Framework

2.3.1 CBME Framework

This section provides an idealized construct of a CBME-based educational framework for preclerkship education.

2.3.1.1 Develop the educational competency framework.

The ILOs – what the learner is capable of doing at the time of graduation – ought to be developed on the basis of the mission. Based on the ILOs, the school identifies the competencies that are necessary to meet those outcomes

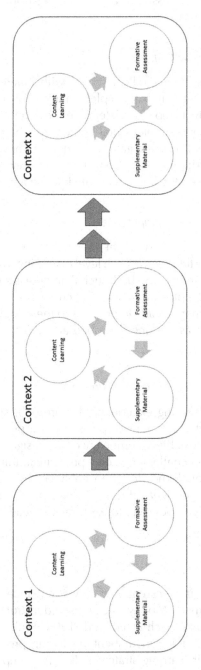

FIGURE 2.7 Progression in demonstrating learning of a competency objective. To move from one context to the next, a learner must demonstrate meeting the established criteria for "passing" the formative assessment.

at the highest level. Institutions then need to articulate what the expectations are for entry into each successive level of training from matriculation to graduation.

2.3.1.2 Matriculant Level Setting

Medical school learners enter medical school with different backgrounds. Thus, consistent with the clinical implementation of mastery learning (McGaghie, 2015), the first step is to determine the level of knowledge and capabilities of the learners. Supplemental content can be part of the initial curriculum to ensure that learners gain the requisite knowledge and skills expected by the faculty. This material also provides a review for those learners who have already achieved the Initial requisite knowledge and skills.

2.3.1.3 Build Progression into Competencies

As described above, institutions ought to determine what the required knowledge, skills, and attitudes are at each level of training. To prepare learners for the next level, competencies are built such that there is a progression from less complex to more complex along learning curves so that at the end of a level of training, the learner is ready to progress to the next. Use of a learning achievement scale, such as the one described above, could help formalize that process.

2.3.1.4 Develop Experiences that Guide Learning

In CBME, the specific learning experience, lecture, lab, small group, etc., is not about the content that is taught, per se. It is a process of providing guidance for the student to achieve competence. The design of the educational session ought to focus on challenging concepts, critical thinking issues, and application of foundational knowledge to enhance the learner's ability to reach competence at the designated level. These activities could also allow learners to demonstrate competence, for example, in leadership, teamwork, and professionalism.

2.3.1.5 Curate Content

To maximize learning, it is essential that we enhance the "Quality of Instruction" and the learner's "Ability to Understand Instruction." As learners. have different learning approaches (Hilliard, 1995; Feeley and Biggerstaff, 2015; Piumatti et al., 2021), it is incumbent that faculty provide learners with resources that meet their learning strategies. It is not simply providing one resource to the learners but to have a variety of resources available. To ensure that the content in the different resources is accurate and meets the learning goals, faculty should review these resources and indicate to learners whether the identified resource is appropriate. This is particularly true where learners find resources on their own. They need feedback to ensure that they can learn how to identify what resources are accurate and appropriate for their learning. This is a form of self-directed learning (Knowles, 1975; Hill et al., 2020).

2.3.1.6 *Ensure Frequent Feedback to Learners and Educators*

A principal approach to continuous quality improvement is the use of Deming's (2018) quality improvement cycle. In this cycle, there is constant review and feedback to improve quality (Wong and Headrick, 2021). The feedback can be course evaluations, faculty reviews, and, most importantly, assessments.

Assessments, particularly formative assessments, provide feedback to both faculty and learners. It tells both groups whether the learner has mastered certain content, concepts, skills, or behaviors. It allows the learners to adjust and adapt their learning so that they can learn what they missed and provide positive reinforcement when they are successful in demonstrating their knowledge and skills. For faculty, it can provide immediate information on where learners are successful and where they are not (Irving, 2020). The faculty can then address the challenges immediately instead of waiting for the subsequent year. This is continuous quality improvement, part of USA accreditation standards for medical school (Commission on Osteopathic College Accreditation, 2023; Liaison Committee on Medical Education, 2023).

2.3.1.7 *Employ Principles of Learning Engineering*

The term "Learning Engineering" was introduced by Simon (1967) in which he envisioned "a team of individuals who *are* professionals in the design of learning environments" (Simon, 1967, pg. 77). A combined group working within the IEEE Industry Connections/Industry Consortium on Learning Engineering (ICICLE) defined learning engineering as "a process and practice that … (1) applies the learning sciences, (2) using human-centered engineering design methodologies, and (3) data-informed decision-making … to support learners and their development" (Goodell, 2023, pg. 10). While generally consisting of a team of learning professionals working with faculty to develop educational experiences, the principles of learning engineering to design appropriate CBME materials can be performed by individuals. The principles are using learning sciences (Goodell et al., 2023), be learner-centered (Thai et al., 2023), and be driven by data analytics (Barrett et al., 2023). Further, view feedback and personalized learning as engineering problems (Barr et al., 2023). These principles are consistent with a CBME approach.

2.3.1.8 Focus on Outcome and Less on Content

As noted above, CBME is a process. Faculty tend to hold onto topics and content due to personal expertise and ideas of their importance. Sometimes, "faculty should be prepared to let go of some things" (Held et al., 2023). In medical education, what is true today may not be true tomorrow. Thus, the focus is on the outcomes necessary to so that the learner can be successful at the next educational level. Learners will also encounter external barrier exams (e.g., USMLE and COMLEX). Thus, development of a CBME curriculum does require consideration of all the subjects that might be on those barrier exams.

2.4 Summary

The fundamental belief on which this chapter is grounded is that there should be one educational approach in medical school – there should not be a dichotomy in the educational approach between the preclerkship years and the clinical education years. As CBME is the predominant model for medical training in clinical training both in UME and GME, it becomes necessary to adapt preclerkship education to that model.

I present a particular approach to accomplish CBME through integration of multiple education theories and concepts. There are many other additional, necessary underlying support systems necessary to enable a CBME program, for example, technology to support learner outcomes tracking, exam outcomes, or other content resources. However, the key principles are that CBME is focused on evidence-based outcomes and individualized to the learner.

Finally, the point of CBME is to enable the learners to be successful in providing good outcomes for their patients. Regardless of educational theory or approach, the goal of preclerkship education must be to enable better outcomes for future patients of our learners.

DISCLOSURE: None.

References

Abeyaratne, C., & Galbraith, K. (2023). A review of entrustable professional activities in pharmacy education. *American Journal of Pharmaceutical Education, 87*(3), 454–462. https://doi.org/10.5688/ajpe8872

Acker, S., Noelke, A., Huckabee, M., & Rieck, K. M. (2021). Development of the proposed 13 entrustable professional activities for physician assistant graduates. *The Journal of Physician Assistant Education, 32*(4), 232–236. https://doi.org/10.1097/jpa.0000000000000387

The AFMC EPA Working Group. (2019). *Afmc entrustable professional activities for the transition from medical school to residency.* The Association of Faculties of Medicine of Canada. http://www.afmc.ca/wp-content/uploads/2022/10/AFMC_Entrustable-Professional-Activities_ EN_Final.pdf

Alexander, N., Maaz, A., Peters, H., & Kottner, J. (2022). Entrustable professional activities in nursing education: A scoping review protocol. *BMJ Open, 12*(10), e061451. https://doi.org/10.1136/bmjopen-2022-061451

American Association of Colleges of Osteopathic Medicine. (2012). *Osteopathic core competencies for medical students.* www.aacom.org/docs/default-source/core-competencies/corecompetencyreport2012.pdf?sfvrsn=4

American Association of Colleges of Osteopathic Medicine. (2016). *Osteopathic considerations for core entrustable professional activities (epas) for entering residency.* www.aacom.org/docs/default-source/old-documents/old-med-ed/core-epas.pdf?sfvrsn=b6145397_2#:~:text=The%20entrustable%20professional%20activities%20,have%20attained%20sufficient%20specific%20competence.

Amiel, J., Ryan, M. S., Andriole, D. A., & Whelan, A. J. (2022). Core entrustable professional activities for entering residency: Summary of the 10-school pilot 2014–2021. https://store.aamc.org/core-entrustable-professional-activities-for-entering-residency-summary-of-the-10-school-pilot-2014-2021.html

Anderson, L. W., Krathwohl, D. R., Airasian, P. W., Cruikshank, K. A., Mayer, R. E., Pintrich, P. R., Raths, J., & Wittrock, M. C. (2001). *A taxonomy for learning, teaching, and assessing. A revision of bloom's taxonomy of educational objectives* (L. W. Anderson & D. R. Krathwohl, Eds.). Longman.

Arunachalam, S., Pau, A., Nadarajah, V. D., Babar, M. G., & Samarasekera, D. D. (2023). Entrustable professional activities in undergraduate dental education: A practical model for development and validation. European Journal of Dental Education, 27(2), 332–342. https://doi.org/10.1111/eje.12809

Association of American Medical Colleges (AAMC). (2014). Core entrustable professional activities for entering residency: Curriculum developers' guide. https://store.aamc.org/downloadable/download/sample/sample_id/63/%20

Association of American Medical Colleges (AAMC). (2022). Diversity, equity, and inclusion competencies across the learning continuum. https://store.aamc.org/diversity-equity-and-inclusion-competencies-across-the-learning-continuum.html

Association of American Medical Colleges (AAMC). (2023). Grading systems used in medical school programs. Association of American Medical Colleges. Retrieved 6/18/2023 from www.aamc.org/data-reports/curriculum-reports/data/grading-systems-used-medical-school-programs

Bandiera, G., Boucher, A., Neville, A., Kuper, A., & Hodges, B. (2013). Integration and timing of basic and clinical sciences education. *Medical Teacher, 35*(5), 381–387. https://doi.org/10.3109/0142159X.2013.769674

Barr, A., Dargue, B., Goodell, J., & Redd, B. (2023). Learning engineering is engineering. In J. Goodell & J. Kolodner (Eds.), *Learning engineering toolkit* (pp. 125–151). Routledge.

Barrett, M., Czerwomski, E., Goodell, J., Jacobs, D., Ritter, S., Sottilare, R., & Thai, K.-P. (2023). Learning engineering uses data (part 2): Analytics. In J. Goodell & J. Kolodner (Eds.), *Learning engineering toolkit* (pp. 175–198). Routledge.

Barsuk, J. H., Cohen, E. R., Wayne, D. B., McGaghie, W. C., & Yudkowsky, R. (2018). A comparison of approaches for mastery learning standard setting. *Academic Medicine, 93*(7), 1079–1084. https://doi.org/10.1097/acm.0000000000002182

Batalden, P., Leach, D., Swing, S., Dreyfus, H., & Dreyfus, S. (2002). General competencies and accreditation in graduate medical education. *Health Affairs, 21*(5), 103–111. https://doi.org/10.1377/hlthaff.21.5.103

Black, P., Harrison, C., Lee, C., Marshall, B., & Wiliam, D. (2004). Working inside the black box: Assessment for learning in the classroom. *Phi delta kappan, 86*(1), 8–21. https://doi.org/10.1177/003172170408600105

Black, P., & Wiliam, D. (2009). Developing the theory of formative assessment. *Educational Assessment, Evaluation and Accountability (Formerly: Journal of Personnel Evaluation in Education), 21*, 5–31. https://doi.org/10.1007/s11 092-008-9068-5

Block, J. H., Airasian, P. W., Carroll, J. B., & Bloom, B. S. (1971). *Mastery learning: Theory and practice*. Holt, Rinehart and Winston.

Bloodgood, R. A., Short, J. G., Jackson, J. M., & Martindale, J. R. (2009). A change to pass/fail grading in the first two years at one medical school results in improved psychological well-being. *Academic Medicine, 84*(5), 655–662. https://doi.org/10.1097/ACM.0b013e31819f6d78

Bloom, B. S. (1968). Learning for mastery. Instruction and curriculum. Regional education laboratory for the Carolinas and Virginia, topical papers and reprints, number 1. In Evaluation comment (Vol. 1, pp. n2).

Bloom, B. S. (1971). Mastery learning. In J. H. Block (Ed.), *Mastery learning: Theory and practice* (pp. 47–63). Holt, Rinehart and Winston, Inc.

Bloom, B. S., Engelhart, M. D., Furst, E. J., Hill, W. H., & Krathwohl, D. R. (1956). *Taxonomy of educational objectives: The classification of educational goals. Handbook 1. Cognitive domain* (B. S. Bloom, Ed.). David McKay Company.

Blumenthal, D. (2002). *Training tomorrow's doctors: The medical education mission of academic health centers*. The Commonwealth Fund. www.commonwealthf und.org/sites/default/files/documents/___media_files_publications_fund_report_ 2002_apr_training_tomorrows_doctors__the_medical_education_mission_of_ academic_health_centers_ahc_trainingdoctors_516_pdf.pdf

Bordage, G. (2009). Conceptual frameworks to illuminate and magnify. *Medical Education, 43*(4), 312–319. https://doi.org/10.1111/j.1365-2923.2009.03295.x

Bramley, A., Forsyth, A., & McKenna, L. (2023). Validity and educational impact of clinical entrustable professional activities linked to the nutrition care process for work-based assessment of entry-level dietetics students: Evaluation of a 3-year implementation study in Australia. *Journal of the Academy of Nutrition and Dietetics, 123*(4), 614–625. https://doi.org/10.1016/j.jand.2022.09.009

Bramley, A. L., Thomas, C. J., Mc Kenna, L., & Itsiopoulos, C. (2021). E-portfolios and entrustable professional activities to support competency-based education in dietetics. *Nursing and Health Sciences, 23*(1), 148–156. https://doi.org/10.1111/ nhs.12774

Branch, W. T. J. (2000). The ethics of caring and medical education. *Academic Medicine, 75*(2), 127–132. https://doi.org/10.1097/00001888-200002000-00006

Branzetti, J., Gisondi, M. A., Hopson, L. R., & Regan, L. (2019). Aiming beyond competent: The application of the taxonomy of significant learning to medical education. *Teaching and Learning in Medicine, 31*(4), 466–478. https://doi.org/10.1080/10401334.2018.1561368

Caccia, N., Nakajima, A., Scheele, F., & Kent, N. (2015). Competency-based medical education: Developing a framework for obstetrics and gynaecology. *Journal of Obstetrics and Gynaecology Canada, 37*(12), 1104–1112. https://doi.org/10.1016/ S1701-2163(16)30076-7

Carraccio, C., Englander, R., Gilhooly, J., Mink, R., Hofkosh, D., Barone, M. A., & Holmboe, E. S. (2017). Building a framework of entrustable professional activities, supported by competencies and milestones, to bridge the educational continuum. *Academic Medicine, 92*(3), 324–330. https://doi.org/10.1097/ACM.000000000 0001141

Carraccio, C., Lentz, A., & Schumacher, D. J. (2023). Dismantling fixed time, variable outcome education: Abandoning 'ready or not, here they come' is overdue. *Perspectives on Medical Education, 12*(1), 68–75. https://doi.org/10.5334/pme.10

Carraccio, C., Wolfsthal, S. D., Englander, R., Ferentz, K., & Martin, C. (2002). Shifting paradigms: From Flexner to competencies. *Academic Medicine, 77*(5), 361–367. https://doi.org/10.1097/00001888-200205000-00003

Carraccio, C. L., Benson, B. J., Nixon, L. J., & Derstine, P. L. (2008). From the educational bench to the clinical bedside: Translating the dreyfus developmental model to the learning of clinical skills. *Academic Medicine, 83*(8), 761–767. https://doi.org/10.1097/ACM.0b013e31817eb632

Carraccio, C. L., & Englander, R. (2013). From Flexner to competencies: Reflections on a decade and the journey ahead. *Academic Medicine, 88*(8), 1067–1073. https://doi.org/10.1097/ACM.0b013e318299396f

Carroll, J. B. (1963). A model of school learning. *Teachers College Record, 64*(8), 1–9. https://doi.org/10.1177/016146816306400801

Carroll, J. B. (1971). Problems of measurement related to the concept of learning for mastery. In J. H. Block (Ed.), *Mastery learning: Theory and practice* (pp. 29–46). Holt, Rinehart and Winston, Inc.

Chatterjee, D., & Corral, J. (2017). How to write well-defined learning objectives. *Journal of Education in Perioperative Medicine, 19*(4), E610.

Chen, H. C., McNamara, M., Teherani, A., ten Cate, O., & O'Sullivan, P. (2016). Developing entrustable professional activities for entry into clerkship. *Academic Medicine, 91*(2), 247–255. https://doi.org/10.1097/acm.0000000000000988

Colbert-Getz, J. M., Lindsley, J., Moore, K. B., Formosa, T., & Pippitt, K. (2023). Promotion of a mastery orientation to learning in medical school: Implementation of the not yet pass grade. *Academic Medicine, 98*(1), 52–56. https://doi.org/10.1097/acm.0000000000005002

Colbert-Getz, J. M., & Shea, J. A. (2021). Three key issues for determining competence in a system of assessment. *Medical Teacher, 43*(7), 853–855. https://doi.org/10.1080/0142159X.2020.1804540

Commission on Osteopathic College Accreditation. (2023). Accreditation of colleges of osteopathic medicine: COM continuing accreditation standards–effective august 1, 2023. https://osteopathic.org/wp-content/uploads/COCA-2023-COM-Continuing-Standards.pdf

Committee on the Health Professions Education Summit. (2003). *Health professions education: A bridge to quality* (A. C. Greiner & E. Knebel, Eds.). National Academy Press. www.nap.edu/catalog/10681.html

Cook, D. A., Brydges, R., Zendejas, B., Hamstra, S. J., & Hatala, R. (2013). Mastery learning for health professionals using technology-enhanced simulation: A systematic review and meta-analysis. *Academic Medicine, 88*(8), 1178–1186. https://doi.org/10.1097/ACM.0b013e31829a365d

Cooke, M., Irby, D. M., & O'Brien, B. C. (2010). *Educating physicians. A call for reform of medical school and residency.* Jossey-Bass.

Cooke, M., Irby, D. M., Sullivan, W., & Ludmerer, K. M. (2006). American medical education 100 years after the Flexner report. *New England Journal of Medicine, 355*(13), 1339–1344. https://doi.org/10.1056/NEJMra055445

Corrigan, C., Moran, K., Kesten, K., Conrad, D., Manderscheid, A., Beebe, S. L., & Pohl, E. (2022). Entrustable professional activities in clinical education: A practical approach for advanced nursing education. *Nurse Educator, 47*(5), 261–266. https://doi.org/10.1097/nne.0000000000001184

Cully, J. L., Schwartz, S. B., Quinonez, R., Martini, A., Klein, M., & Schumacher, D. J. (2023). Development of entrustable professional activities for post-doctorate pediatric dentistry education. *Journal of Dental Education, 87*(1), 6–17. https://doi.org/10.1002/jdd.13096

Cusimano, M. D. (1996). Standard setting in medical education. *Academic Medicine, 71*(10), S112–S120. https://doi.org/10.1097/00001888-199610000-00062

Custers, E. J. F. M. (2010). Long-term retention of basic science knowledge: A review study. *Advances in Health Sciences Education, 15*(1), 109–128. https://doi.org/10.1007/s10459-008-9101-y

Custers, E. J. F. M., & ten Cate, O. T. J. (2011). Very long-term retention of basic science knowledge in doctors after graduation. *Medical Education, 45*(4), 422–430. https://doi.org/10.1111/j.1365-2923.2010.03889.x

Cutrer, W. B., Miller, B., Pusic, M. V., Mejicano, G., Mangrulkar, R. S., Gruppen, L. D., Hawkins, R. E., Skochelak, S. E., & Moore, D. E. J. (2017). Fostering the development of master adaptive learners: A conceptual model to guide skill acquisition in medical education. *Academic Medicine, 92*(1), 70–75. https://doi.org/10.1097/acm.0000000000001323

Cutrer, W. B., Pusic, M., Gruppen, L. D., Hammoud, M. M., & Santen, S. A. (2019). *The master adaptive learner.* Elsevier Health Sciences.

Cutrer, W. B., Spickard, W. A., Triola, M. M., Allen, B. L., Spell, N., Herrine, S. K., Dalrymple, J. L., Gorman, P. N., & Lomis, K. D. (2021). Exploiting the power of information in medical education. *Medical Teacher, 43*(sup2), S17–S24. https://doi.org/10.1080/0142159X.2021.1925234

Deci, E. L., & Ryan, R. M. (2012). Self-determination theory. In P. A. M. V. Lange, A. W. Kruglanski, & E. T. Higgins (Eds.), *Handbook of Theories of Social Psychology: Volume 1* (pp. 416–437). SAGE Publications Ltd. https://doi.org/10.4135/9781446249215

de Graaf, J., Bolk, M., Dijkstra, A., van der Horst, M., Hoff, R. G., & ten Cate, O. (2021). The implementation of entrustable professional activities in postgraduate medical education in the Netherlands: Rationale, process, and current status. *Academic Medicine, 96*(7S), S29–S35. https://doi.org/10.1097/acm.0000000000004110

Deming, W. E. (2018). *The new economics for industry, government, education.* MIT Press.

Deng, F., Gluckstein, J. A., & Larsen, D. P. (2015). Student-directed retrieval practice is a predictor of medical licensing examination performance. *Perspectives on Medical Education, 4*(6), 308–313. https://doi.org/10.1007/s40037-015-0220-x

Dominguez, I., & Zumwalt, A. C. (2020). Integrating the basic sciences in medical curricula: Focus on the basic scientists. *Advances in Physiology Education, 44*(2), 119–123. https://doi.org/10.1152/advan.00172.2019

Dreyfus, H. L., & Dreyfus, S. E. (1986). *Mind over machine: The power of human intuition and expertise in the age of the computer.* Basil Blackwell.

Edgar, L., McLean, S., Hogan, S. O., Hamstra, S., & Holmboe, E. S. (2020). The Milestones guidebook, version 2020. www.acgme.org/Portals/0/MilestonesGuidebook.pdf?ver=2020-06-11-100958-330

Ehlinger, C., Fernandez, N., & Strub, M. (2023). Entrustable professional activities in dental education: A scoping review. *British Dental Journal, 234*(3), 171–176. https://doi.org/10.1038/s41415-023-5503-8

Englander, R., Cameron, T., Ballard, A. J., Dodge, J., Bull, J., & Aschenbrener, C. A. (2013). Toward a common taxonomy of competency domains for the health professions and competencies for physicians. *Academic Medicine, 88*(8), 1088–1094. https://doi.org/10.1097/ACM.0b013e31829a3b2b

Englander, R., Frank, J. R., Carraccio, C., Sherbino, J., Ross, S., & Snell, L. (2017). Toward a shared language for competency-based medical education. *Medical Teacher, 39*(6), 582–587. https://doi.org/10.1080/0142159X.2017.1315066

Eno, C., Correa, R., Stewart, N. H., Lim, J., Westerman, M. E., Holmboe, E. S., & Edgar, L. (2020). *Milestones guidebook for residents and fellows.* www.acgme.org/Portals/0/PDFs/Milestones/MilestonesGuidebookforResidentsFellows.pdf

Feeley, A.-M., & Biggerstaff, D. L. (2015). Exam success at undergraduate and graduate-entry medical schools: Is learning style or learning approach more important? A critical review exploring links between academic success, learning styles, and learning approaches among school-leaver entry ("traditional") and graduate-entry ("nontraditional") medical students. *Teaching and Learning in Medicine, 27*(3), 237–244. https://doi.org/10.1080/10401334.2015.1046734

Fink, L. D. (2003). What is significant learning. University of Oklahoma Significant Learning Website, Program for Instructional Innovation at the University of Oklahoma. Retrieved 5/14/2020, from www.wcu.edu/Webfiles/PDFs/facultycenter_SignificantLearning.pdf

Flexner, A. (1910). *Medical education in the United States and Canada: A report to the Carnegie foundation for the advancement of teaching.* D. B. Updike.

Forehand, M. (2010). Bloom's taxonomy. *Emerging Perspectives on Learning, Teaching, and Technology, 41*(4), 47–56. https://cmapspublic3.ihmc.us/rid=1FPRRBRBK-1V1PZ0J-2JPL/Blooms%20revised%20Taxonomy.pdf

Frank, J. R., & Danoff, D. (2007). The CanMEDS initiative: Implementing an outcomes-based framework of physician competencies. *Medical Teacher, 29*(7), 642–647. https://doi.org/10.1080/01421590701746983

Frank, J. R., Mungroo, R., Ahmad, Y., Wang, M., De Rossi, S., & Horsley, T. (2010a). Toward a definition of competency-based education in medicine: A systematic review of published definitions. *Medical Teacher, 32*(8), 631–637. https://doi.org/10.3109/0142159X.2010.500898

Frank, J. R., Snell, L. S., ten Cate, O., Holmboe, E. S., Carraccio, C., Swing, S. R., Harris, P., Glasgow, N. J., Campbell, C., Dath, D., Harden, R. M., Iobst, W., Long, D. M., Mungroo, R., Richardson, D. L., Sherbino, J., Silver, I., Taber, S., Talbot, M., & Harris, K. A. (2010b). Competency-based medical education: Theory to practice. *Medical Teacher, 32*(8), 638–645. https://doi.org/10.3109/0142159X.2010.501190

Frenk, J., Chen, L., Bhutta, Z. A., Cohen, J., Crisp, N., Evans, T., Fineberg, H., Garcia, P., Ke, Y., Kelley, P., Kistnasamy, B., Meleis, A., Naylor, D., Pablos-Mendez, A., Reddy, S., Scrimshaw, S., Sepulveda, J., Serwadda, D., & Zurayk, H. (2010). Health professionals for a new century: Transforming education to strengthen health systems in an interdependent world. *Lancet, 376*(9756), 1923–1958. https://doi.org/10.1016/s0140-6736(10)61854-5

Gifford, K. A., Thoreson, L., Burke, A. E., Lockspeiser, T. M., Lockwood, L. Z., Reed, S., Schumacher, D. J., & Mahan, J. D. (2021). Describing overarching curricular goals for individualized education. *Teaching and Learning in Medicine, 33*(3), 282–291. https://doi.org/10.1080/10401334.2020.1835665

Goodell, J. (2023). What is learning engineering. In *Learning engineering toolkit* (pp. 5–25). Routledge.

Goodell, J., Kolodner, J., & Kessler, A. (2023). Learning engineering applies the learning sciences. In J. Goodell & J. Kolodner (Eds.), *Learning engineering toolkit* (pp. 47–82). Routledge.

Griswold-Theodorson, S., Ponnuru, S., Dong, C., Szyld, D., Reed, T., & McGaghie, W. C. (2015). Beyond the simulation laboratory: A realist synthesis review of clinical outcomes of simulation-based mastery learning. *Academic Medicine, 90*(11), 1553–1560. https://doi.org/10.1097/acm.0000000000000938

Guevara, M., Grewald, Y., Hutchinson, K., Amoateng-Adjepong, Y., & Manthous, C. (2011). Individualized education plans in medical education. *Connecticut Medicine, 75*(9), 537–540.

Guskey, T. R. (2023). *Implementing mastery learning*, 3rd edition. Corwin.

Hagopian, E. J. (2020). Liver ultrasound: A key procedure in the surgeon's toolbox. *Journal of Surgical Oncology, 122*(1), 61–69. https://doi.org/10.1002/jso.25908

Haines, S. T., Pittenger, A. L., Gleason, B. L., Medina, M. S., & Neely, S. (2018). Validation of the entrustable professional activities for new pharmacy graduates. *American Journal of Health-System Pharmacy, 75*(23), 1922–1929. https://doi.org/10.2146/ajhp170815

Haines, S. T., Pittenger, A. L., Stolte, S. K., Plaza, C. M., Gleason, B. L., Kantorovich, A., McCollum, M., Trujillo, J. M., Copeland, D. A., Lacroix, M. M., Masuda, Q. N., Mbi, P., Medina, M. S., & Miller, S. M. (2017). Core entrustable professional activities for new pharmacy graduates. *American Journal of Pharmaceutical Education, 81*(1), S2. https://doi.org/10.5688/ajpe811S2

Hamza, D. M., Hauer, K. E., Oswald, A., van Melle, E., Ladak, Z., Zuna, I., Assefa, M. E., Pelletier, G. N., Sebastianski, M., Keto-Lambert, D., and Ross, S. (2023). Making sense of competency-based medical education (CBME) literary conversations: A BEME scoping review: BEME Guide No. 78. *Medical Teacher, 45*(8), 802–815. https://doi.org/10.1080/0142159X.2023.2168525

Harden, R. (2000). The integration ladder: A tool for curriculum planning and evaluation. *Medical Education, 34*, 551–557. https://doi.org/10.1046/j.1365-2923.2000.00697.x

Harden, R. M. (2001). AMEE guide no. 21: Curriculum mapping: A tool for transparent and authentic teaching and learning. *Medical Teacher, 23*(2), 123–137. https://doi.org/10.1080/01421590120036547

Harden, R. M. (2002). Learning outcomes and instructional objectives: Is there a difference? *Medical Teacher, 24*(2), 151–155. https://doi.org/10.1080/0142159022020687

Harden, R. M. (2007). Learning outcomes as a tool to assess progression. *Medical Teacher, 29*(7), 678–682. https://doi.org/10.1080/01421590701729955

Harden, R. M., Crosby, J. R., & Davis, M. H. (1999a). AMEE guide no. 14: Outcome-based education: Part 1-an introduction to outcome-based education. *Medical Teacher, 21*(1), 7–14. https://doi.org/10.1080/01421599979969

Harden, R. M., Crosby, J. R., Davis, M. H., & Friedman, R. (1999b). AMEE guide no. 14: Outcome-based education: Part 5-from competency to meta-competency: A model for the specification of learning outcomes. *Medical Teacher, 21*(6), 546–552. https://doi.org/10.1080/01421599978951

Harden, R. M., and Laidlaw, J. M. (2021). *Essential skills for a medical teacher: An introduction to teaching and learning in medicine* (3rd ed.). Elsevier Health Sciences.

Harris, K. A., Nousiainen, M. T., & Reznick, R. (2020). Competency-based resident education-the Canadian perspective. *Surgery, 167*(4), 681–684. https://doi.org/10.1016/j.surg.2019.06.033

Harris, P., Snell, L., Talbot, M., & Harden, R. M. (2010). Competency-based medical education: Implications for undergraduate programs. *Medical Teacher, 32*(8), 646–650. https://doi.org/10.3109/0142159X.2010.500703

Harvey, A., Paget, M., McLaughlin, K., Busche, K., Touchie, C., Naugler, C., & Desy, J. (2023). How much is enough? Proposing achievement thresholds for core epas of graduating medical students in Canada. *Medical Teacher, 45*(9), 1054–1060. https://doi.org/10.1080/0142159X.2023.2215910

Heeneman, S., Oudkerk Pool, A., Schuwirth, L. W. T., van der Vleuten, C. P. M., & Driessen, E. W. (2015). The impact of programmatic assessment on student learning: Theory versus practice. *Medical Education, 49*(5), 487–498. https://doi.org/10.1111/medu.12645

Held, N., Jimenez, S., Lockspeiser, T., & Adams, J. E. (2023). Designing a shortened preclinical basic science curriculum: Expert-derived recommendations. *Academic Medicine, 98*(8), 922–928. https://doi.org/10.1097/acm.0000000000005221

Hernández-Torrano, D., Ali, S., & Chan, C.-K. (2017). First year medical students' learning style preferences and their correlation with performance in different subjects within the medical course. *BMC Medical Education, 17*(1), 131. https://doi.org/10.1186/s12909-017-0965-5

HHMI, & AAMC. (2009). Scientific foundations for future physicians. https://store.aamc.org/downloadable/download/sample/sample_id/207/

Hill, M., Peters, M., Salvaggio, M., Vinnedge, J., & Darden, A. (2020). Implementation and evaluation of a self-directed learning activity for first-year medical students. *Medical Education Online, 25*(1), 1717780. https://doi.org/10.1080/10872981.2020.1717780

Hilliard, R. I. (1995). How do medical students learn: Medical student learning styles and factors that affect these learning styles. *Teaching and Learning in Medicine, 7*(4), 201–210. https://doi.org/10.1080/10401339509539745

Holmboe, E. S., Sherbino, J., Long, D. M., Swing, S. R., & Frank, J. R. (2010). The role of assessment in competency-based medical education. *Medical Teacher, 32*(8), 676–682. https://doi.org/10.3109/0142159X.2010.500704

Holmes, W., Bialik, M., & Fadel, C. (2023). Artificial intelligence in education. In C. Stückelberger & P. Duggal (Eds.), *Data ethics: Building trust: How digital technologies can serve humanity* (pp. 621–653). Globethics Publications. https://doi.org/10.58863/20.500.12424/4276068

Iliya, A. (2014). Formative and summative assessment in educational enterprise. *Journal of Education and Practice, 5*(20), 111–117.

Irby, D. M., Cooke, M., & O'Brien, B. C. (2010). Calls for reform of medical education by the Carnegie foundation for the advancement of teaching: 1910 and 2010. *Academic Medicine, 85*(2), 220–227. https://doi.org/10.1097/ACM.0b013e3181c88449

Irving, K. E. (2020). Technology-assisted formative assessment. In M. Khosrow-Pour, S. Clarke, M. E. Jennex, & A.-V. Anttiroiko (Eds.), *Learning and performance assessment: Concepts, methodologies, tools, and applications* (pp. 435–453). IGI Global.

Jape, D., Zhou, J., & Bullock, S. (2022). A spaced-repetition approach to enhance medical student learning and engagement in medical pharmacology. *BMC Medical Education, 22*(1), 337. https://doi.org/10.1186/s12909-022-03324-8

Jensen, J. K., Dyre, L., Jørgensen, M. E., Andreasen, L. A., & Tolsgaard, M. G. (2018). Simulation-based point-of-care ultrasound training: A matter of competency rather than volume. *Acta Anaesthesiologica Scandinavica, 62*(6), 811–819. https://doi.org/10.1111/aas.13083

Kang, S. H. K. (2016). Spaced repetition promotes efficient and effective learning: Policy implications for instruction. *Policy Insights from the Behavioral and Brain Sciences, 3*(1), 12–19. https://doi.org/10.1177/2372732215624708

Karpinski, J., & Frank, J. R. (2021). The role of EPAs in creating a national system of time-variable competency-based medical education. *Academic Medicine, 96*(7S), S36–S41. https://doi.org/10.1097/acm.0000000000004087

Khalil, M. K., Giannaris, E. L., Lee, V., Baatar, D., Richter, S., Johansen, K. S., & Mishall, P. L. (2021). Integration of clinical anatomical sciences in medical education: Design, development and implementation strategies. *Clinical Anatomy, 34*(5), 785–793. https://doi.org/10.1002/ca.23736

Kibble, J. D. (2017). Best practices in summative assessment. *Advances in Physiology Education, 41*(1), 110–119. https://doi.org/10.1152/advan.00116.2016

Knowles, M. (1975). *Self-directed learning.* Follet.

Kogan, J. R., Whelan, A. J., Gruppen, L. D., Lingard, L. A., Teunissen, P. W., & ten Cate, O. (2018). What regulatory requirements and existing structures must change if competency-based, time-variable training is introduced into the continuum of medical education in the United States? *Academic Medicine, 93*(3S), S27–S31. https://doi.org/10.1097/acm.0000000000002067

Kooloos, J. G. M., Bergman, E. M., Scheffers, M., Schepens-Franke, A. N., & Vorstenbosch, M. (2020). The effect of passive and active education methods applied in repetition activities on the retention of anatomical knowledge. *Anatomical Sciences Education, 13*(4), 458–466. https://doi.org/10.1002/ase.1924

Krathwohl, D. R. (2002). A revision of Bloom's taxonomy: An overview. *Theory Into Practice, 41*(4), 212–218. https://doi.org/10.1207/s15430421tip4104_2

Krathwohl, D. R., Bloom, B. S., & Masia, B. B. (1956). *Taxonomy of educational objectives. The classification of educational goals. Handbook ii. Affective domain.* David McKay Company.

Kulasegaram, K. M., Martimianakis, M. A., Mylopoulos, M., Whitehead, C. R., & Woods, N. N. (2013). Cognition before curriculum: Rethinking the integration of basic science and clinical learning. *Academic Medicine, 88*(10), 1578–1585. https://doi.org/10.1097/ACM.0b013e3182a45def

Larsen, T. M., Endo, B. H., Yee, A. T., Do, T., & Lo, S. M. (2022). Probing internal assumptions of the revised Bloom's taxonomy. *CBE—Life Sciences Education, 21*(4), ar66. https://doi.org/10.1187/cbe.20-08-0170

Li, S.-T. T., & Burke, A. E. (2010). Individualized learning plans: Basics and beyond. *Academic Pediatrics, 10*(5), 289–292. https://doi.org/10.1016/j.acap.2010.08.002

Liaison Committee on Medical Education. (2023). Functions and structure of a medical school: Standards for accreditation of medical education programs leading to the MD degree. https://lcme.org/wp-content/uploads/2023/03/2024-25-Functions-and-Structure_2023-03-21.docx

Lok, B., McNaught, C., & Young, K. (2016). Criterion-referenced and norm-referenced assessments: Compatibility and complementarity. *Assessment and*

Evaluation in Higher Education, 41(3), 450–465. https://doi.org/10.1080/02602 938.2015.1022136

Ma, T. P., & ten Cate, O. (2023). Entrustable professional activities: A model for job activity competency framework with microcredentials. *International Journal of Information and Learning Technology, 40*(4), 317–333. https://doi.org/10.1108/IJILT-05-2022-0108

MacLeod, A. (2011). Caring, competence and professional identities in medical education. *Advances in Health Sciences Education, 16*(3), 375–394. https://doi.org/10.1007/s10459-010-9269-9

Marinelli, J. P., Hwa, T. P., Lohse, C. M., & Carlson, M. L. (2022). Harnessing the power of spaced repetition learning and active recall for trainee education in otolaryngology. *American Journal of Otolaryngology, 43*(5), 103495. https://doi.org/https://doi.org/10.1016/j.amjoto.2022.103495

Markee, J. E. (1968). Changing teaching practices in individualized curricula. In J. P. Lysaught (Ed.), *Individualized instruction in medical education: Proceedings of the third Rochester conference on self-instruction in medical education* (pp. 11–23). University of Rochester.

Mayer, R. E. (2010). Applying the science of learning to medical education. *Medical Education, 44*(6), 543–549. https://doi.org/10.1111/j.1365-2923.2010.03624.x

McGaghie, W. C. (2015). Mastery learning: It is time for medical education to join the 21st century. *Academic Medicine, 90*(11), 1438–1441. https://doi.org/10.1097/acm.0000000000000911

McGaghie, W. C., Issenberg, S. B., Barsuk, J. H., & Wayne, D. B. (2014). A critical review of simulation-based mastery learning with translational outcomes. *Medical Education, 48*(4), 375–385. https://doi.org/10.1111/medu.12391

McGaghie, W. C., Sajid, A. W., Miller, G. E., & Telder, T. V. (1978). *Competency-based curriculum development in medical education*. World Health Organization. https://apps.who.int/iris/handle/10665/39703

McNeir, G. (1993). Outcomes-based education: Tool for restructuring (0095-6694). Oregon School Study Council. http://files.eric.ed.gov/fulltext/ED357457.pdf

Meyer, E. G., Chen, H. C., Uijtdehaage, S., Durning, S. J., & Maggio, L. A. (2019). Scoping review of entrustable professional activities in undergraduate medical education. *Academic Medicine, 94*(7), 1040–1049. https://doi.org/10.1097/acm.0000000000002735

Miller, G. E. (1990). The assessment of clinical skills/competence/performance. *Academic Medicine, 65*(9), S63–S67. https://journals.lww.com/academicmedicine/Fulltext/1990/09000/The_assessment_of_clinical.45.aspx

Moen, R., & Norman, C. (2006). Evolution of the PDCA cycle. In *Proceedings of the 7th ANQ congress*. https://elfhs.ssru.ac.th/phusit_ph/pluginfile.php/48/block_html/content/Moen-Norman-2009%20PDCA.pdf

Morcke, A. M., Dornan, T., & Eika, B. (2013). Outcome (competency) based education: An exploration of its origins, theoretical basis, and empirical evidence. *Advances in Health Sciences Education, 18*(4), 851–863. https://doi.org/10.1007/s10459-012-9405-9

Mueller, V., Morais, M., Lee, M., & Sherbino, J. (2022). Implementation of entrustable professional activities assessments in a Canadian obstetrics and gynecology residency program: A mixed methods study. *Canadian Medical Education Journal, 13*(5), 77–81. https://doi.org/10.36834/cmej.72567

Mulder, H., ten Cate, O., Daalder, R., & Berkvens, J. (2010). Building a competency-based workplace curriculum around entrustable professional activities: The case of physician assistant training. *Medical Teacher, 32*(10), e453–e459. https://doi.org/10.3109/0142159X.2010.513719

Murre, J. M., & Dros, J. (2015). Replication and analysis of Ebbinghaus' forgetting curve. *PLoS One, 10*(7), e0120644.

Nabishah, M., Ab, N., & Salam, A. (2011). Standard setting for assessment of basic medical science modules. *Procedia-Social and Behavioral Sciences, 18*, 118–121. https://doi.org/10.1016/j.sbspro.2011.05.017

Nara, N., Suzuki, T., & Tohda, S. (2011). The current medical education system in the world. *Journal of medical and dental sciences, 58*(2), 79–83. https://doi.org/10.11480/jmds.580207

Newton, P. M., Da Silva, A., & Peters, L. G. (2020). A pragmatic master list of action verbs for Bloom's taxonomy [Brief Research Report]. *Frontiers in Education, 5.* https://doi.org/10.3389/feduc.2020.00107

Nousiainen, M. T., Bardana, D., Gofton, W., Broekhuyse, H. M., & Kraemer, W. (2022). Creating a national competency-based curriculum for orthopaedic surgery residency: The Canadian experience. *JB JS Open Access, 7*(1). https://doi.org/10.2106/jbjs.Oa.21.00131

Nousiainen, M. T., Mironova, P., Hynes, M., Glover Takahashi, S., Reznick, R., Kraemer, W., Alman, B., & Ferguson, P. (2018). Eight-year outcomes of a competency-based residency training program in orthopedic surgery. *Medical Teacher, 40*(10), 1042–1054. https://doi.org/10.1080/0142159X.2017.1421751

O'Dowd, E., Lydon, S., O'Connor, P., Madden, C., & Byrne, D. (2019). A systematic review of 7 years of research on entrustable professional activities in graduate medical education, 2011–2018. *Medical Education, 53*(3), 234–249. https://doi.org/10.1111/medu.13792

Oluwabunmi O.-O., E., Adisa, A. O., Olopade, F. E., Lawal, T. A., Hammad, N., Iputo, J. E., & Scott-Emuakpor, A. B. (2024). Medical education in sub-Saharan Africa. *Fundamentals and frontiers in medical education and decision-making: Innovation, implementation, and translational research.* Routledge.

Østergaard, M. L., Rue Nielsen, K., Albrecht-Beste, E., Kjær Ersbøll, A., Konge, L., & Bachmann Nielsen, M. (2019). Simulator training improves ultrasound scanning performance on patients: A randomized controlled trial. *European Radiology, 29*(6), 3210–3218. https://doi.org/10.1007/s00330-018-5923-z

Pangaro, L., & ten Cate, O. (2013). Frameworks for learner assessment in medicine: AMEE guide no. 78. *Medical Teacher, 35*(6), e1197–e1210. https://doi.org/10.3109/0142159X.2013.788789

Pawlina, W. (2009). Basic sciences in medical education: Why? How? When? Where? *Medical Teacher, 31*(9), 787–789. https://doi.org/10.1080/01421590903183803

Pereira, A. G., Woods, M., Olson, A. P. J., van den Hoogenhof, S., Duffy, B. L., & Englander, R. (2018). Criterion-based assessment in a norm-based world: How can we move past grades? *Academic Medicine, 93*(4), 560–564. https://doi.org/10.1097/acm.0000000000001939

Piumatti, G., Abbiati, M., Gerbase, M. W., & Baroffio, A. (2021). Patterns of change in approaches to learning and their impact on academic performance among medical students: Longitudinal analysis. *Teaching and Learning in Medicine, 33*(2), 173–183. https://doi.org/10.1080/10401334.2020.1814295

Pusic, M., Pecaric, M., & Boutis, K. (2011). How much practice is enough? Using learning curves to assess the deliberate practice of radiograph interpretation.

Academic Medicine, 86(6), 731–736. https://doi.org/10.1097/ACM.0b013e318 2178c3c

Pusic, M. V., Boutis, K., Hatala, R., & Cook, D. A. (2015). Learning curves in health professions education. *Academic Medicine, 90*(8), 1034–1042. https://doi.org/ 10.1097/acm.0000000000000681

Pusic, M. V., Kessler, D., Szyld, D., Kalet, A., Pecaric, M., & Boutis, K. (2012). Experience curves as an organizing framework for deliberate practice in emergency medicine learning. *Academic emergency medicine, 19*(12), 1476–1480. https:// doi.org/10.1111/acem.12043

Reed, D. A., Shanafelt, T. D., Satele, D. W., Power, D. V., Eacker, A., Harper, W., Moutier, C., Durning, S., Massie, F. S. J., Thomas, M. R., Sloan, J. A., & Dyrbye, L. N. (2011). Relationship of pass/fail grading and curriculum structure with well-being among preclinical medical students: A multi-institutional study. *Academic Medicine, 86*(11), 1367–1373. https://doi.org/10.1097/ACM.0b013 e3182305d81

Reed, T., Pirotte, M., McHugh, M., Oh, L., Lovett, S., Hoyt, A. E., Quinones, D., Adams, W., Gruener, G., & McGaghie, W. C. (2016). Simulation-based mastery learning improves medical student performance and retention of core clinical skills. *Simulation in Healthcare, 11*(3), 173–180. https://doi.org/10.1097/sih.00000 00000000154

Rivera-Lares, K., Stamate, A., & Della Sala, S. (2022). The cognitive concept of forgetting. In S. Della Sala (Ed.), *Encyclopedia of behavioral neuroscience*, 2nd edition (pp. 432–442). Elsevier. https://doi.org/https://doi.org/10.1016/B978-0-12-819641-0.00155-9

Robbins, B. D., Tomaka, A., Innus, C., Patterson, J., & Styn, G. (2008). Lessons from the dead: The experiences of undergraduates working with cadavers. *Omega (Westport), 58*(3), 177–192. https://doi.org/10.2190/om.58.3.b

Rubin, P., & Franchi-Christopher, D. (2002). New edition of Tomorrow's Doctors. *Medical Teacher, 24*(4), 368–369. https://doi.org/10.1080/0142159021000000816

Ryan, M. S., Blood, A. D., Park, Y. S., & Farnan, J. M. (2022). Competency-based frameworks in medical school education programs: A thematic analysis of the academic medicine snapshots, 2020. *Academic Medicine, 97*(11S), S63–S70. https://doi.org/10.1097/acm.0000000000004912

Ryan, M. S., Lomis, K. D., Deiorio, N. M., Cutrer, W. B., Pusic, M. V., & Caretta-Weyer, H. A. (2023). Competency-based medical education in a norm-referenced world: A root cause analysis of challenges to the competency-based paradigm in medical school. *Academic Medicine, 98*(11), 1251–1260. https://doi.org/10.1097/ acm.0000000000005220

Schoenherr, J. R & Beaudoin, J. (2024). Medical pluralism in East Asian medical education: The evolving landscape of health professions education in East Asia. In Schoenherr, J. R. (ed.), *Fundamentals and frontiers in medical education and decision-making: Innovation, implementation, and translational research.* (pp. XX–YY). Routledge.

Schoenherr, J. R., & Hamstra, S. J. (2024). Validity in health professions education: From assessment instruments to program innovation and evaluation. In Schoenherr, J. R. & McConnell, M. (eds.), *Fundamentals and frontiers in medical education: Educational theory and psychological practice: Innovation, implementation, and translational research.* Routledge.

Schoenherr, J. R., Mahias-Ito, Y., & Li, X. Y. (2024). Collective competence and social learning in the health professions: Learning, thinking, and deciding in groups. In Schoenherr, J. R. (ed.), *Fundamentals and frontiers in medical education and decision-making: Innovation, implementation, and translational research.* Routledge.

Schoenherr, J. R. & McConnell, M. (2024). Human-centered design in health professions education: Informing competency-based education with psychological science. In Schoenherr, J. R. & McConnell, M. (eds.), *Fundamentals and frontiers in medical education: Educational theory and psychological practice.* Routledge.

Schultz, K., & Griffiths, J. (2016). Implementing competency-based medical education in a postgraduate family medicine residency training program: A stepwise approach, facilitating factors, and processes or steps that would have been helpful. *Academic Medicine, 91*(5), 685–689. https://doi.org/10.1097/acm.0000000000001066

Schumacher, D. J., Englander, R., & Carraccio, C. (2013). Developing the master learner: Applying learning theory to the learner, the teacher, and the learning environment. *Academic Medicine, 88*(11), 1635–1645. https://doi.org/10.1097/ACM.0b013e3182a6e8f8

Schumacher, D. J., Kinnear, B., Carraccio, C., Holmboe, E., Busari, J. O., van der Vleuten, C., and Lingard, L. (2024). Competency-based medical education: The spark to ignite healthcare's escape fire. *Medical Teacher, 46*, 140–146. https://doi.org/10.1080/0142159X.2023.2232097

Schwinn, D. A., Cooper, C. S., & Robillard, J. E. (2019). Putting students at the center: Moving beyond time-variable one-size-fits-all medical education to true individualization. *Advances in Medical Education and Practice, 10*, 109–112. https://doi.org/10.2147/AMEP.S187946

Scriven, M. (1967). The methodology of evaluation. In R. Stake (Ed.), *Perspectives of curriculum evaluation.* Rand McNally and Company.

Sherbino, J., Bandiera, G., Doyle, K., Frank, J. R., Holroyd, B. R., Jones, G., Norum, J., Snider, C., & Magee, K. (2020). The competency-based medical education evolution of Canadian emergency medicine specialist training. *Canadian Journal of Emergency Medicine, 22*(1), 95–102. https://doi.org/10.1017/cem.2019.417

Shumway, J. M., & Harden, R. M. (2003). AMEE guide no. 25: The assessment of learning outcomes for the competent and reflective physician. *Medical Teacher, 25*(6), 569–584. https://doi.org/10.1080/0142159032000151907

Simon, H. A. (1967). The job of a college president. *Educational Record, 48*(1), 68–78.

Simpson, J. G., Furnace, J., Crosby, J., Cumming, A. D., Evans, P. A., David, M. F. B., Harden, R. M., Lloyd, D., McKenzie, H., McLachlan, J. C., McPhate, G. F., Percy-Robb, I. W., & MacPherson, S. G. (2002). The Scottish doctor—Learning outcomes for the medical undergraduate in Scotland: A foundation for competent and reflective practitioners. *Medical Teacher, 24*(2), 136–143. https://doi.org/10.1080/01421590220120713

Smith, S. R., Goldman, R. E., Dollase, R. H., and Taylor, J. S. (2007). Assessing medical students for non-traditional competencies. *Medical Teacher, 29*(7), 711–716. https://doi.org/10.1080/01421590701316555

Soetikno, R., Asokkumar, R., McGill, S. K., & Kaltenbach, T. (2020). Simulation-based mastery learning for practicing gastroenterologists-renewed importance in the era of Covid-19. *American Journal of Gastroenterology, 115*(9), 1380–1383. https://doi.org/10.14309/ajg.0000000000000788

Spies, L. A., & Feutz, K. (2023). Developing and implementing entrustable professional activities to prepare global nurses. *Journal of Transcultural Nursing, 34*(1), 100–105. https://doi.org/10.1177/10436596221125896

Spring, L., Robillard, D., Gehlbach, L., & Moore Simas, T. A. (2011). Impact of pass/fail grading on medical students' well-being and academic outcomes. *Medical Education, 45*(9), 867–877. https://doi.org/10.1111/j.1365-2923.2011.03989.x

Stamy, C. D., Schwartz, C. C., Phillips, D. A., Ajjarapu, A. S., Ferguson, K. J., & Schwinn, D. A. (2018). Time-variable medical education innovation in context. *Advances in Medical Education and Practice, 9*, 469–481. https://doi.org/10.2147/AMEP.S163984

Stanny, C. J. (2016). Reevaluating Bloom's taxonomy: What measurable verbs can and cannot say about student learning. *Education Sciences, 6*(4), 37. www.mdpi.com/2227-7102/6/4/37

Swart, A. J., & Venter, M. (2018). Regular self-assessments in a learning management system negates the Ebbinghaus forgetting curve. 47th Annual Conference of the Southern African Computer Lecturers' Association (SACLA 2018), Harbour Island, Gordon's Bay, South Africa.

Swing, S. R. (2007). The ACGME outcome project: Retrospective and prospective. *Medical Teacher, 29*(7), 648–654. https://doi.org/10.1080/01421590701392903

Tamblyn, R. (1999). Outcomes in medical education: What is the standard and outcome of care delivered by our graduates? *Advances in Health Sciences Education, 4*(1), 9–25. https://doi.org/10.1023/A:1009893715930

ten Cate, O. (2005). Entrustability of professional activities and competency-based training [Article]. *Medical Education, 39*(12), 1176–1177. https://doi.org/10.1111/j.1365-2929.2005.02341.x

ten Cate, O. (2017). Competency-based postgraduate medical education: Past, present and future. *GMS Journal for Medical Education, 34*(5), Doc69. https://doi.org/10.3205/zma001146

ten Cate, O. (2019a). An updated primer on entrustable professional activities (EPAs). *Revista brasileira de educação médica, 43*(1 suppl 1), 712–720. https://doi.org/10.1590/1981-5271v43suplemento1-20190238.ing

ten Cate, O. (2019b). When I say … Entrustability. *Medical Education, 54*, 103–104. https://doi.org/10.1111/medu.14005

ten Cate, O. (2022). How can entrustable professional activities serve the quality of health care provision through licensing and certification? *Canadian Medical Education Journal, 13*(4), 8–14. https://doi.org/10.36834/cmej.73974

ten Cate, O., Carraccio, C., Damodaran, A., Gofton, W., Hamstra, S. J., Hart, D., Richardson, D., Ross, S., Schultz, K., Warm, E., Whelan, A., & Schumacher, D. J. (2021). Entrustment decision making: Extending Miller's pyramid. *Academic Medicine, 96*(2), 199–204. https://doi.org/10.1097/acm.0000000000003800

ten Cate, O., Chen, H. C., Hoff, R. G., Peters, H., Bok, H., & van der Schaaf, M. (2015). Curriculum development for the workplace using entrustable professional activities (EPAs): AMEE guide no. 99. *Medical Teacher, 37*(11), 983–1002. https://doi.org/10.3109/0142159X.2015.1060308

ten Cate, O., Gruppen, L. D., Kogan, J. R., Lingard, L. A., & Teunissen, P. W. (2018). Time-variable training in medicine: Theoretical considerations. *Academic Medicine, 93*(3S), S6–S11. https://doi.org/10.1097/acm.0000000000002065

ten Cate, O., Hart, D., Ankel, F., Busari, J., Englander, R., Glasgow, N., Holmboe, E., Iobst, W., Lovell, E., Snell, L. S., Touchie, C., Van Melle, E., Wycliffe-Jones, K., & Collaborators, on behalf of the International Competency-Based Medical Education Collaborators (2016). Entrustment decision making in clinical training. *Academic Medicine, 91*(2), 191–198. https://doi.org/10.1097/acm.0000000000001044

ten Cate, O., & Schumacher, D. J. (2022). Entrustable professional activities versus competencies and skills: Exploring why different concepts are often conflated. *Advances in Health Sciences Education: Theory and Practice, 27*(2), 491–499. https://doi.org/10.1007/s10459-022-10098-7

ten Cate, O., Snell, L., & Carraccio, C. (2010). Medical competence: The interplay between individual ability and the health care environment. *Medical Teacher, 32*(8), 669–675. https://doi.org/10.3109/0142159X.2010.500897

ten Cate, O., & Taylor, D. R. (2021). The recommended description of an entrustable professional activity: AMEE guide no. 140. *Medical Teacher, 43*(10), 1106–1114. https://doi.org/10.1080/0142159X.2020.1838465

Tewksbury, L. R., Carter, C., Konopasek, L., Sanguino, S. M., & Hanson, J. L. (2018). Evaluation of a national pediatric subinternship curriculum implemented through individual learning plans. *Academic Pediatrics, 18*(2), 208–213. https://doi.org/10.1016/j.acap.2017.11.009

Thai, K.-P., Craig, S. D., Goodell, J., Lis, J., Schoenherr, J. R., & Kolodner, J. (2023). Learning engineering is human-centered. In J. Goodell & J. Kolodner (Eds.), *Learning engineering toolkit* (pp. 83–123). Routledge.

Thomas, P. A. (2016). Goals and objectives … focusing the curriculum. In P. A. Thomas, D. E. Kern, M. T. Hughes, & B. Y. Chen (Eds.), *Curriculum development for medical education* (pp. 50–64). Johns Hopkins University Press.

Triola, M. M., & Burk-Rafel, J. (2023). Precision medical education. *Academic Medicine, 98*(7), 775–781. https://doi.org/10.1097/acm.0000000000005227

Turnbull, J. M. (1989). What is… normative versus criterion-referenced assessment. *Medical Teacher, 11*(2), 145–150. https://doi.org/10.3109/01421598909146317

Van Melle, E., Frank, J. R., Holmboe, E. S., Dagnone, D., Stockley, D., Sherbino, J., & Collaborators, on behalf of the International Competency-Based Medical Education Collaborators (2019). A core components framework for evaluating implementation of competency-based medical education programs. *Academic Medicine, 94*(7), 1002–1009. https://doi.org/10.1097/acm.0000000000002743

Venosa, A. R., Baroneza, J. E., & Fernandes, R. A. F. (2024). Medical education in Brazil: A history of an evolving pluralistic healthcare system. In Schoenherr, J. R. & McConnell, M. M. (eds.), *Fundamentals and frontiers in medical education and decision-making*. Routledge.

Watson, A., Leroux, T., Ogilvie-Harris, D., Nousiainen, M., Ferguson, P. C., Murnahan, L., & Dwyer, T. (2021). Entrustable professional activities in orthopaedics. *JBJS Open Access, 6*(2), e20.00010. https://doi.org/10.2106/jbjs.Oa.20.00010

Weggemans, M. M., Custers, E. J. F. M., & ten Cate, O. T. J. (2017). Unprepared retesting of first year knowledge: How much do second year medical students remember? *Medical Science Educator, 27*(4), 597–605. https://doi.org/10.1007/s40670-017-0431-3

White, C. B., Gruppen, L. D., & Fantone, J. C. (2013). Self-regulated learning in medical education. In *Understanding medical education* (pp. 201–211). https://doi.org/https://doi.org/10.1002/9781118472361.ch15

Wijnen-Meijer, M., Burdick, W., Alofs, L., Burgers, C., & ten Cate, O. (2013). Stages and transitions in medical education around the world: Clarifying structures and terminology. *Medical Teacher, 35*(4), 301–307. https://doi.org/10.3109/0142159X.2012.746449

Wijnen-Meijer, M., van den Broek, S., Koens, F., & ten Cate, O. (2020). Vertical integration in medical education: The broader perspective. *BMC Medical Education, 20*(1), 509. https://doi.org/10.1186/s12909-020-02433-6

Wiliam, D. (2010). An integrative summary of the research literature and implications for a new theory of formative assessment. In H. L. Andrade & G. J. Cizek (Eds.), *Handbook of formative assessment* (pp. 18–40). Routledge.

Winters, R. S. (2002). *Score normalization as a fair grading practice.* https://files.eric.ed.gov/fulltext/ED470592.pdf

Wollstein, Y., & Jabbour, N. (2022). Spaced effect learning and blunting the forgetfulness curve. *Ear, Nose & Throat Journal, 101*(9_suppl), 42S–46S. https://doi.org/10.1177/01455613231163726

Wong, B. M., & Headrick, L. A. (2021). Application of continuous quality improvement to medical education. *Medical Education, 55*(1), 72–81. https://doi.org/10.1111/medu.14351

World Health Organization. (2022). Global competency framework for universal health coverage. World Health Organization. www.who.int/publications/i/item/9789240034686

Yap, M., Reddy, K., & Poh, C. (2023). Transition from existing systems to competency-based medical education (CBME) anchored on entrustable professional activities (EPAs): The Singapore experience [part 1]. Retrieved 4/12/2023 from https://icenetblog.royalcollege.ca/2023/01/12/transition-from-existing-systems-to-competency-based-medical-education-cbme-anchored-on-entrustable-professional-activities-epas-the-singapore-experience-part-1/

Yeh, D. D., & Park, Y. S. (2015). Improving learning efficiency of factual knowledge in medical education. *Journal of Surgical Education, 72*(5), 882–889. https://doi.org/10.1016/j.jsurg.2015.03.012

Yudkowsky, R., Park, Y. S., Lineberry, M., Knox, A., & Ritter, E. M. (2015). Setting mastery learning standards. *Academic Medicine, 90*(11), 1495–1500. https://doi.org/10.1097/acm.0000000000000887

3

VALIDITY IN HEALTH PROFESSIONS EDUCATION

From Assessment Instruments to Program Innovation and Evaluation

Jordan Richard Schoenherr and Stanley J. Hamstra

The changing context and demands of health professions education (Dunn, 2010; Gruppen et al., 2017; Irby, 2003, 2016; Mclean, 2008; Tolsgard et al., 2020; van Gaalen et al., 2021; Williams, 2019) requires a new approach to developing, implementing, and evaluating training programs as well as the courses and training sessions that define them. While the promise of learning analytics (LA; Bilgic, et al., 2024) and artificial intelligence (AI; Schoenherr & Michael, 2024; Wartman & Coombs, 2018) in health professions education looms large, the efficacy of AI is based on identifying and measuring competencies and providing feedback that is timely and intelligible to learners. With the introduction of competency-based educational frameworks in North America by the Accreditation Council for Graduate Medical Education (ACGME) in the United States and the Royal College of Physicians and Surgeons in Canada, learning institutions are required to demonstrate that they are providing a comprehensive program of education. The shift away from apprenticeship model (e.g., Frank, 2010; Hamdorf, 2000) has promoted the development of standardized training tasks for education and assessment (Brownell Anderson, 2009; May, 2009).

As health professions education has matured as an interdisciplinary field, it has sought out appropriate criteria to promote the development of competencies in a principled manner that ensures consistency for learners (Miller, 1990; Swanson, 1995; Wass, 2001). The nature of these criteria has remained a matter of considerable debate even in areas as specific as surgical education (e.g., Elliott, 2010; Grierson, 2014; Hamstra, 2014) and as general as simulation studies (Schoenherr & Hamstra, 2017). Moreover, the need to implement these training procedures given the demands of the curriculum must prompt educators and researchers to revisit ways of designing and

DOI: 10.4324/9781003316091-4

implementing their learning objectives (Ross, 2013; Schoenherr, 2024b). As extant projects and programs reduce the degrees of freedom of task developers (Cook, 1986), we must acknowledge the importance of the programmatic context for any educational intervention and assessment method. These concerns are reflected in the shift toward a programmatic-level evaluation of health professions education initiatives (van der Vleuten & Schuwirth, 2005; van der Vleuten et al., 2012). Moreover, the need for patient safety as well as accountability and defensibility of decisions that are based on information from assessment necessitates the consideration of numerous activities to effectively assess learning across competencies.

In this chapter, we outline a two-dimensional program evaluation framework that provides meaningful conceptual distinctions between criteria used in task development (construct validity) and that used in program evaluation (implementation validity). We first provide a review of major construct validity frameworks and the relationship between those provided by Messick (1995) and Kane (1992, 2001) as they can inform medical education task development (Cook, 2006). Paralleling observations in the literature on translational research in biomedical sciences (e.g., Rubio et al., 2010; Woolf, 2008; for a review, see Schoenherr, 2024a), we argue that providing evidence for construct validity does not imply that the task or program can be implemented in an organizational context. Implementation requires a wholly different set of considerations (Leonard-Barton, 1988). Similarly, whereas simply demonstrating that a task can be implemented in no way implies that it has construct validity and should be used within a program. To account for this additional dimension of task evaluation, we introduce the concept of *implementation validity*, the extent to which a coherent, evidence-based argument can be made for particular educational intervention or assessment method being useful in a particular institutional context. These two dimensions of validity should be viewed as orthogonal to one another, each defined by mutually exclusive sources of evidence. Our account rests on the assumption that both forms of validity are necessary when examining tasks in the context of a program (for related views, see Rossi, 2004; van der Vleuten & Schuwirth, 2005). When we have significant evidence for both construct validity and implementation validity, this supports the claim that a simple training task, assessment instrument, or complex simulation can function in the ecology of an institution's education and training programs.

3.1 Design Considerations for Task Validation in Health Professions Education

The incorporation of educational theory to support clinical training is a comparatively recent development relative to the instructional methods used to train physicians (e.g., Flexner, 1910/1960). For instance, instruction in surgical skills was previously guided by the "see one, do one, teach one" approach and characterized by an apprenticeship model wherein a student would learn directly from a surgeon (e.g., Halsted, 1904). In the early history of the healthcare professions, such a model was compatible with the social context and resources available at that time (e.g., Conrad, 1995; Duffin, 1999; Waddington, 2011). Similarly, there has been considerable focus on the integration of "high fidelity" simulations into training programs despite the high cost and limited evidence supporting their widespread use (Matsumoto et al., 2002; Norman et al., 2012; Schoenherr & Hamstra, 2017). On the side of program evaluation, LA faces many of these same challenges as educators and program developers must ensure that the analytic and visualization techniques are valid (Bilgic, et al., 2024). Thus, considering both the extent to which a training or assessment method[1] effectively imparts knowledge and how they fit into a curriculum requires independent methods of evaluation in the healthcare professions.

3.1.1   The Two Validities of Program Evaluation

The psychometric literature that is often used to justify assessment instruments in health professions education is populated with different forms of "validity" (Schoenherr & Hamstra, 2016). For instance, *face validity* is typically defined as the superficial adequacy of a measurement instrument, procedure, or test in measuring a construct (cf., Nevo, 1985), whereas *convergent validity* is evidenced when multiple assessment methods measure the same trait, ability, etc. (e.g., simulated patients, OSCEs, and MCQs) producing similar scores while *divergent validity* is observed when the variation between two scores is unrelated to one another thereby suggest the measurement of independent traits (Gravetter & Forzano, 2016). Complementing (and conflicting) with these forms of validity are many others (Anastasi, 1986; Angoff, 1988; Clark & Watson, 1995; Wainer & Braun, 1988).

In contrast to these approaches to conceptualizing validity, Messick (1989, 1995) presented a comprehensive validity framework which instead assumes that there is only a single form of validity: *construct validity* (Cronbach & Meehl, 1955; cf. Borsboom et al., 2004). Researchers must formulate hypotheses and seek out types of validity evidence that cumulatively suggest the degree of construct validity for a given intervention or assessment scale (Schoenherr, 2024c). For instance, if a simulation intervention increases a learner's performance on a defined set of skills (e.g., communication and medical expertise) and increases their confidence (cf. Schoenherr et al., 2024), this might be taken as evidence for its construct validity. For this reason, considerable research in the health professions education literature has been directed toward demonstration of construct validity of tasks (Cook & Beckman, 2006).

Program evaluation has an equivalent depth of considerations (e.g., Rossi, 2004; Stufflebaum, 2001). In program evaluation, while *construct validity is necessary, it is not in itself sufficient* to ensure that educational interventions, assessment methods, LA, etc. are effectively implemented in a particular context. Thus, while the adoption of a well-defined notion of construct validity is required to develop and evaluate tasks, curriculum developers must additionally consider another feature of their environment: the curriculum provided by an institution and its organizational context (e.g., van der Vleuten & Schuwirth, 2005; Ross, 2013). How tasks fit into a curriculum from a programmatic level reflects the "fitness of purpose" of the set of individual tasks for the attainment of institutional learning objectives (e.g., van der Vleuten & Schuwirth, 2005; van der Vleuten et al., 2012; for related comments, see Hamstra, 2014). While a task might reflect the best design principles (e.g., Norman, 1988/2013; Norman, 1999), tasks can be misaligned with the context, thereby requiring further modification (Leonard-Barton, 1988, 1992), informed by means of studying and interpreting feedback (Brown & Kiernan, 2001; Richards, 2011). For instance, while studies might suggest that a particular simulation promotes learning, simply using the same simulation techniques does not guarantee that it will produce the same outcomes if an institution does not have the appropriate resources to support its use. This is analogous to assuming that a plug from North America will fit into a socket in Europe.

If construct validity and implementation validity represent two independent selection criteria for educational innovations, then each aspect of the curriculum must have distinct sources of evidence that are identifiable. To ensure that appropriate skills and knowledge are acquired by the learners, educational innovations must be considered in terms of construct validity. In contrast, to ensure that educational innovations are compatible with the human and financial resources and educational objectives embodied by an institution's curriculum, educational innovations must be considered in terms of how they are implemented in a programmatic context. Thus, in the same manner as construct validity, we suggest that clinicians and educators must ensure that their tasks have *implementation validity*.

In the following section, we outline two facets of construct validity (Messick, 1989, 1995; Kane, 1992, 2001) used in the field of health professions education and develop an analogous method for the examination of implementation validity. Together, these two sources of validity will determine the fit of educational innovations in a program evaluation space.

3.1.1.1 *Construct Validity: Defining Skills, Selecting Learners, and Designing Tasks*

The extent to which assessment techniques promote the development of the underlying skill of interest can be understood in terms of construct validity

(Cronbach, 1989; Cronbach & Meehl, 1955). In general, construct validity represents the degree to which performance on a task can be interpreted as reflecting a hypothetical ability, process, or skill (cf. Borsboom et al., 2004). Rather than an all-or-none property, validity can be considered in terms of a continuous value determined by the amount of available converging evidence (Campbell, 1959, 1988; Messick, 1989, 1995). This general approach to isolating independent sources of evidence for a validity argument will also be critical to an understanding of implementation validity.

To provide greater empirical and theoretical integration, Messick (1989, 1995) urged researchers and educators to consider both the properties of the educational intervention and assessment instruments as well as how they were used in the context of an organization (for an account specific to healthcare professions education, see Cook & Beckman, 2006).[2] He proposed a two-dimensional framework wherein designers considered the bases of the task and instrumentation (evidence and consequences) and how the task was interpreted and used (see Table 3.1). A key issue faced by many in healthcare professions education is how to adapt existing assessment methods that already have considerable validity evidence supporting their use. Not all these tasks might be relevant or have utility for health professions education programs. For instance, a task might reliably assess learners' auditory short-term memory capacity or tactile sensitivity when performing an examination, yet this evidence might not be relevant to determining whether HCPs have attained a sufficient level of competency (Ma, 2024).

Evidence for Construct Validity. When evaluating an educational innovation, Messick identified six sources of evidence required to establish construct validity in a controlled setting: content, response process, internal structure, relations to other variables, generalizability, and the social consequences of testing. The content of an assessment instrument can be understood in terms of whether it completely represents the construct being considered. The response process requires an understanding of the underlying affective and sensory-motor responses, reasoning, and decision-making, as well as communication skills used to complete a diagnosis or procedure. When applied to surgical skills, an educational intervention or assessment task

TABLE 3.1 Facets of Construct Validity

	Test Interpretation	Test Use
Evidential Basis	Construct Validity (CV)	CV + Relevance/Utility
Consequential Basis	CV + Value Implications (VI)	CV + R/U + VI + Social Consequences

Source: Adapted from Messick (1995).

that requires the same response processes would include the diagnosis of a condition, use of anatomical landmarks, and motor coordination. Taken together, the extent to which content and responses process jointly determine the construct validity of the task can be understood in terms of the functional task alignment (Hamstra, 2014), which represents the extent to which a task can achieve the learning objectives of the educator (Schoeneherr & Hamstra, 2017; cf. Grierson, 2014).

The dimension of internal structure presents limits on the applications of the concept of construct validity when assessing educational interventions. Namely, whereas assessment instruments can be designed to reflect several facets of the underlying constructs that have a specific relationship to one another, educational interventions need not be similarly designed. An educator could, in principle, develop a task to train learners but without any consideration of how various features of the task relate to one another, e.g., performance might improve in a virtual reality simulator without understanding what visualization, psychomotor, or reasoning processes have changed. As we noted above, when researchers and educators have little *a priori* information concerning the nature of a skill, it will be difficult to design a task that discriminates between novice and experts on specific skills or subtasks. Neither is it necessary for an educator to monitor the learner and provide feedback formally or informally. Educational interventions exist that represent standalone exercises for self-learning without any information on performance. In such cases, evidence for internal structure would be absent. Otherwise, when available, evidence that the internal structure adequately conforms of operationalization of a competency can be obtained.

Complementing internal structure, evidence describing the relationship with other variables represents the associations between a task or measurement instrument with other existing measurement instruments or novel tasks that should be related. The extent to which the performance on a task relates to other outcomes is crucial to determining a training procedure's effectiveness. In the case of surgical skills, results on a task trainer should show a positive relationship with patient outcomes in the operating room independently of whether the task has similarities with the operative environment. For instance, performance in a particular task need not be related to a clinician's ability to effectively communicate with a patient. Another task can be designed to directly promote a learner's understanding of a particular domain or assess the development of a skill. While the goal of health professions education is to integrate these skills in the clinic or operating room, the independent development of individual skills will allow for more targeted feedback and the reduction of confounds in developing separate skills.

The two remaining sources of evidence are related to the broader function of a task: the extent to which an assessment instrument is calibrated to assess

TABLE 3.2 Examples of Sources of Evidence for Construct Validity for Tasks in Medical Education

Source of Evidence	Description of Evidence	Example 1: OSCE	Example 2: Virtual Reality Trainer
Content	The features of the instrument adequately represent a construct.	OSCEs feature a sampling of high-frequency procedures and live patients mimicking symptoms.	The VR trainer represents all relevant affordances of a surgical procedure including visual and haptic cues.
Response Process	The affective, behavioral, and cognitive processes used in the task are comparable to those in the target environment.	Learners must process multiple symptoms to identify relevant and irrelevant cues, provide appropriate treatment, as well as act with professionalism.	Learners are presented with the appropriate responses given the choices they make, with changes in physiology and anatomy.
Internal Structure	Items have adequate reliability and a factor structure that supports the construct.	Each station in an OSCE assesses a different competence reliably.	The VR trainer is capable of varying features of a surgical procedure.
Relations to Other Variables	Performance in the task is highly correlated to similar tasks and uncorrelated to dissimilar tasks.	OSCE performance can be related to clinical performance.	Performance in VR training is associated with simpler tasks (e.g., suturing, laparoscopic box trainers).
Generalizability	The scores obtained by the instrument are calibrated to discriminate learner performance at different contexts and at different institutions.	Learners' rate of learning in Institution A and Institution B that are otherwise matched for equipment and training, reach milestones at similar rates.	Learners across institutions demonstrate the same gains in performance when using the trainer.
Consequences	The scores obtained in the task have implications for the learners' performance in the program and accreditation.	Learners might learn to take the test rather than the general content knowledge and skills.	Use of the VR trainer is seen as a prestigious form of education activity, privileging institutions and learners who have access to this technology.

Note: The table follows Messick's (1995) validity framework.

competency in multiple contexts (generalizability) and the social consequences of a task. Generalizability is arguably a key source of evidence in validating competency-based education in the health professions. For instance, competencies, milestones, and entrustable professional activities (EPA; Ma, 2024) should be assessed in a standardized manner across institutions. This is the basis for accreditation. The development of assessment instruments must take into consideration individual differences that can be observed within an institution and over the course of training. Generalizability evidence reinforces the need to evaluate assessment instruments in multi-site trials and periodically evaluate their efficacy to ensure that they are well-calibrated to differentiate learner performance. The importance of generalizability is also evidenced in the so-called replication crisis in the social sciences wherein large-scale attempts to replicate research results from studies have often met with failure (Amrhein et al., 2019; Anderson & Maxwell, 2017; Maxwell et al., 2015; Schooler, 2014; Shrout & Rodgers, 2018).[3] Health professions education will likely face similar challenges if research is limited to a single site or conducted in homogenous cultures. However, as we note below, a failure to replicate results outside of an institution is only problematic to the extent that programmatic context is ignored in other institutions.

Constructing Validity Arguments. Evidence alone is not sufficient to demonstrating that an educational task is adequate and relevant. While implicit in Messick's framework, Kane (1992, 2001) emphasizes that evidence is used to make inferences and that these inferences must be clearly defined. In his argument-based approach to validity, validity is understood in terms of how evidence is interpreted as representing a construct rather than being an intrinsic property of the test instrument. For instance, while performance on a "high fidelity" simulator might suggest that a learner can perform a procedure, the simulator might be presented in an environment that has minimal noise and distractions. Thus, despite the available evidence, it would not be a reasonable inference that performance on the task will necessarily transfer to a realistic context with intermittent noise and distractions such as a real operating or emergency room. Rather than reflecting disparate perspectives, we consider Messick (1989, 1995) and Kane (1992, 2001) to be focusing complementary determinants of construct validity: sources of evidence and how they are used in inferential arguments.

Values and Social Consequences. Evidence of the content, response processes, internal structure and relationship to other variables, and generalizability address the features of educational interventions and assessment instruments. Crucially, Messick (1989, 1995) additionally emphasized the importance of considering the value implications and social consequences of assessment on the organization and the learner. This critical insight echoes a recognition in the literature that teaching and assessment are value-laden (Ghaye & Ghaye, 1998; Whitehead, 1989). Educators must select information that is accurate and relevant, acknowledging their role as stewards of learners' understanding and their prospects. Each stage of a selection process narrows the number of potential candidates who are being considered (i.e., phased-narrowing; Levin et al., 1995) thereby representing a value judgment (Thorngate, 1988; Thorngate et al., 2010). For instance, a summative assessment instrument could be used to determine whether a learner passes or fails a course, determining whether they have a sufficient level of competency to continue training or engage in practice.

Empirical results support these claims. Studies of candidate selection have observed that the adoption of inclusion or exclusion criteria can change who is selected. For instance, Levin et al. (2001) found that when evaluators used inclusion criteria, they selected fewer candidates than evaluators who used exclusion criteria (also see, Heller et al., 2002). Complementing these results, other studies have demonstrated that not only does the adoption of inclusion criteria result in smaller sets of options, but confidence and quality of the consideration set also increase (Goodman & Reczek, 2021; Sokolova & Krishna, 2016; for research on individual differences, see Levin et al., 2000). Moreover, as the pool of candidates narrows, it becomes progressively more difficult to identify assessment criteria that can differentiate candidates based on their competencies (Thorngate, 1988). These considerations also affect other aspects of health professions education (for example in patient selection for teaching, see Gierk & Harendza, 2012). As chapters in this series demonstrate, external social structures and the embedded values can affect the composition of who enters the healthcare professions (see, Venosa et al., 2024; Khan, 2024; Schoenherr, 2024d).

3.1.1.2 Evidence for Implementation Validity: Programmatic Context and Task Alignment

While establishing the construct validity of a task is crucial to selecting among alternative educational interventions and assessment instruments, it should not be overextended and used as a catch-all term (Borsboom et al., 2004). Rather, the extent to which a task has been effectively implemented within a curriculum or programmatic context must independently be evaluated. We refer to this dimension of program evaluation as *implementation validity*. While we examine implementation in the context of program evaluation in health professions education, implementation issues reflect general concerns as researchers attempt to translate the research from basic scientific research to directly inform clinical research (e.g., patient care or public health strategies; Drolet & Lorenzi, 2011; Rubio et al., 2010; Schoenherr, 2024b).

Implementation validity requires an understanding of the system in which an educational innovation is being used and implemented. Context is defined as the physical, financial, and social features of an environment that have a strong direct or indirect effect on the conduct of a program such as equipment, facilities, personnel, and overall security of financial resources. These attributes are properties of the program rather than that of educational innovations and learners. Similarly, construct validity considers whether a construct is adequately reflected in the task one has designed. It does not consider whether this is the most efficient means to do so. For instance, "high fidelity" simulation might promote learning of a skill; however, it is not necessarily the case that they are either necessary or sufficient (Matsumoto et al., 2002; Norman et al., 2012; Schoeneherr & Hamstra, 2017). Following from this perspective, Messick's framework leaves unaddressed the feasibility of a task in terms of a comparison of the required time commitment on the part of learners and clinicians, the short- and long-run financial commitment of educational institutions, and the extent to which a task is integrated into the curriculum. Thus, implementation validity requires the development of a validity argument supported by distinct sources of evidence (Kane, 1992, 2001).

To identify potential sources of evidence to support implementation validity, we must consider validity more generally and what kinds of evidence are not considered in present formulations of construct validity. Whereas construct validity requires examining assumptions and the inferences made about how performance relates to a hypothetical entity, implementation validity requires considering whether inferences concerning resources and curriculum are sound. Implementation validity requires the consideration of the context in which a program is being developed (Palumbo, 1989; Scheirer, 1987; Weiss, 1997) and the extent to which the tasks and courses under development are compatible with this institutional system (e.g., Cook, 1986; Ross, 2013). For instance, Leonard-Barton (1988) suggested that developers must avoid a misalignment in terms of an organization's technical capabilities and capacity, the infrastructure that supports delivery, and the values of an organization. Leonard-Barton (1992) has further suggested that innovation within an organization is determined by the core capabilities of an organization. These capabilities can be understood in terms of four dimensions: employee knowledge and skills, technical systems, managerial systems, and the values and norms. Implementation can be understood in similar terms although the feasibility of a task will also be constrained by financial concerns.

The discourses on implementation and innovation suggest another dimension along which a task can be understood. In a comparable manner to Messick's (1995) framework, sources of evidence can be identified to demonstrate the extent to which a task has implementation validity (see Table 3.3). Implementation validity requires that there is sufficient financial (financial support), administrative, and personnel support within an institution

TABLE 3.3 Sources of Evidence for Implementation Validity

Source of Evidence	Description	Example 1: OSCE	Example 2: VR Trainer
Financial Support	After the features of the task have been clearly outlined (e.g., facilities, personnel), the total costs have been identified for each task and can be supplied by the program's current available funding.	In general, OSCEs have become widely integrated into programs thereby ensuring they have a stable financial base. The costs of conducting OSCEs are not inexpensive.	Following the initial investment in task development, the VR trainer will not require funding in the immediate future. Software updates, technical support, replacement of parts, and maintenance might require additional funding.
Program Support	The staff needed to administer, assess, and support a task are clearly defined and there is a reasonable degree of retention in skilled positions.	When established, OSCEs are typically provided full institutional support in coordinating their delivery.	Enough knowledgeable staff are required to set up and maintain the equipment, access, and interpret the data.
Availability of Material Resources	A program has readily accessible resources to successfully implement a task in terms of its content, e.g., materials, specimens, actors.	While specialized OSCEs can require any kind of supplementary material resources, standard OSCEs require readily available material resources.	Unlike traditional training devices (e.g., cadaveric, synthetic tissues), no material is required on an ongoing basis.
Task Dependencies	When assessed over the long run, qualified personnel and financial resources are sufficiently stable that multiyear projections can be made for task delivery.	The presentation of typical cases within the OSCEs indicates that there are few if any task dependencies when conducted inside the context of a hospital.	Once set-up is complete, the VR trainer can be situated alongside other training activities until the equipment or exercise becomes obsolete.

Relation to Other Educational Innovations	The purpose of the task and its assessment is clearly defined relative to other tasks within a program such that it fills a gap in the curriculum while ensuring that there is little redundancy.	Relative to other aspects of program, OSCEs provide a uniquely structured, formal, summative assessment tasks.	Relative to simulated patients, synthetic tissues, etc., the VR trainer can allow a learner to develop visuo-spatial reasoning skills by integrating skills that would otherwise require cadavers or live patients.
Program Integration	The task is explicitly situated within the program in terms of the time when it will be provided to learners, the assessment outcomes that are expected to directly relate to the program of study, the task serves the community of learners and health seekers, and whether the assessment is formative or summative.	OSCEs are generally integrated within the existing curriculum relative to didactic modules and technical skills training.	The VR trainer is developed as an educational intervention which includes a formative assessment component. It can also be adapted as a summative feature of a course to assess whether learners should be permitted to perform operations on live patients.

to sustain the program (program support), demonstrating that adequate materials and personnel resources are available (availability of material resources), that there is prospective continuity in delivering the program given the competencies of educators at an institution (task dependency), that a task is clearly defined in relation to others and enables the development of competencies (relation to other tasks), and that the educational intervention or assessment instrument is effectively integrated within the curriculum (program integration; van der Vleuten & Schuwirth, 2005). Demonstrating that an assessment or instructional activity has these features provides evidence for implementation validity. The claim that a measure of implementation validity can be obtained by accumulating evidence requires clearly demarcated sources of evidence that differentiate it from construct validity. We consider the six sources of evidence for implementation validity and how they can be used to create a program evaluation framework.

Financial Support. A topic that has recently garnered considerable discussion is how to assess the financial feasibility of a task. This relates to our notion of evidence for financial support. Financial support is defined as the immediate and short-term sources of funding that are available to task developers. This includes grant and institutional funding that is available to allocate to a task or its associated program. Recent work in the context of health professions education has also highlighted the need for considering the feasibility of program delivery in terms of costs (Ker, 2010; Zendejas et al., 2012). Studies have begun to consider various aspects of the costs of simulation (e.g., Goova, 2008; Matsumoto et al., 2002). Each of these provides evidence that can be used to make an argument for implementation validity. For instance, in a broad review, Zendejas et al. (2012) identified costs in terms of equipment and materials, personnel, facilities, required client inputs (i.e., financial opportunity costs), as well as others including information technology and communication. Where costs are clearly understood such as when a task is embedded within an established curriculum, this will provide a clear source of evidence for a task's implementation validity. However, initially, the invention and development of education innovations will not likely be associated with a stable financial base and will likely lack an adequate administrative infrastructure for long-term delivery. Educational innovators must also be mindful that development is a continuing process that occurs in discrete steps that lessen in frequency after the implementation of a technology (Tyre & Orlikowski, 1994). Larger adaptation cycles will consist of developing technology, adjusting performance criteria, and modifying the delivery system within the organizational context (Leonard-Barton, 1988). For instance, the introduction of AI (Schoenherr & Michael, 2024) and LA (Bilgic et al., 2024) will likely be defined by such adaptation cycles given that these methods require integration of various datasets, learning technologies and methodologies, and visualization techniques to support programs that are constantly changing.

Program Support. While human resources are often constrained by financial resources, they are determined by a unique set of factors and have historically been an overlooked facet of program delivery (Peterson, 1988). Organizational positions typically represent a stable feature of a program (e.g., an administrative assistant or technician will be assigned to a program) because of prior financial commitments. There is, however, no guarantee that the organization will retain any given individual. For instance, innovation studies have repeatedly demonstrated the importance of organizational leadership (Kesting et al., 2015; Lee et al., 2020). Considerations of retention thereby define a critical feature of task delivery and its prospective integration within an organization (e.g., Porter, 1973; Rhodes, 2002). Employee retention in the health professions is affected by a number of factors including empowerment and job satisfaction (Waldman, 2004; Wagner et al., 2010).

The independence of human resources from financial resources can also be illustrated by considering volunteers. Volunteers can be comparatively unskilled (e.g., inexperienced volunteers and research assistants) or highly skilled (e.g., retired academics and nurses, engineers). The voluntary nature of their contribution is a critical feature of any program that comes to rely on their input. For instance, volunteers might normally be tasked with set-up, cleaning, or other tasks. If they are absent, other personnel must provide additional support taking them away from other tasks. Formally, Peterson and Bickman (1988) have suggested that the measurement of personnel can be considered in terms of global features (e.g., composition, background, and size), proficiency and productivity, motivation and satisfaction with the work environment, and congruency of personal beliefs and program objectives. While this level of analysis might not always be appropriate or feasible, it highlights the need for a number of factors subsumed within this single source of evidence.

Availability of Material Resources. While financial and human resources represent clear limitations on the development of a task and its provision within a program, the availability of materials used in a task also presents a unique source of variation. First, it should be noted that not all materials are associated with financial resources. Especially in the context of medicine and surgery, medical equipment suppliers will often donate materials that can be used to train learners. Similarly, hospitals can also supply surplus or outdated materials (Gable et al., 2020). Neither of these sources of material incurs a cost to the program, making this approach more sustainable (Wu & Cerceo, 2021). Thus, a consideration of supply chains in health care is a necessary feature of any effective educational program in the healthcare professions

(Chen, 2013). Similarly, while availability could be framed in terms of the personnel costs associated with preparation of the specimen, it should be noted that even if there are no restrictions on personnel costs, certain training activities would be infeasible if specimens simply were not available.

Materials used in many tasks can also be understood in terms of a continuum of preparedness. One end of this continuum is defined by task trainers which are designed as standalone educational interventions or assessment instruments that need little or no modification. On the other end of this continuum are tasks that require that a supply of limited materials is obtained for their conduct. For instance, learners might be trained by using a simulation mannequin that comes to a training center without the need for further modification. Alternatively, *ex vivo* organic specimens might be available in large numbers but might require considerable preparation. Other factors affect the availability of materials as well. For instance, some surgical training tasks might require live animal models or human remains (cadavers), the availability of which is restricted due to ethical concerns (Schoenherr, 2022). While the use of technologies such as AI and virtual reality might address these needs, they are associated with their own material concerns, e.g., software compatibility, database storage, obsolescence, and equipment degradation.

Task Dependencies. While program support considers the global features of a program's personnel, some tasks are dependent on specific individuals for their continued provision. For example, leaders and task designers as well as qualified support staff who have highly developed technical skills provide expertise that cannot be easily replaced. For instance, the use of AI for training and assessment (Schoenherr & Michael, 2024) or LA for program evaluation requires specific expertise (Bilgic, et al., 2024). The extent to which any given task requires any individual or individuals will be an important determinant of task dependency. This is especially problematic if external organizations (e.g., private organizations) are providing support as they are subject to their own decision-making process, e.g., discontinuing a product and/or support, restructuring, or dissolution. The greater the dependency, the less evidence there is to support the continued implementation of a task. Thus, the greater the formal infrastructure that supports an educational innovation and the more clearly defined its goals, the less likely it will be dependent on individuals (Peterson, 1988). Educational innovations that are designed as standalone educational interventions or assessment instruments decrease task dependency. Similarly, tasks that are supported by a managerial system that has developed to support a particular task (Leonard-Barton, 1992) should also reduce the dependency of a task on any given individual. Task dependencies can also be understood in terms of the sources of funding. Even if funding has been received on an annual basis, education innovators must be mindful that these conditions can change at any time and should develop tasks accordingly.

This point becomes a critical concern if the source of funding is associated with a project leader or task designer who subsequently leaves the project.

Relations to Other Educational Innovations. Even when designed on an *ad hoc* basis, educational innovations are neither designed nor administered in a vacuum. Educational innovators should always seek to operationalize a learning objective into a physical (behavior) or mental (cognitive) activity that learners and educators can engage in. Relations to other educational innovations can be understood as the extent to which an educational innovation provides a unique training or assessment opportunity for learners, educators, and program administrators. Educational interventions that are not redundant will provide learners with the opportunity to become accustomed to a new procedure or acquired new knowledge in a safe environment or assessment instruments that are designed to detect the extent to which learners have mastered a skill. Such tasks have the most potential to contribute to a program, although their success will need to be assessed in terms of construct validity. Similarly, whether formative or summative tasks are required will also necessitate a consideration of other available educational innovations for learning, assessment, and evaluation, respectively. Relation to other educational innovations differs from the concept of relations to other variables in Messick's framework in that, at a programmatic level, the learning outcomes of an educational innovation will not necessarily be understood. Here, gaps are identified within a program and educational innovation are seen as addressing these gaps to a greater or lesser extent.

Program Integration. Considering when an educational intervention or assessment should be presented and to whom represents a final dimension of implementation validity: program integration. Curriculum developers must consider when learners receive training in terms of their level of skill, characteristics of the learners that will receive it, whether it serves the community of learners and health seekers, and the specificity of the educational innovation (Schoenherr, 2022b). Learners might simply complete a rotation to gain experience in an area of clinical practice. Rather than mastery, educators might simply want to provide learners with a set of tasks that are representative of the area of practice. For instance, curriculum developers might believe that technical skills (Abdo et al., 2024) or EPAs (Ma, 2024) should be taught to students but leave the exact means to do so underspecified for educators.

The more specific the educational innovation, the more highly integrated it is within a program. Highly specified tasks will consider the nature (e.g., a laparoscopic training to practice a laparoscopic cholecystectomy, an assessment scale for point-of-care ultrasound, training in diagnostic abilities of AI in radiology) and timing (e.g., the second block of a rotation) of an educational intervention or assessment. Specificity, however, should be concerned not with the detail as they can be left to others concerned with construct validity. For underspecified tasks, while there is overt recognition that some activity is required, no specific task might be acknowledged as meeting these requirements. Thus, tasks provided in an unsystematic *ad hoc* manner will have no program integration.

Tasks that are integrated within a program will be defined in terms of their placement with the learners' educational experience, build skills that have been recognized as beneficial to their performance, and have the legitimacy of formal support from the institution. Compatibility with the values of an organization will also be an important determinant of implementation (Leonard-Barton, 1992). In an educational setting, values cannot be considered solely in terms of an institution's administration. Rather, as user participation is critical to successful task development (Ives, 1984), learner feedback is essential to understanding the efficacy of integration of a task within the curriculum.

The sources of evidence that can be used to demonstrate implementation validity highlight the need to analyze tasks at a level of analysis beyond learner performance. Following Leonard-Barton (1992) remarks in the context of innovation implementation, we suggest that the greater alignment between the educational intervention or assessment instrument and the sources of evidence, the more likely the task will have an enduring impact on the curriculum. This approach necessitates a macroscopic perspective of a task within the context of an institution's program while also considering how educators and learners perceive the task. For instance, in addition to developing a program that conforms to the best available knowledge to optimize learners' performance, Ross et al. (2013) have claimed that the perception of the involvement of preceptors in a program is also critical. We would go further and claim that explicit institutional support is critical not only in terms of obtaining funding but by demonstrating to educators and learners that such programs are integrated within the curriculum and are a worthwhile use of their time. Without integration, learners will be less likely to see the connections between areas of instruction and will fail to obtain the breadth of possible educational insight.

3.2   Ecological Optimization of Tasks as Determined by Construct and Implementation Validity

Translational research requires the use of basic research findings to inform patient-centered and population-level research (e.g., Rubio et al., 2010; Schoenherr & McConnell, 2024). Here, we have operationalized this process by considering independent sources of evidence for both construct validity and implementation validity, reflecting two orthogonal evaluation dimensions. When considered together, the extent to which a task is well adapted to the educational objectives within a program (i.e., construct validity) as well as the program structure and resources (i.e., implementation validity) provide an effective means of describing and evaluate an educational program. Tasks that have considerable evidence for both construct and implementation validity are *ecologically optimal*. Below, we demonstrate how these two dimensions allow for a consideration of a program as well as providing an example of how individual tasks can be assessed.

To illustrate the properties of ecological optimality of an element of the curriculum, we will consider three potential scenarios that could occur in an evaluation space. We define an evaluation space as a two-dimensional space defined by the degree to which a task has construct and implementation validity (Figure 3.1). Educational or assessment programs can be plotted in terms of their individual tasks, with each task assigned a value in terms of the extent to which it has construct validity and implementation validity. When evidence is available, it can reflect quantitative, weighted scores or the judgment of experts (van der Vleuten et al., 2012; van der Vleuten, 1996). Again, as we note above, educational interventions will not necessarily have

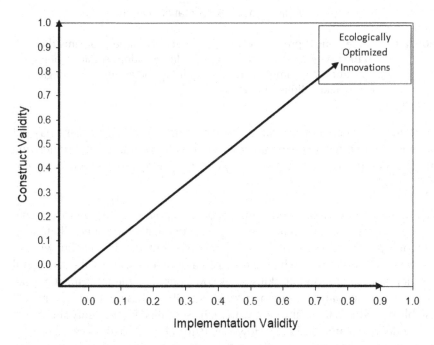

FIGURE 3.1 Two-dimensional program evaluation space. Evidence is obtained and interpreted by researchers and experts, making an argument for validity. Evidence is gathered separately for construct and implementation validity dimensions. High levels of evidence for both forms of validity define programmatically optimized tasks.

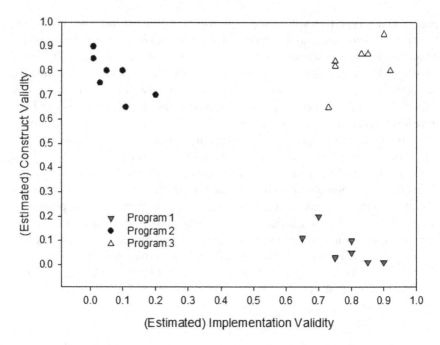

FIGURE 3.2   A theoretical program evaluation space for three programs differing in their degrees of construct and implementation validity. Conjointly, construct and implementation validity determine the degree of ecological validity of a program.

all forms of evidence supporting their construct validity if the task has not been developed for assessment or that little is known about the underlying mental operation of the task. We briefly consider these three kinds of programs (Figure 3.2).

Type 1 Programs. Medical education programs could purchase instructional software and simulators in addition to hiring dedicated and specially trained support staff, resulting in a high degree of implementation validity but without considering the extent to which these tasks are directed toward the successful development of appropriate skills and knowledge, i.e., the tasks meet a weak criterion of "face validity" but their construct validity has not been adequately established. This is likely the case with many so-called high-fidelity simulators (Schoenherr & Hamstra, 2017). However, in the absence of direct evidence for their effectiveness, programs of these types are vulnerable to being effective in principle but not in practice.

Type 2 Programs. The introduction of competency-based health professions education has been the catalyst for the rigorous testing and development of training tools and assessment instruments. Researchers in health professions education have focused on the development of skills and knowledge by considering affective, cognitive, and social aspects of performance resulting in sets of tasks with a high degree of construct validity. Presently, the literature is beginning to swell with innovations that have considerable construct validity supporting their adoption in the programmatic context. If health professions educators fail to consider *specifically* how these innovations can be implemented within the context of their institution, construct validity on its own might not translate into reliable gains in learner outcomes at the programmatic level. Specifically, a leader in the healthcare professions might propose and adopt an instrument and monitor the program within which it is embedded. If they depart, new leadership and staff might not understand the relationship of an instrument to organizational resources, resulting in the loss of implementation validity. In the absence of knowledge of a tasks roles in a program this might also lead to reduction in the construct validity a specific context: a task could continue to be used without evaluating whether it was still effective in assessing the competency of learners.

Type 3 Programs. The negative examples of Type 1 and Type 2 Programs underscore the importance of effective programs that consider both evidence for construct validity and implementation validity. This requires effective knowledge translation from the domain the educational innovation was developed within to the specific organizational context (Schoenherr & Hamstra, 2017; Schoenherr, 2024b), while also ensuring that healthcare professionals who administer the program are aware of the organizational resources required to maintain the program and how the educational and assessment instruments relate to one another. A number of these tools will then reflect a program that has a large number of ecologically optimized tasks as it provides sustainable, curriculum-integrated training opportunities for learners while ensuring the effective development of key clinical competencies (Program 3). In this case, neglecting either the evidence for construct validity or the evidence for implementation validity can threaten the efficacy of a health professions education program.

While we have presented construct and implementation validity as orthogonal dimensions, there can be dependencies between the two dimensions. A clear instance of this is the use of Problem-Based Learning (PBL). Kwan (2019) describes how PBL faced issues when it was implemented in East Asian countries. Specifically, due to differences in educational traditions, language, and the limited number of qualified educators (Schoenherr & Beaudoin, 2024), PBL was often adopted, modified, and then rejected. Thus, despite the construct validity for PBL to occupy a useful programmatic niche, inappropriate implementation reduced the validity evidence to support its use in the East Asian institutions that adopted it.

3.3 Conclusions

Recent concerns over the appeals to "high fidelity" simulation as a panacea for training in health professions education (Hamstra, 2014; Schoenherr & Hamstra, 2017) highlight the need to consider the learning objectives of educators and how they align with an institution's curriculum. Although the objective of this review is to demonstrate the need to distinguish between the extent to which educational interventions like simulation have evidence for their construct validity and implementation validity, the ideal use of the evaluation space framework we have developed is at a programmatic level. The introduction of competency-based education in the United States (AGCME) and Canada (RCPSC) will require that programs, not individual tasks, be examined to determine whether they allow for the development of competencies. For instance, the CanMEDS Physician Competency Framework requires that physicians are medical experts, communicators, collaborators, scholars, managers, professionals, and health advocates. No tasks alone can assess these competencies, nor do we feel that any one task should be designed to do so. This is a principal difficulty of the misuse of quantitative evidence (Schoenherr & Hamstra, 2016) and "high fidelity" simulators (Schoenherr & Hamstra, 2017). Task and curriculum designers must acknowledge that they require a representative sample of tasks to determine a learner's competency in a given area. Even in an ecological setting, a clinician's competencies will not be effectively sampled. Thus, tasks need to be devised to focus on one facet of a competency while being able to control others – experimentally or statistically. These individual tasks must be developed while acknowledging gaps within the current curriculum while being mindful of the available resources and consistency of delivery over multiple years. The present framework should aid in adopting this approach as it provides an overview of how elements of a program are associated together. It will enable educators and task developers to situate simulation rather than using it as a standalone learning and assessment instrument.

Like Messick's construct validity framework, the implementation validity framework we have outlined is meant to be used to assess any educational activity or assessment instrument and evaluate its implementation (and de-implementation) within any institutional context. As institutions begin to adopt AI and machine learning (ML), healthcare professionals and administrators must also consider the construct and implementation validity of these systems. Despite the potential benefits of AI and ML, we must be equally cautious. As trials with IBM Watson Medical demonstrate, implementation of

AI and ML can be associated with problems: in addition to HCPs having little experience using these systems, a failure to understand their operations can lead to mistrust in their recommendations. Conversely, HCPs might use these systems despite having little knowledge of the datasets used to train these systems, how they arrive at recommendations, or how to interpret their results (Schoenherr, 2021b, 2022b, 2022c; Schoenherr & Michael, 2024). Whether considering the assessment of learners or the provision of medical advice, we must consider the implementation validity of these systems. Specifically, we must consider whether institutions maintain the requisite competencies to implement, maintain, and de-implement these systems.

Notes

1 Collectively referred to as educational innovation in the remainder of this chapter.
2 In contrast to Messick's framework, their review does not distinguish generalizability as a sixth form of validity evidence. It instead includes it as a facet of internal structure.
3 Here, the "crisis" is largely a function of *some* failures to replicate. In many cases, it might very well be the case that situational or cultural factors were not accounted for and that the effects are simply far less robust than initial studies imply.

References

Abdo, S., Elliot, L., Micallef, J., Sivanathan, M., & Dubrowski, A. (2024). Optimizing psychomotor skills acquisition in healthcare simulation through knowledge mobilization. In Schoenherr, J. R. & McConnell, M. M. (eds.) *Fundamentals and Frontiers in Medical Education and Decision-Making: Educational Theory and Psychological Practice*. New York: Routledge.

Amrhein, V., Trafimow, D., & Greenland, S. (2019). Inferential statistics as descriptive statistics: There is no replication crisis if we don't expect replication. *The American Statistician*, 73(sup1), 262–270.

Anastasi, A. (1986). Evolving concepts of test validation. *Annual Review of Psychology*, 37, 1–16.

Anderson, S. F., & Maxwell, S. E. (2017). Addressing the "replication crisis": Using original studies to design replication studies with appropriate statistical power. *Multivariate Behavioral Research*, 52, 305–324.

Angoff, W. H. (1988). Validity: An evolving concept. In Wainer H. & Braun H. I. (eds.) *Test Validity* (pp. 19–32). Hillsdale: Lawrence Erlbaum Associates.

Bilgic, E., Chen, D. M., & Chan, T. (2024). Implementation of learning analytics in medical education: Practical considerations. In Schoenherr, J. R. & McConnell, M. M. (eds.) *Fundamentals and Frontiers in Medical Education and Decision-Making: Educational Theory and Psychological Practice*. New York: Routledge.

Borsboom, D., Mellenbergh, G. J., & van Heerden, J. (2004). The concept of validity. *Psychological Review*, 111, 1061–1071.

Brown, J., & Kiernan, N. E. (2001). Assessing the subsequent effect of a formative evaluation on a program. *Evaluation and Program Planning*, 24, 129–143.

Brownell Anderson, M. S. (2009). Growing use of standardized patients in teaching and evaluation in medical education. *Teaching and Learning in Medicine*, 6, 15–22.

Campbell, D. T. (1959). Convergent and discriminant validity by the multitrait multimethod matrix. *Psychological Bulletin*, 56, 81–105.

Campbell, D. T. (1988). *Methodology and Epistemology for Social Science: Selected Papers* (pp. 315–333). Chicago: University of Chicago Press.

Chen, D. Q. (2013). Enhancing hospital supply chain performance: A relational view and empirical test. *Journal of Operations Management*, 31, 39–408.

Clark, L. A., & Watson, D. (1995). Constructing validity: Basic issues in objective scale development. *Psychological Assessment*, 7, 309–319.

Conrad, L. I. (1995). *The Western Medical Tradition: 800 BC to AD 1800, Volume 1.* Cambridge: Cambridge University Press.

Cook, D. A. (2006). Current concepts in validity and reliability for psychometric instruments: Theory and application. *The American Journal of Medicine*, 119, e7–e16.

Cook, T. D. (1986). Program evaluation: The worldly science. *Annual Review of Psychology*, 37, 193–232.

Cronbach, L. J. (1989). Construct validation after thirty years. In Linn, R. L. (ed.) *Intelligence: Measurement Theory and Public Policy* (pp. 147–171). Urbana: University of Illinois Press.

Cronbach, L. J., & Meehl, P. E. (1955). Construct validity in psychological tests. *Psychological Bulletin*, 52, 281–302.

Drolet, B. C., & Lorenzi, N. M. (2011). Translational research: understanding the continuum from bench to bedside. *Translational Research*, 157, 1–5.

Duffin, J. (1999). *History of Medicine*. Toronto: University of Toronto Press.

Dunn, M. B. (2010). Institutional logics and institutional pluralism: The contestation of care and science logics in medical education, 1967–2005. *Administrative Science Quarterly*, 55, 114–149.

Elliott, D. H. (2010). Goal-directed aiming: Two components but multiple processes. *Psychological Bulletin*, 136, 1023.

Flexner, A. (1910/1960). *Medical Education in the United States and Canada. Bulletin Number Four.* New York: Carnegie Foundation for the Advancement of Teaching.

Frank, J. R. (2010). Competency-based medical education: Theory to practice. *Medical Teacher*, 32, 638–645.

Gable, B., Ballas, D., & Ahmed, R. A. (2020). Enhancing simulation education using expired materials. *BMJ Simulation & Technology Enhanced Learning*, 6, 129–131.

Ghaye, A., & Ghaye, K. (1998). *Teaching and Learning through Critical Reflective Practice*. London: David Fulton.

Gierk, B., & Harendza, S. (2012). Patient selection for bedside teaching: Inclusion and exclusion criteria used by teachers. *Medical Education*, 46, 228–233.

Goodman, J. K., & Reczek, R. W. (2021). Choosing what to choose from: Preference for inclusion over exclusion when constructing consideration sets from large choice sets. *Journal of Behavioral Decision Making*, 34, 85–98.

Goova, M. T. (2008). Implementation, construct validity, and benefit of a proficiency-based knot-tying and suturing curriculum. *Journal of Surgical Education*, 65, 309–315.

Gravetter, F. J., & Forzano, L. A. B. (2016). *Research Methods for the Behavioral Sciences*, 5th edition. Stamford: Cengage Learning.

Grierson, L. E. (2014). Information processing, specificity of practice, and the transfer of learning: Considerations for reconsidering fidelity. *Advances in Health Science Education*, 19, 281–289.

Gruppen, L., Frank, J. R., Lockyer, J., Ross, S., Bould, M. D., Harris, P., ... & ICBME Collaborators. (2017). Toward a research agenda for competency-based medical education. *Medical Teacher*, 39, 623–630.

Halsted, W. S. (1904). The training of the surgeon. *Bulletin of John Hopkins Hospital*, 15, 267–276.

Hamdorf, J. M., &. Hall, J. (2000). Acquiring surgical skills. *British Journal of Surgery*, 87, 28–37.

Hamstra, S. J. (2014). Reconsidering fidelity in simulation-based training. *Academic Medicine*, 89, 387–392.

Heller, D., Levin, I. P., & Goransson, M. (2002). Selection of strategies for narrowing choice options: Antecedents and consequences. *Organizational Behavior and Human Decision Processes*, 89, 1194–1213.

Irby, D. M. (2003). Educational innovations in academic medicine and environmental trends. *Journal of General Internal Medicine*, 18, 370–376.

Irby, D. M. (2016). Parting the clouds: Three professionalism frameworks in medical education. *Academic Medicine*, 91, 1606–1611.

Ives, B. & Olson, M. H. (1984). User involvement and MIS success: A review of research. *Management Science*, 30, 586–603.

Kane, M. T. (1992). An argument-based approach to validity. *Psychological Bulletin*, 112, 527–535.

Kane, M. T. (2001). Current concerns in validity theory. *Journal of Educational Measurement*, 38, 319–342.

Ker, J. H. (2010). Cost-effective simulation. In Walsh K. (ed.) *Cost Effectiveness in Medical Education* (pp. 61–71). Oxon: Radcliffe.

Kesting, P., Ulhøi, J. P., Song, L. J., & Niu, H. (2015). The impact of leadership styles on innovation – A review. *Journal of Innovation Management*, 3, 22–41.

Khan, K. (2024). Inequality and social mobility in the medical professions in India: Career availability and vulnerabilities. In Schoenherr, J. R. (ed.) *Fundamentals and Frontiers in Medical Education and Decision-Making: Innovation, Implementation, and Translational Research*. New York: Routledge.

Kwan, C. Y. (2019). A thorny path: I developmental course of problem-based learning for health sciences education in Asia. *Advances in Health Sciences Education*, 24, 893–901.

Lee, A., Legood, A., Hughes, D., Tian, A.W., Newman, A., & Knight, C. (2020). Leadership, creativity and innovation: A meta-analytic review. *European Journal of Work and Organizational Psychology*, 29, 1–35.

Leonard-Barton, D. (1988). Implementation as mutual adaptation of technology and organization. *Research Policy*, 17, 251–267.

Leonard-Barton, D. (1992). Core capabilities and core rigidities: A paradox in managing new product development. *Strategic Management Journal*, 13, 111–125.

Levin, I. P., Huneke, M. E., & Jasper, J. D. (2000). Information processing at successive stages of decision making: Need for cognition and inclusion–exclusion effects. *Organizational Behavior and Human Decision Processes*, 82, 171–193.

Levin, I. P., & Jasper, J. D. (1995). Phased narrowing: A new process tracing method for decision making. *Organizational Behavior and Human Decision Processes*, 64, 1–8.

Levin, I. P., Prosansky, C. M., Heller, D., & Brunick, B. M. (2001). Prescreening of choice options in 'positive' and 'negative' decision-making tasks. *Journal of Behavioral Decision Making*, 14(4), 279–293.

Ma, T. (2024). Considerations for implementation of a competency-based education program for preclerkship courses. In Schoenherr, J. R. & McConnell, M. M. (eds.) *Fundamentals and Frontiers in Medical Education and Decision-Making: Educational Theory and Psychological Practice*. New York: Routledge.

Matsumoto, E. D. (2002). The effect of bench model fidelity on endourological skills: A randomized controlled study. *Journal of Urology*, 167, 1243–1247.

Maxwell, S. E., Lau, M. Y., & Howard, G. S. (2015). Is psychology suffering from a replication crisis? What does "failure to replicate" really mean? *American Psychologist*, 70, 487–498.

May, W. P. (2009). A ten-year review of the literature on the use of standardized patients in teaching and learning: 1996–2005. *Medical Teacher*, 31, 487–492.

Mclean, M. C. (2008). Faculty development: Yesterday, today and tomorrow. *Medical Teacher*, 30, 555–584.

Messick, S. (1989). Meaning and values in test validation: The science and ethics of assessment. *Educational Researcher*, 18, 5–11.

Messick, S. (1995). Validation of inferences from persons' responses and performances as scientific inquiry into score meaning. *American Psychologist*, 50, 741–749.

Miller, G. E. (1990). The assessment of clinical skills/competence/performance. *Academic Medicine*, 65, S63–S67.

Nevo, B. (1985). Face validity revisited. *Journal of Educational Measurement*, 22, 287–293.

Norman, D. A. (1988/2013). *The Design of Everyday Thing*. New York: Basic Books.

Norman, D. A. (1999). Affordance, conventions, and design. *Interactions*, 6, 38–43.

Norman, G., Dore, K., & Grierson, L. (2012). The minimal relationship between simulation fidelity and transfer of learning. *Medical Education*, 46, 636–647.

Palumbo, D. J. (1989). Implementation theory and the theory-driven approach to validity. *Evaluation and Program Planning*, 12, 337–344.

Peterson, K. A. (1988). Program personnel: The missing ingredient in describing the program environment. In J. Kendon, Roberts-Gray, C. & Roberts-Gray, C. (eds.) *Evaluating Program Environments* (pp. 83–92). San Francisco: Jossey-Bass, Inc.

Peterson, K. A., & Bickman, L. (1988). Program personnel: The missing ingredient in describing the program environment. *New Directions for Program Evaluation*, 1988(40), 83–92.

Porter, L. W. (1973). Organizational, work, and personal factors in employee turnover and absenteeism. *Psychological Bulletin*, 80, 151–176.

Rhodes, L. &. Eisenberger, R. (2002). Perceived organizational support: A review of the literature. *Journal of Applied Psychology*, 87, 698–714.

Richards, G. & DeVries, I. (2011). Revisiting formative evaluation: dynamic monitoring for the improvement of learning activity design and delivery. In *Proceedings of t^he 1st International Conference on Learning Analytics and Knowledge LAK '11*, ACM (pp. 157–162). New York: ACM.

Ross, S. P. (2013). The impact of varying levels of implementation fidelity on resident perceptions of assessment innovation. *Journal of Graduate Medical Education*, 5, 711.

Rossi, P. H. (2004). *Evaluation: A Systematic Approach*. Thousand Oaks, CA: SAGE Publications.

Rubio, D. M., Schoenbaum, E. E., Lee, L. S., Schteingart, D. E., Marantz, P. R., Anderson, K. E., ... & Esposito, K. (2010). Defining translational research: Implications for training. *Academic Medicine*, 85(3), 470–475.

Scheirer, M. A. (1987). Program theory and implementation theory: Implications for evaluators. In Bickman, L. (ed.) *New Directions for Program Evaluation, Vol. 33: Using Program Theory in Evaluation* (pp. 40–68). San Francisco: Jossey-Bass.

Schoenherr, J. R. (2021a). Designing ethical agency for adaptive instructional systems: The FATE of learning and assessment. In *International Conference on Human-Computer Interaction* (pp. 265–283). Springer International Publishing.

Schoenherr, J. R. (2021b). Trust and explainability in A/IS-mediated healthcare: Operationalizing the therapeutic alliance in a distributed system. In *2021 IEEE International Symposium on Technology and Society (ISTAS)* (pp. 1–8). IEEE.

Schoenherr, J. R. (2022a). Learning engineering is ethical. In *Learning Engineering Toolkit* (pp. 201–228). Routledge.

Schoenherr, J. R. (2022b). *Ethical Artificial Intelligence from Popular to Cognitive Science: Trust in the Age of Entanglement*. Routledge.

Schoenherr, J. R. (2022c). Folkmedical technologies and the sociotechnical systems of healthcare. *IEEE Technology and Society Magazine*, 41(3), 38–49.

Schoenherr, J. R. (2024a). Translational and implementation process. In Eltorai, A. E. M., Bakal, J. A., Toms, S. A., & Ahmad, M. (eds.) *Translational Neurosurgery*. Springer.

Schoenherr, J. R. (2024b). Innovation and implementation in health professions education and healthcare delivery. In Schoenherr, J. R. (ed.), *Fundamentals and Frontiers in Medical Education and Decision-Making: Innovation, Implementation, and Translational Research*. Routledge.

Schoenherr, J. R. (2024c). Hypothesis testing and error. In Eltorai, A. E. M., Bakal, J. A., Toms, S. A., & Ahmad, M., *Translational Neurosurgery*. Springer.

Schoenherr, J. R. (2024d). The development and dynamics of Mayan healthcare systems: A socioecological approach. In Schoenherr, J. R. (ed.), *Fundamentals and Frontiers in Medical Education and Decision-Making: Innovation, Implementation, and Translational Research*. Routledge.

Schoenherr, J. R., & Hamstra, S. J. (2016). Psychometrics and its discontents: An historical perspective on the discourse of the measurement tradition. *Advances in Health Science Education*, 21, 1–11.

Schoenherr, J. R., & Hamstra, S. J. (2017). Beyond fidelity: Deconstructing the seductive simplicity of fidelity in simulator-based education in the health care professions. *Simulation in Healthcare*, 12, 117–123.

Schoenherr, J. R., & Le-Bouar, C. (2024). Fundamentals of persuasive health communication: Representing, communicating, and distributing health information. In Schoenherr, J. R. (ed.) *Fundamentals and Frontiers in Medical Education and Decision-Making: Innovation, Implementation, and Translational Research*. New York: Routledge.

Schoenherr, J. R. & McConnell, M. (2024). Human-centered design in health professions education: Informing competency-based education with psychological science. In Schoenherr, J. R. & McConnell, M. (eds.), *Fundamentals and frontiers in medical education: Educational theory and psychological practice*. Routledge.

Schoenherr, J. R., & Michael, K. (2024). AI-Based technologies in the healthcare ecosystem: Applications in medical education and decision-making. In Schoenherr, J. R. (ed.), *Fundamentals and Frontiers in Medical Education and Decision-Making: Innovation, Implementation, and Translational Research*. Routledge.

Schoenherr, J. R., Chiou, E., & Goldshtein, M. (2024). Building trust with the ethical affordances of education technologies: A sociotechnical systems perspective. In *Putting AI in the Critical Loop* (pp. 127–165). Academic Press.

Schoenherr, J. R., Waechter, J., & Lee, C. H. (2024). Quantifying expertise in the healthcare professions: Cognitive efficiency and metacognitive calibration. In Schoenherr, J. R. & McConnell, M. M. (eds.) *Fundamentals and Frontiers in Medical Education and Decision-Making: Educational Theory and Psychological Practice*. New York: Routledge.

Schooler, J. W. (2014). Metascience could rescue the 'replication crisis'. *Nature*, 515, 9–9.

Shrout, P. E., & Rodgers, J. L. (2018). Psychology, science, and knowledge construction: Broadening perspectives from the replication crisis. *Annual Review of Psychology*, 69, 487–510.

Sokolova, T., & Krishna, A. (2016). Take it or leave it: How choosing versus rejecting alternatives affects information processing. *Journal of Consumer Research*, 43, 614–635.

Stufflebaum, D. L. (2001). Evaluation models. *New Directions for Evaluation*, 89, 7–98.

Swanson, D. B. (1995). Performance-based assessment: Lessons from the health professions. *Educational Researcher*, 24, 5–11.

Thorngate, W. (1988). On the evolution of adjudicated contests and the principle of invidious. *Journal of Behavioral Decision Making*, 1, 5–15.

Thorngate, W., Dawes, R. M., & Foddy, M. (2010). *Judging Merit*. London: Psychology Press.

Tolsgaard, M. G., Boscardin, C. K., Park, Y. S., Cuddy, M. M., & Sebok-Syer, S. S. (2020). The role of data science and machine learning in health professions education: Practical applications, theoretical contributions, and epistemic beliefs. *Advances in Health Sciences Education*, 25, 1057–1086.

Tyre, M. J., & Orlikowski, W. J. (1994). Windows of opportunity: Temporal patterns of technological adaptation in organizations. *Organization Science*, 5, 98–118.

van der Vleuten, C. et al. (2012). A model for programmatic assessment fit for purpose. *Medical Teacher, 34*, 205–214.

van der Vleuten, C. P. (1996). The assessment of professional competence: developments, research and practical implications. *Advances in Health Sciences Education*, 1, 41–67.

van der Vleuten, C. P., & Schuwirth, L. W. (2005). Assessment of professional competence: From methods to programmes. *Medical Education*, 39, 309–317.

van der Vleuten, C. P., Schuwirth, L. W., Driessen, E. W., Dijkstra, J., Tigelaar, D., Baartman, L. K., & Van Tartwijk, J. (2012). A model for programmatic assessment fit for purpose. *Medical Teacher, 34*, 205–214.

van Gaalen, A. E., Brouwer, J., Schönrock-Adema, J., Bouwkamp-Timmer, T., Jaarsma, A. D. C., & Georgiadis, J. R. (2021). Gamification of health professions education: A systematic review. *Advances in Health Sciences Education*, 26, 683–711.

Venosa, A. R., Baroneza, J. E., & Fernandes, R. A. F (2024). Medical education in Brazil: A history of an evolving pluralistic healthcare system. In Schoenherr, J. R. (ed.) *Fundamentals and Frontiers in Medical Education and Decision-Making: Innovation, Implementation, and Translational Research*. New York: Routledge.

Waddington, K. (2011). *An Introduction to the Social History of Medicine*. New York: Palgrave Macmillan.

Wagner, J. I J., et al. (2010). The relationship between structural empowerment and psychological empowerment for nurses: A systematic review. *Journal of Nursing Management*, 18, 448–462.

Wainer, H., & Braun, H. I. (Eds.) (1988). *Test Validity*. Hillsdale: Lawrence Erlbaum Associates.

Waldman, J. D. (2004). The shocking cost of turnover in health care. *Health Care Management Review*, 29, 2–7.

Wartman, S. A., & Combs, C. D. (2018). Medical education must move from the information age to the age of artificial intelligence. *Academic Medicine*, 93, 1107–1109.

Wass, V. V. (2001). Assessment of clinical competence. *Lancet*, 357, 945–949.

Weiss, C. H. (1997). How can theory-based evaluation make greater headway? *Evaluation Review*, 21, 501–524.

Whitehead, J. (1989) Creating a living educational theory from questions of the kind, 'How do I improve my practice?'. *Cambridge Journal of Education*, 19(1), 41–52.

Williams, P. (2019). Does competency-based education with blockchain signal a new mission for universities? *Journal of Higher Education Policy and Management*, 41, 104–117.

Woolf, S. H. (2008). The meaning of translational research and why it matters. *JAMA*, 299, 211–213.

Wu, S., & Cerceo, E. (2021). Sustainability initiatives in the operating room. *The Joint Commission Journal on Quality and Patient Safety*, 47, 663–672.

Zendejas, B. et al. (2012). Cost: The missing outcome in simulation-based medical education research: A systematic review. *Surgery*, 153, 160–176.

4

IMPLEMENTATION OF LEARNING ANALYTICS IN MEDICAL EDUCATION

Practical Considerations

Elif Bilgic, Daisy Minghui Chen, and Teresa Chan

4.1 Definitions, Concepts, and Theories about Learning Analytics

Learning analytics (LA) has evolved remarkably over the past decade, with increasing use of data and technical tools to address educational issues, including improving learning experiences for various learning trajectories and informing evidence-based policy and decision-making with the intended objectives (Knight & Buckingham Shum, 2017; Selwyn & Gašević, 2020). Across stakeholders at different levels, there is growing interest in communicating among different LA applications with their own robust data models and scale of implementation, within given domains and contexts (Thoma, Caretta-Weyer et al., 2021). However, there remain challenges moving from designing and developing closed and deterministic LA solutions into more complex and connected ones. Therefore, we often face the tension between a desire to deploy LA to reach as many users as possible and that of making large impact on learning improvement for specific target users or skill development (Knight & Buckingham Shum, 2017).

The potential challenges and tension have been observed and described in the field of medical education, with a discussion of the concerns of utilization of large datasets from competency-based medical education (CBME) by Thoma, Ellaway et al. (2021). In particular, they depicted a possible utopian scenario that draws on the integrated analytics to link trainee assessment data from medical education to clinical practices and all the way to the clinical outcomes of the healthcare by mining multiple data sources from CBME. They adapted and proposed principles for an ethical framework for LA applied to CBME built upon the principles of LA that have been developed in the broader

DOI: 10.4324/9781003316091-5

fields of education and computer science. As such, we will discuss and review the basic concept of LA in general and the way in which researchers propose theoretical underpinnings for practical LA applications in medical education.

4.1.1   Definition of Learning and Learning Analytics

LA must be embedded within broader approaches to education. Learning can be conceptualized as a developmental progress comprising sequential tasks, resources, and support that teachers design and provide for learners in the specified learning environments. Multiple metatheoretical models exist that account for the learning process. In contrast to simple information transmission approach that assume that educators merely encode information that is decoded by learners (see Schoenherr & Le-Bouar, 2024), constructivism assumes that learners do not passively receive information during the learning process. Instead, they play active roles in knowledge construction and engage in the meaning negotiation process through interacting with peers, reflecting upon learning experiences, and incorporating new information into their prior knowledge. Hence, the goal of LA is to accurately capture and represent the process of learning. It must enable the measurement, collection, analysis, and interpretation of learning data to gain insights to improve learning and the sociotechnical educational contexts in which it occurs (Knight & Buckingham Shum, 2017; Selwyn & Gašević, 2020).

4.1.2   Learning Analytics in Medical Education

To achieve the meaningful learning improvement and decision-making through the use of LA, much of the work from LA research indicated the importance of theories and models for guiding the development of LA approaches, techniques, and artifacts that mediate the relationships among educational stakeholders, including educators, learners, policymakers, and researchers (Knight & Buckingham Shum, 2017). There are similar insights into LA in medical education that are informed by Chan et al. (2018), advocating the need for integrating theories into the educationally informative analytics for CBME-based training and learning. To cope with the challenges of LA utilization in the CBME systems, Thoma, Ellaway et al. (2021) argued that the LA development and implementation should continue within the guidance of the principles for an ethical framework. For example, trainees should be the co-designers and co-operators of the LA systems, which should be considered a moral practice to gain deep understanding of learning for the benefit of the trainees, institutions, and patients. Similarly, Martinez-Maldonado et al. (2021) proposed a conceptual model that integrates LA and learning theory to inform the human-centered design system, which aims to support collaboration for learners in the medical learning context. The operationalized model proposed in their research depicts how theory and analytics close the loop by enabling the co-design of LA tool under the authentic settings to improve the effectiveness of group learning.

Various authors have argued that by designing LA artifacts (e.g., the LA systems and tools), the data itself becomes meaningful by considering the underlying theoretical and practical assumptions around the motivations for their use, in what way do we define the objectives of learning and align assessment design to demonstrate the outcomes. Hall et al. (2021) proposed that the CBME outcome taxonomy model can be adopted to guide the design of LA systems from three-domain outcomes: focus (educational, clinical), level (macro, meso, or micro), and timeline (training, transition to practice, practice). In addition, the "six W" questions designed by Knight and Buckingham Shum (2017) also provide fine-grained guidance in the development of LA. The conceptual framework of a digitally integrated DDO (deliberately developmental organization) into CBME helps conceptualize and facilitate the integration of digitized assessment data into longitudinal coaching, promotions, and faculty development (Thoma, Caretta-Weyer, et al., 2021). And let's not forget the stakeholders who interact with the systems – Martinez-Maldonado et al. (2021) elicit the multiple roles in their model, emphasizing the essential connection and communication of various stakeholders by capturing their understanding of learning and assessment goals, as well as their data needs and requirements.

In this book chapter, we provide a broad review of LA within the context of medical education. In Sections 1 and 2, we consider various LA systems and tools articulating different foci underpinned by theoretical frameworks that address the objectives, system design, methods, and stakeholders. In Section 3, we examine the critical roles of medical educators in LA. In Section 4, we identify the dilemmas and controversies for LA that follow from the connectivity and integration of LA solutions into educational practices. Finally, Section 5 considers the numerous future opportunities for LA in medical education.

4.1.3 A Systems Approach to Learning Analytics

LA can be implemented across multiple systems within medical education. Table 4.1 provides a summary of the systems (see Section 2 for a detailed explanation). However, while LA might be introduced into the systems independently to assess and inform educational practices within a given domain, they can function within a common environment that intersects the systems. For example, medical students and residents are trained together and observed/assessed by the same faculty in the same context where patient care happens. Thus, educators and administrators who seek to adopt LA must consider the complexities that stem from the systems being linked together,

TABLE 4.1 Overview of the Systems in Which LA Can Be Implemented

Component	Admissions	Undergraduate Medical Education (UGME)	Postgraduate Medical Education (PGME)	Continuing Professional Development (CPD)	Health Systems
Back end: What is in the Database?	- Prior education data (e.g., undergraduate) - Standardized test scores (e.g., MCAT) - Grade point average (GPA) - Reference letters - Letters of intent - Interview scores - Demographic data of applicants	- Medical school admissions data - Standardized test scores - Simulation-based assessment (SBA) (e.g., Objective Structured Clinical Examinations [OSCE]) - Workplace-based assessment (WBA) - Demographic data of students	- CaRMS data - Standardized test scores - SBA (e.g., OSCE) - WBA (e.g., Entrustable Professional Activity (EPA) assessments, In-training Assessment Reports [ITERs]) - Demographic data of trainees	- Billing data - Demographic data of faculty and trainees - WBA and SBA scores faculty provided to trainees	- Aggregate healthcare data, clinical outcomes data (e.g., complication rates), patient-oriented outcomes data (e.g., patient satisfaction, patient-reported outcomes) - Billing data - Lawsuit data
Data Entry Encounters	- Application systems (e.g., Ontario Medical School Application Service)	- Mobile application for WBA entry - Linkage with learning management system for test score entry	- Observed assessment entry applications, mobile or web-based (e.g., one45, MedSIS)	- WBA/SBA entry applications, mobile or web-based (e.g., one45, MedSIS)	- Electronic health record
Teacher Applications	N/A	- Track trainees who need remediation or enrichment - Trends in trainee progress	- Track trainees who need remediation or enrichment - Trends in trainee progress	- Track one's own assessment progress (e.g., trends in scores assigned, expiration of initiated assessments)	N/A

(Continued)

TABLE 4.1 (Continued)

Component	Admissions	Undergraduate Medical Education (UGME)	Postgraduate Medical Education (PGME)	Continuing Professional Development (CPD)	Health Systems
Learner Applications	N/A	- Track one's own progress - Set goals	- Track one's own progress (e.g., number of EPA assessments received, EPA assessment scores) - Set goals	N/A	N/A
Front end: Dashboard displays	- Trends in applicant test scores across the years - Trends in applicant pool	- Progress testing trajectory - Rotation comments and WBA/SBA scores	- Progress testing trajectory - Rotation/EPA comments and other WBA/SBA scores	- Rotation/EPA comments and other WBA/SBA scores provided to trainees - Trends in faculty assessment practices	- Trends in clinical outcomes, patient-oriented outcomes, cost, and lawsuits
System Leader Applications	- Evaluation of admissions process based on aggregate trends (e.g., applicant scores, applicant pool demographics)	- Program evaluation based on aggregate trends (e.g., pass rates, time to completion of portfolios)	- Program evaluation based on aggregate trends (e.g., pass rates, completion of stages of training)	- Program evaluation of faculty performance and engagement in UGME and PGME	- Health system evaluation for patient safety concerns (e.g., complication rates)

e.g., interoperability – ability of multiple systems to exchange and use information that has been exchanged (Bates & Samal, 2018).

Assessments and LA: In considering the validity of LA, we must first consider the kind of assessment that LA is being used to support. Assessments can be *formative or low-stakes*, directed toward providing feedback to support continuous learning, or *summative or high-stakes*, directed toward decision-making regarding performance and readiness for next stage of training (Epstein, 2007; Lockyer et al., 2017). In CBME, there is increasing emphasis on frequent formative assessments, with the written and verbal feedback that the faculty provide playing a central role in the growth of the trainees. However, summative decisions are made by competence committees (CCs) by combining multiple formative assessments (Acai et al., 2021; Holmboe et al., 2010; Van Melle et al., 2019). The use of LA is subject to the same consideration of validity theory (e.g., Schoenherr & Hamstra, 2024). When assessments are conducted for either purpose, it is important to consider (a) who will be conducting the assessments (e.g., the raters), (b) what metrics will be used, (c) how often the assessments will be conducted, (d) who will be assessed, and (e) where will assessments take place, among other considerations, that will all come together and help educators make sense of trainee performance and progress. Educators can use LA to interpret the assessment data for both formative and summative purposes (e.g., analyze and visualize trends in trainee progress for an entrustable professional activity [EPA] – observable sets of knowledge, skills, and attitudes that represent core competencies of a discipline that are assessed to ensure that, by the end of training, a trainee is ready for independent practice; see Ma 2024) across a rotation and within a stage of training (Hennus et al., 2022; Holmboe et al., 2010; Sherbino et al., 2021; ten Cate et al., 2021; Thoma, Bandi et al., 2020).

Underlying Assumptions and Conceptual Frameworks of LA: Traditionally, LA has been rooted in post-positivist epistemology, but with the introduction of qualitative comments in medical education, LA has been increasingly constructivist (Chan et al., 2018; Hodges, 2013). With post-positivism, there is an emphasis on psychometrics and a singular truth, and that no assessment and analysis would be complete without reliability and other psychometric analysis. The idea here is that assessments are seen as high-stakes, and they become more reliable with a higher number of assessment data points, with rater training and with a major emphasis on standardized assessment conditions (Hodges, 2013). However, in the medical education context, variability in diagnosis, patient care setting, education setting, and trainee abilities required to perform clinical tasks are a part of real practice, which cannot be standardized. Additionally, the feedback that the raters provide would be as important as the score they assign on an assessment tool to optimize trainee learning, which goes against the high-stakes emphasis of post-positivism (Thoma, Ellaway, et al., 2021). Hence, with constructivism, there is an understanding that there are multiple truths (rather than a singular truth) to be uncovered and that trainees and faculty create their own knowledge and skills through (a) emphasis on assessment and feedback, (b) trainees' usage of the faculty feedback they receive to optimize their learning, (c) faculty's usage of the assessment and feedback they provide for continuing professional development (CPD), and (d) tailoring assessment and learning opportunities to the needs of the stakeholders (Dagnone et al., 2021; Hall et al., 2021; Van Melle et al., 2019). One of the emphases with constructivism and LA is the notion of self-regulated, individualized learning that facilitates healthcare trainees/professionals participating across the systems. The assessment and learning are self-paced and flexible to fulfill the authentic needs of trainees and faculty, whereby through using LA, evidence of progress can be understood, effective feedback and interventions could be designed where needed, and progress based on these changes can be re-evaluated.

4.2   The Role of Learning Analytics in Medical Education

Medical education represents a process, wherein criteria with established validity evidence are developed to identify and select a subset of trainees to progress onward within a program (Schoenherr & Hamstra, 2024). This section will contextualize ways in which LA can be used within multiple levels of medical education, starting from admissions to CPD, as well as within the health systems (Table 4.1).

4.2.1   Admissions

Medical school admissions usually require applicants to fulfill certain criteria that are outlined by each school and to submit documentation that show that they have fulfilled the requirements of each school (Cleland et al., 2023). Some of the information that is in the application package might include the Medical College Admission Test (MCAT) scores, the year(s) MCAT was taken, grade point average (GPA) in the undergraduate program, letter of intent (LI), curriculum vitae (CV), reference letters (RL), among other information. Once the applications are received, the written information (e.g., LI, CV, and RL) can be assigned a score based on the assessment criteria established by the school. Therefore, when the admissions committee is reviewing files and making decisions about who will be admitted, they have several narrative and numeric information to work with.

Standardized test scores, GPA, written documents, interview scores, science prerequisites, and demographics information, such as undergraduate institution, and various social identity variables such as gender, disability, membership in a minority group reflect data points that can be inputs for LA and used to facilitate the admissions process (Fong et al., 2009; Oladokun et al., 2008). Each of these data provides valuable information for the admissions committee. However, the high volume of applications received by medical schools makes it challenging to synthesize and interpret the data. To overcome this challenge, LA could allow the admissions committee to process, visualize, and interpret the large dataset in a feasible and meaningful way. For example, LA can be used by the committee for data visualization to allow for the efficient review of trends in applicant scores compared to other applicants and criteria set by the school, but also across the years. LA can also be important for the identification and quantification of applicants from various equity-seeking groups, and if the school has been implementing initiatives to support applicants from these groups, then LA can be used to visualize and quantify the impact of the initiatives on the applicant pool (Joy, 2022). Not only can LA be used within a single institution, but admissions committees from multiple institutions could combine their efforts and create an aggregated dataset to visualize trends across institutions in regard to both applicants and acceptances.

4.2.2 Undergraduate Medical Education

As medical students progress through their medical school curriculum, they receive many types of assessments that become a part of their student portfolios. These include their workplace-based assessments (WBAs; e.g., mini-clinical evaluation exercises, end of rotation assessments), assessments in the simulation setting (simulation-based assessments (SBA); e.g., objective structured clinical examinations), and standardized knowledge exam scores (Berendonk et al., 2018; Dong et al., 2012). Outside of these, undergraduate medical education (UGME) could have access to the students' pre-medicine scores through the admissions package. Finally, programs could collect equity, diversity, and inclusion (EDI)-related information from each student but also have information on various red flags that might be present per student (e.g., due to unprofessional behavior). Therefore, within UGME, we have many data points for each student that could span the timeline of pre-medicine and during medical school that provide distinctive kinds of information. Nonetheless, all these data can conceivably be merged into an aggregated dataset, and with LA, this large dataset can be visualized and interpreted at both the program level and for faculty/teacher members and students.

For *students*, LA can be used by each student to understand and track their own progress in terms of their performances in the knowledge and observed assessments (WBA and SBA) over time. With the support of the senior trainees and/or faculty, students can use this information to set short- and long-term goals. Students can also use LA to track their progress in relation to their classmates at an aggregate level. Additionally, students could include the visuals created through LA as a part of their Canadian Resident Matching Service (CaRMS) application package, to show their progress over time, which could be a valuable addition to the CaRMS application. For *faculty/educators*, especially at the committee level where decisions about students are made, LA can be used to track trainee progress but also easily identify students who need remediation or enrichment and track their progress accordingly (Prieto-Alvarez et al., 2018; Saqr et al., 2017). Additionally, students also provide written feedback to the faculty about their teaching that goes into the faculty portfolio. Therefore, at the UGME level of teaching, faculty could leverage LA to better understand the quantity and quality of their feedback and track their own progress. At the program level, *program evaluation* can be conducted based on the aggregate data trends that are generated through LA, including understanding trends in pass rates and time to completion of portfolios. Additionally, if there are concerns with red flags, programs could use LA to try to understand why certain red flags occurred and whether there are any program level concerns over EDI such as unconscious biases that need to be investigated further (Brown et al., 2020).

4.2.3 Postgraduate Medical Education

Given that the educational paradigm at the postgraduate medical education (PGME) level is shifting from an apprenticeship model toward an outcomes-based CBME model that focuses on development of skills through progressively sequenced learning experiences and competency acquisition evaluated through programmatic assessment (Ma, 2024; Schoenherr, Mahias-Ito, & Li, 2024), there have been major changes in the frequency and types of assessments that create exciting opportunities for implementing LA (Frank et al., 2017; Hsu et al., 2021; LoGiudice et al., 2022; ten Cate & Scheele, 2007; Touchie & ten Cate, 2016).

Outside of the traditional knowledge-focused testing of CBME (Witheridge et al., 2019), WBAs – (assessments conducted through direct observation of residents in the clinical setting [Marty et al., 2023]) have predominantly focused on EPA assessments, which are formative in nature and meant to enhance feedback provided to trainees through a focus on assessment *for* learning (Lockyer et al., 2017; ten Cate & Schumacher, 2022). Within CBME, EPA assessments are designed to be frequent, context-specific, and timely assessments of observable behaviors that collect a wide range of different snapshots of trainees' competency development, ensuring the acquisition of the necessary skillsets for effective and safe patient care (David et al., 2021; Jeyalingam et al., 2022; ten Cate et al., 2020; Woods et al., 2022). Additionally, outside of the workplace, there has been an increased emphasis on assessing individuals in the simulation setting through the usage of any type of simulation representative of the authentic training environments (Croft et al., 2020; Jeyalingam et al., 2022; ten Cate et al., 2021). As such, with CBME, there has been a major increase in the number and diversity of assessment data available per resident, and LA could play an important role in processing and understanding the vast amount of data by conducting a variety of analyses and visualizations to present the assessment data in a way that informs resident learning, the normative evaluation of individual programs, and the improvement of the assessment system by the specialty committee (Chan et al., 2018).

Within the residency programs themselves, including in CCs, LA can be used to understand progress of trainees per EPA, rotation, and stage (Goldhamer et al., 2022). Additionally, since the Royal College of Physicians and Surgeons of Canada (RCPSC) has outlined specific number of assessments that need to be completed for a given EPA with a certain entrustment level, LA could be used to understand trends around (a) number of assessments needed for each EPA versus how many completed so far, (b) different EPAs that are assessed in a given rotation versus EPAs that were assigned to a specific rotation to be completed, (c) which faculty has completed the EPA assessments in which context, and (d) number of assessments completed by faculty and scores they assign in each assessment (e.g., concept of hawk [raters that give more difficult marks] versus dove [easy going raters that tend to give easier marks]), among others (Thoma, Bandi et al., 2020; Yilmaz, Carey et al., 2022). Additionally, programs could make associations between test scores, EPA assessment scores, faculty variabilities, among others to make predictions or gather insights. Programs could also gain a better understanding of the diversity of experiences of competence by design (CBD) within their program, potentially identifying EDI-related challenges, including any conscious or unconscious biases (both gender- and race-based), and serve as a starting point for more detailed analysis of the impact of CBME on educational outcomes. If data can be aggregated at the national level, visual assessment dashboards can be generated, and programs could explore in depth their aggregated assessment data, compare their data to other programs and institutions nationally, determine areas where improvements are required, and take concrete actions (Thoma, Hall et al., 2020).

At the resident level, LA can be used by residents to understand their individual progress for each EPA, including whether they have fulfilled the assessment requirements (Carey et al., 2020). Additionally, LA could help them understand which EPAs are mapped to which rotations and whether they were able to complete the necessary EPA assessments for the rotations they completed. Outside of the EPA assessments, they could also better understand their standardized exam progress. Therefore, through LA, residents can more easily keep track of their progress across many data points as they receive many assessments over the course of their residency.

4.2.4   *Continuing Professional Development*

A distinguishing feature of contemporary education practices in the health professions is the recognition that learning is a lifelong process. Healthcare professionals must continue to engage in educational and other professional activities including workshops related to giving quality feedback and assessment and being effective mentors. Additionally, there is a lot of data that is already accrued at the PGME level, with residents needing many assessments from faculty, and through LA, by using the same data that is already collected, we could create CPD opportunities (Yilmaz et al., 2021).

At the faculty level, LA could help faculty track how many assessments they have completed to date overall and, by residency level, how many initiated assessments have expired, their scoring patterns (e.g., whether they tend to score residents at the higher or lower end of the scale), and the quality of their written feedback (e.g., number of words and whether their feedback is constructive). Additionally, CCs could use LA to track faculty involvement with and completion of trainee assessments (Acai et al., 2021; Cheung et al., 2022; Thoma, Bandi, et al., 2020). For example, CC could determine (a) which faculty are completing how many EPA assessments in relation to their practice routines, (b) which faculty are easy versus hard raters, and (c) how many days it takes each faculty to complete assessments. Once these trends are identified, CCs and programs could work together to determine improvement strategies for the program, with educational initiatives targeted toward faculty (Yilmaz, Carey, et al., 2022).

With the advent of new medical phenomena (e.g., emerging diseases) and also advancements in technology (e.g., artificial intelligence [AI]; see Schoenherr & Michael, 2024), the landscape of CPD is ripe for the entry of bundled learning opportunities like microcredentials. Microcredentials are small-scale competency-based credentials that are becoming progressively more common across the private and the public sectors. They engage in assisting those seeking to upskill in a focused area (much like CBME) and likely hold the key to linking CBME with the world of CPD (Hunt et al., 2019). Crucial for effectively integrating microcredentials into the healthcare professions will be the plan to harness the power of LA to assist with determining the pathway for a professional, but also to engage in generating useful data for individuals to close the knowing-doing gap. As in any area of education, the incorporation of microcredentials into CBME must proceed with caution to ensure that the development and implementation of microcredentials within the applied health professions are highly robust (Peppler-Beechey & Weingarten, 2021).

4.2.5   *Health Systems*

Health systems that intersect with academia (e.g., academic hospitals), and where both patient care and research and trainee education take place, are unique environments that come together as a learning organization (Gordon, 2022). Outside of the various trainee data that is collected, at the hospital level, especially with the implementation of electronic health records, there are many data points that get captured, including aggregate healthcare data (e.g., clinical outcomes data), billing data, and lawsuits. The thousands of data points collected by these systems can be aggregated, analyzed, and visualized, to explore multiple health system level trends such as types and number of procedures being performed within a specific timeframe and number and types of patient safety concerns (e.g., latent safety threats, high levels of complications for a specific procedure, and specific contexts where certain complications occur [e.g., in the intensive care unit, in the emergency department]). Hence, LA can be used to identify gaps in programs and practices within and across health systems, as Schoenheer and Hamstra (2024) have alluded. For example, when specific trends are identified within a health system, then further explorations can be done to understand why these trends are observed and educational interventions such as interdisciplinary *in-situ* simulation sessions can be developed and implemented. Ultimately, evidence is accumulated to assess the human, financial, and material resources of a system, and LA can be used as one variable in a more complex calculus around operationalized programmatic vulnerabilities and gaps.

4.3   Role of the Medical Educator in Learning Analytics

The opportunities of LA in medical education appear limitless. However, their effective implementation must ensure that medical educators are actively engaged in the process of helping their institution create, regulate, and use LA databases and implementation strategies. Below, we will describe various considerations that should be taken into account to successfully implement and use LA.

4.3.1   Composition of the LA Team

4.3.1.1   Development Team

The development and administration of any program requires that teams are created and sustained that have the appropriate competencies (Schoenherr & Hamstra, 2024). LA requires the accurate and complete collection of data, analyses that can include descriptive statistics and predictive models, and visualization that provide stakeholders with insights concerning these patterns and predictions. LA teams should be minimally composed of computer programmers, lawyers, data managers, administrators, and ethics/data compliance/data security officers. Ideally, LA development teams should be directed toward user-engaged co-design, which could involve numerous stakeholders including trainees, frontline physicians, program directors (PDs), and other "end users" of LA outputs (Prieto-Alvarez et al., 2018; Thoma, Ellaway et al., 2021).

The introduction of AI and LA into medical education requires a further extension of interprofessional and multidisciplinary teams. In a study that explored and defined new CBME-related roles and competencies for administrative staff and faculty (Yilmaz et al., 2023), a major theme was related to assessment system facilitators, including the need for (a) assessment process and systems designers, who are responsible for programming/designing assessment systems and/or instruments, (b) CBME analytics/data support staff, who are responsible for performing data analytics and assist in leading the development of analytics that support CBME, and (c) information technology (IT) leads, who are responsible for the e-portfolio or electronic curriculum/assessment system. These teams might be further supplemented with learning engineers who have competencies within the domains of AI and machine learning.

4.3.1.2 Stakeholders

Beyond the development team, numerous stakeholders with diverse motivations, competencies, and roles must also be involved as they will make use of LA by interpreting patterns and making decisions for education and healthcare at the level of individuals, programs, and institutions. Stakeholders could include trainees, frontline physicians, CC members, PDs, curriculum leads, department chairs, and associate chairs of education. Due to differences in their objectives and professional training, each stakeholder will approach LA from different perspectives. Stakeholders must be capable of understanding how data was collected, processed, and presented for decision-making, as the interpretation of visualizations based on LA will be heavily dependent on stakeholder competencies and their understanding of the LA processes (Bakharia et al., 2016; Lockyer et al., 2013). Hence, it is imperative to make stakeholder intentions explicit both in the modeling and in the stakeholder-facing interface for all stakeholders to make sense of the complex data underpinning the assessments suggested by the interface (Martinez-Maldonado et al., 2021).

4.3.2 The Method and Timing of Medical Educator Involvement

Medical educators can assist with LA during four stages (see Figure 4.1): data generation, prototyping and design, policy and ethics, and data interpretation. We provide a brief summary of each of these stages and the opportunities they present below.

Where Medical Educators Can Help

Data Generation

Frontline clinician teachers are often the source of much of the data collection required for generating learning analytics. Workplace-based observations are made and entered into EPAs.

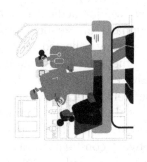

Prototyping & Design

Frontline faculty should make sure they coordinate and provide feedback to systems designers to ensure user-experiences are understood.

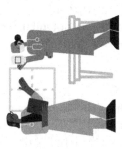

Policy & Ethics

Leaders & policy makers need to consider implementation of quality assurance and monitoring systems to ensure the quality of the inputs and outputs of LA.

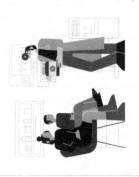

Data Interpretation

There are descriptive, explanatory, predictive, and evaluative LA, all of which have different usages that require different types of data, different LA techniques, and lead to different outcomes and interpretation.

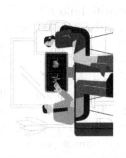

FIGURE 4.1 Infographic regarding the involvement of a medical educator in the learning analytics process.

4.3.2.1 Frontline Data Collection

Medical educators often simultaneously hold the roles of teacher, clinical supervisors, and assessors (Li et al., 2021). This means that they generate the bulk of the assessment data (Acai et al., 2019; Yilmaz et al., 2023). In other settings, teachers or senior residents often engage heavily in providing feedback or grading students (Schiff et al., 2017). However, the data and the end analysis will only be useful and accurate if the assessments are conducted properly (Chan et al., 2018). Consequently, frontline faculty and educators need to be trained to ensure that they can effectively document their observations and insights about trainee performances. In addition, if there are missing data or data is subject to biases (e.g., nonrandom selection), steps need to be taken to determine what information is missing, how to address the missing/biased data, and any potential negative consequences that might arise from the missing/biased data (Chan et al., 2017).

4.3.2.2 Prototyping and Design

The development of prototypes must be human-centered and guided by considerations of the end-users (Thai et al., 2022). For this initial phase of LA, the development team should explore the types of data available, which data should be used, and the LA techniques that should be selected, based on the goals for developing and using LA (Chan et al., 2018). Extensive assessment data is collected as a part of CBME requirements. Frontline faculty should make sure they coordinate and provide feedback to systems designers to ensure user experiences are understood. Prototype development should begin with relatively simple prototypes, with the goal of making the purpose of LA concrete, allowing for stakeholder engagement. Through rapid iterations, prototypes can be developed and tested until the kinds of analytics, interface, and other output can be used by all stakeholders. These activities have the added benefit of increasing engagement and acceptance at all levels.

4.3.2.3 LA Techniques and Interpretation

Until recently, LA was not feasible within medical education. With the introduction of CBME and its emphasis on frequent assessments, large quantities of assessment data are now being collected, creating opportunities for implementing LA to guide assessment decisions. There are descriptive, explanatory, predictive, and evaluative LA, all of which have different usages that require different types of data, different LA techniques, and lead to different outcomes and interpretations (Chan et al., 2018). For example, descriptive LA can be used to characterize past performance data, whereas explanatory LA is to identify causal relationships between constructs within a dataset. Ideally, once the initial prototyping phase has concluded, institutions should engage large groups of stakeholders to actively use the data within their professional training/practice, share aggregated patterns with colleagues, and publish the datasets in peer-reviewed journals. By promoting the use of LA techniques and interpretation, a clearer shared understanding can be gained about the objectives and practices of medical education.

4.3.2.4   Policy Development and Ethics

Though LA can be a very effective approach for visualizing and interpreting data, LA is ultimately dependent on the quality of the data that is collected, the LA techniques that are chosen, and how that data is used to inform decision-making. Consequently, the development team and stakeholders, such as CC leads and PDs, will need to consider implementation of quality assurance and monitoring systems to ensure the quality of the inputs and outputs of LA. This is especially important given that the assessment data interpretations will have positive or negative social consequences for the people or systems the LA was focused on (e.g., consequences for trainees, consequences for faculty) (Chan et al., 2018). For example, identifying struggling residents and directing them to complete remediation would be valuable to ensure that we are graduating residents who will safely take care of patients. However, this might have negative consequences for the residents themselves whereby their confidence in their practices might decrease, affecting their future performance.

Beyond LA, there is a broad recognition that biases can be found in large datasets. If left uncorrected, these biases can be perpetuated. Biases are not always self-evident, instead they can often reflect latent variables that are left undefined or unlabeled within a dataset (see Schoenherr & Michael, 2024). Within medical education, these EDI issues could include gender bias (e.g., female trainees being rated differently than male trainees) or racial bias. Anyone who is involved in the development and interpretation of large datasets through LA should be aware of the potential pitfalls due to the data itself and various implicit and hidden biases that can be present. Additionally, there are recommendations for data sharing that all individuals developing or using LA should abide by, including the *Data-Sharing in Canadian Medical Education Research: Consensus Recommendations and Principles for Governance* that outline risks and benefits of multi-institutional and data-driven medical education research and provide recommendations for the ethical use of education data (Chahine et al., 2018; Grierson et al., 2022). The main recommendations from the consensus document include (a) establishing a governance body that includes representation from all relevant stakeholders, ensuring appropriate research process (e.g., transparency, informed consent, respect for data sovereignty, and ethical review), (b) involving a data management facility that will be trusted with technical and procedural aspects of data sharing, and (c) using best practices to manage data, including a clear outline of institutional strategies, developing data management plans, and contemplating data deposits (Grierson et al., 2022).

4.4 Dilemmas and Controversies

The opportunities provided by LA for medical education are paralleled with a variety of challenges and depend on the extent that educators, administrators, and other stakeholders understand their properties and the appropriate usage context. Here, we briefly consider the dilemmas and controversies associated with LA.

4.4.1 Learning Analytics Literacy and Sustainability

Though LA includes psychometric techniques (Schoenherr & Hamstra, 2016), much of the field of LA is relatively new. Many medical educators will have completed training in an era before LA and fluency with LA was expected of them. As such, although there are new roles that are emerging within our field to support LA heavy areas (e.g., CBME; [Carney et al., 2023; Yilmaz et al., 2023]), the training opportunities around LA are still sparse in higher education and specifically medical education (Selwyn & Gašević, 2020; Tolsgaard et al., 2023). Indeed, it will likely be sometime before LA is meaningfully integrated into the medical professions curriculum such that competencies in using these techniques can be effectively assessed.

As the field of medical education creates more data, we are beginning to recognize how costly these systems are to design, test, implement, and update. We must train a cadre of new faculty members and administrative experts to engage in the business of creating LA platforms and maintaining databases. Moreover, as systems are first brought into the LA world, capital investments must be made in training staff, faculty members, and existing trainees about how to operate within these systems. Finally, to maintain these systems in terms of their relevance and abilities, we must find a way to make these human-and-technology systems sustainable through increased investment from universities and training programs. Without continual system updates, improvements, and innovations, these systems and processes will surely stagnate over time.

4.4.2 Meta-Raters and Differences in the Eyes of the Beholders

With increasing data, there is an exponential increase in the way that multiple educators might view, handle, and analyze the data. Research thus far has already shown that when given the same performance, raters might see and rate a given performance differently (Chan et al., 2021; Kogan et al., 2011).

Gingerich et al. (2014) describe this as the meaningful idiosyncrasy of raters. When taken one step further, the aggregate ratings must be analyzed and interpreted by other "meta-raters", such as those on a CC or programmatic assessment committee (Acai et al., 2019; Chan et al., 2018; Chan et al., 2020; Chan et al., 2017). Despite the introduction of more data, subjective elements of assessment will continue to play a role: When there are multiple layers of rating and analysis, then LA data can manifest in conflict. Chan et al. (2021) have explored this issue in depth in a recent conceptual review. They considered whether there might be conflicting data within a pool of data around a certain individual's performance and whether two faculty meta-raters within a committee view a trainee's progression in two disparate ways (one sees slow growth; the other is worried the trainee has stagnated).

To combat differences in data analytics competencies, adopting human-centered design approaches has been found to be helpful (Martinez-Maldonado et al., 2021). In medical education, design-based research (DBR) techniques are increasingly being used to help create better user interfaces to ease the strain of data interpretation. The work of Thoma and colleagues seeks to bring in these techniques, and this team has shown that DBR can clarify the needs of a wide range of end-users for the data analytics of CBME (Carey et al., 2020; Thoma, Bandi, et al., 2020; Yilmaz et al., 2021; Yilmaz, Carey et al., 2022). Pivoting datasets is very common outside of medical education, but it is prudent to consider the ramifications of harnessing data collected for one use (e.g., assessment of trainees) to generate new insights (e.g., faculty teaching quality). Careful consideration of how we fold in policies and procedures that allow for LA to be used efficiently but also to ensure that they are not misused will be something we must consider going forward.

4.4.3   Biases in Modeling

LAs are highly dependent on the data that is presented – and especially those models that are built around black box machine learning algorithms (MLAs) can often build in predictions and analytics that propel certain biases within the system. With the evolution of infamous large language models (LLMs) like ChatGPT, it seems clear that algorithms are on the rise (Chary et al., 2019). Within medical education, early adopters have been reporting inferential AI-driven analysis of data (natural language processing [NLP], MLA for surveillance) (Ariaeinejad et al., 2017; James et al., 2021; Winkler-Schwartz et al., 2019; Yilmaz, Jurado Nunez et al., 2022). NLP is a subfield of AI that focuses on the interaction between human language and computers. It comprises a wide range of tasks from language understanding, speech recognition to information extraction and classification, with the goal of generating useful and meaningful knowledge to humans. In the medical education context, NLP helps analyze the narrative feedback from the clinical assessment of the trainees' performance, transcribed patient-provider interactions, or other clinical documentations (Chary et al., 2019; Yilmaz, Jurado Nunez et al., 2022). An MLA is a type of AI designed to learn from data for analysis and prediction based on the patterns found in the datasets, in the manner of supervised, unsupervised, or semi-supervised. MLA is used to enhance human decision-making and reduce the workload of large narrative datasets, for example, analyzing student performance data and providing personalized feedback and recommendations (Winkler-Schwartz et al., 2019).

The great promise of harnessing MLA and NLP to analyze data, of course, is that there is a marked increase in the burden of assessment data for both faculty and trainees in the modern age (Acai et al., 2019; Burm et al., 2020; Ott et al., 2022). CBME has been seen to be the cause of much of this, and MLA/NLP techniques may prove to be a solution. However, we must be wary of how these algorithms will ultimately influence the judgment and inferences of the decision makers (e.g., meta-raters within a CC).

We must also be cognizant that many of these algorithms, if agnostically applied, may build in the biases that already exist within a system. Specifically, MLA/NLP techniques have been shown to replicate human biases (e.g., racism, misogyny), simply because those who build the models and the human datasets that are used to train the models are prone to these human fallibilities. Ruha Benjamin has previously written extensively around this in her book, *Race after Technology: Abolitionist Tools for the New Jim Code* (Benjamin, 2019). As we apply these models in medical education (and indeed in healthcare writ large), we must be cognizant of our own unperceived biases, which may disproportionately affect certain individuals within our system. As a corollary, if done correctly, harnessing MLA/NLP to *detect* biases against certain groups would be possible as well.

4.4.4 Beyond Physician-Generated Data

In an era where medical schools are increasingly asked to be socially accountable, engaging other healthcare professionals, patients, and families will be crucial for engaging in the future. While interprofessional work has become a standard practice in most medical schools, incorporating non-physician healthcare providers into assessment teams and harnessing their observations to generate LA has not yet been fully realized. There are some clear found pilots that examine this (Echeverria et al., 2019), but in most environments, we are losing much data by not involving non-physicians in the assessment of our trainees, especially in the workplace.

There are also great opportunities to link trainee data to patient outcomes – and some fascinating early work is being done to examine the challenging measurement issues that occur within the workplace to ensure we can tease apart trainee versus faculty member contributions to care. Sebok-Syer and colleagues have been examining how we can tease apart the interdependence of trainees with their faculty supervisors or their healthcare teams (Sebok-Syer et al., 2023; Sebok-Syer et al., 2020) within the clinical sphere. Schumacher and colleagues are exploring the nature of resident-sensitive quality measures (RSQM), which would be specific clinical metrics that are more attributable to trainee performance than other clinical outcome measures (Kinnear et al., 2021; Petosa et al., 2021; Schumacher, Holmboe et al., 2020; Schumacher, Martini, Holmboe et al., 2020; Schumacher et al., 2019; Schumacher, Martini, Sobolewski et al., 2020; Smirnova et al., 2023).

To fulfill the promise of going beyond physician-generated data to link learning outcomes and analytics to patient-oriented outcomes/analytics within healthcare systems, designers will have to tackle some wicked problems (Chahine et al., 2018; Thoma, Ellaway et al., 2021). A key challenge will be in the linkage between such datasets in a manner that protects both patients and trainees but allows for these analyses to occur. Policies and procedures that consider the ethical implications of this work will be key.

4.5 Future Opportunities

There is growing interest in shifting the assessment for licensure from high-stakes, summative assessments to greater integration of training programs and clinical practices through formative assessments to fulfill the promise of CBME (Chan et al., 2022; Thoma et al., 2022). Ideally, CBME assessment data can be collected and utilized at different levels to improve learning and inform decisions for coaching, promotions, and progression that could lead to the transformation of oversight and accreditation processes. The integrated model aims at increasing trainees' clinical autonomy and their ownership of clinical outcomes while they are participating in stages of competency-based assessments and eventually fostering medical practitioners' lifelong learning skills and improvements throughout their careers (Goldhamer et al., 2022). However, there are predictable discrepancies in the use of data for different purposes and domains within the healthcare system, for example, the low levels of adoption of digitalized datasets for faculty development compared to the resident development (Miller et al., 2022). The lack of digitalized data from single or multiple data points could fail the developmental process for the integration among different domains.

To respond to the needs of integrated solutions, we have reviewed the LA systems in Section 2, by not only focusing on learning needs of UGME and PGME, but also turning our attention to the CPD and health systems. The review shows how the designs and implementations of LA innovations that are better aligned with underlying educational theories and models would bring positive impact to targeted users – to support and foster their practices through evidence-based and reflective learning trajectories for personal growth. However, we also observed that the LA innovations are yet to be widely and formally adopted in different levels due to the heavy demand for fundamental and structural support needed for LA implementation (Selwyn & Gašević, 2020). In particular, LA has not yet come to fruition in the WBAs and learning that is based within the health systems for clinicians and faculties, though small-scale pilot research work has been done, including the implementation of practice-based feedback and support mechanisms for audit and feedback (Kamhawy et al., 2021), assessment data as measure of faculty performance (Thoma, Caretta-Weyer et al., 2021), and data dashboards to visualize and inform the faculty development programs (Yilmaz et al., 2021).

The adoption of a mix of traditional and emerging LA methods has been proved and widely used in other fields, with the possibility of transferring the LA innovations into medical education for UGME and PGME (Martinez-Maldonado et al., 2021), as well as CPD – faculty teaching evaluation, research productivity, and clinical performance (Yilmaz et al., 2021), and health systems – clinical and patient-oriented outcomes (Chan et al., 2018; Thoma, Ellaway et al., 2021). Concerns that may lead to misinterpretation and bias have been discussed in Section 4, including insufficient training support, idiosyncrasy of raters, limitation of modeling, and evolving data points. As such, focusing on training outcomes, we argue that LA development should work backward from the goal, with the following recommended practices.

First, the determination of a set of well-defined LA indicators and metrics would serve as a key enabler for a meaningful implementation of LA. The indicators and their observable metrics could be used to identify and connect basic data points for informing higher level object measurement, which is usually unobservable and highly sophisticated. For example, at the individual learning level, Martinez-Maldonado et al. (2021) have mapped the physiological and positioning data to the clinical resuscitation protocol within a group of nursing learners, with the aim to improve their collaborative problem solving skills. At the program level, Goldhamer et al. (2022) identified the need for the CC to review and synthesize multi-source data including formative and summative assessments to generate programmatic trends and progression in terms of the competency-based advancement.

Second, it is evident from Sections 2 and 3 that stakeholders from different LA systems play crucial roles in bringing the learning context into the development of LA and making decisions upon the results of LA. To fulfill the quest of building an integrated LA solution to utilize data fully and effectively across participating institutions and programs, Thoma, Caretta-Weyer et al. (2021) considered CBME as the catalyst for organizational change across different levels (individual, program, and system) within medical education.

The success of the changes – achieving the ultimate goals of learning – would rely on the social-technical transitions, including the embracement of a culture of lifelong learning for all healthcare professionals (Thoma et al., 2022), commitment to honest feedback (Thoma, Caretta-Weyer et al., 2021), as well as technical infrastructure for enabling scalable and sustainable organizational changes. The sociotechnical change can be achieved through multilevel leaderships across the medical education system to ensure that the alignment between the goals and implementation strategies is achieved. As such, systematic changes can be tough to mediate the relationships between educators, learners, policymakers, and researchers if we proceed without investment in staff training of data literacy, human-centered design environment, and other forms of support for the non-technical issues. Thus, we argue that adopting modern educational theories that could possibly help comprehend the complexity of learning can serve as fundamental lenses and languages to conceptualize and monitor different stages of LA development and deployment, in order to drive the power of LA to improve evidence-based learning and decision-making.

References

Acai, A., Cupido, N., Weavers, A., Saperson, K., Ladhani, M., Cameron, S., & Sonnadara, R. R. (2021). Competence committees: The steep climb from concept to implementation. *Med Educ, 55*(9), 1067–1077. https://doi.org/10.1111/medu.14585

Acai, A., Li, S. A., Sherbino, J., & Chan, T. M. (2019). Attending emergency physicians' perceptions of a programmatic workplace-based assessment system: The McMaster modular assessment program (McMAP). *Teach Learn Med, 31*(4), 434–444. https://doi.org/10.1080/10401334.2019.1574581

Ariaeinejad, A., Samavi, R., Chan, T. M., & Doyle, T. E. (2017). A performance predictive model for emergency medicine residents. Proceedings of the 27th Annual International Conference on Computer Science and Software Engineering. Markham, Ontario, Canada.

Bakharia, A., Corrin, L., Barba, P. d., Kennedy, G., Gašević, D., Mulder, R., Williams, D., Dawson, S., & Lockyer, L. (2016). A conceptual framework linking learning design with learning analytics. Proceedings of the Sixth International Conference on Learning Analytics & Knowledge. Edinburgh, United Kingdom. https://doi.org/10.1145/2883851.2883944

Bates, D. W., & Samal, L. (2018). Interoperability: What is it, how can we make it work for clinicians, and how should we measure it in the future? *Health Serv Res, 53*(5), 3270–3277. https://doi.org/10.1111/1475-6773.12852

Benjamin, R. (2019). *Race after Technology: Abolitionist Tools for the New Jim Code.* Polity Press.

Berendonk, C., Rogausch, A., Gemperli, A., & Himmel, W. (2018). Variability and dimensionality of students' and supervisors' mini-CEX scores in undergraduate medical clerkships – A multilevel factor analysis. *BMC Med Educ, 18*(1), 100. https://doi.org/https://dx.doi.org/10.1186/s12909-018-1207-1

Brown, M. E. L., Hunt, G. E. G., Hughes, F., & Finn, G. M. (2020). 'Too male, too pale, too stale': A qualitative exploration of student experiences of gender bias within medical education. *BMJ Open, 10*(8), e039092. https://doi.org/10.1136/bmjopen-2020-039092

Burm, S., Sebok-Syer, S. S., Van Koughnett, J. A., & Watling, C. J. (2020). Are we generating more assessments without added value? Surgical trainees' perceptions of and receptiveness to cross-specialty assessment. *Perspect Med Educ, 9*(4), 201–209. https://doi.org/10.1007/s40037-020-00594-0

Carey, R., Wilson, G., Bandi, V., Mondal, D., Martin, L. J., Woods, R., Chan, T., & Thoma, B. (2020). Developing a dashboard to meet the needs of residents in a competency-based training program: A design-based research project. *Can Med Educ J, 11*(6), e31–e45. https://doi.org/10.36834/cmej.69682

Carney, P. A., Sebok-Syer, S. S., Pusic, M. V., Gillespie, C. C., Westervelt, M., & Goldhamer, M. E. J. (2023). Using learning analytics in clinical competency committees: Increasing the impact of competency-based medical education. *Med Educ Online, 28*(1), 2178913. https://doi.org/10.1080/10872981.2023.2178913

Chahine, S., Kulasegaram, K. M., Wright, S., Monteiro, S., Grierson, L. E. M., Barber, C., Sebok-Syer, S. S., McConnell, M., Yen, W., De Champlain, A., & Touchie, C. (2018). A call to investigate the relationship between education and health outcomes using big data. *Acad Med, 93*(6), 829–832. https://doi.org/10.1097/acm.0000000000002217

Chan, T., Oswald, A., Hauer, K. E., Caretta-Weyer, H. A., Nousiainen, M. T., Cheung, W. J., & Collaborators, I. (2021). Diagnosing conflict: Conflicting data, interpersonal conflict, and conflicts of interest in clinical competency committees. *Med Teach, 43*(7), 765–773. https://doi.org/10.1080/0142159X.2021.1925101

Chan, T., Sebok-Syer, S., Thoma, B., Wise, A., Sherbino, J., & Pusic, M. (2018). Learning analytics in medical education assessment: The past, the present, and the future. *AEM Educ Train, 2*(2), 178–187. https://doi.org/10.1002/aet2.10087

Chan, T. M., Dowling, S., Tastad, K., Chin, A., & Thoma, B. (2022). Integrating training, practice, and reflection within a new model for Canadian medical licensure: A concept paper prepared for the Medical Council of Canada. *Can Med Educ J, 13*(4), 68–81. https://doi.org/https://doi.org/10.36834/cmej.73717

Chan, T. M., Sebok-Syer, S. S., Sampson, C., & Monteiro, S. (2020). The quality of assessment of learning (qual) score: Validity evidence for a scoring system aimed at rating short, workplace-based comments on trainee performance. *Teach Learn Med, 32*(3), 319–329. https://doi.org/10.1080/10401334.2019.1708365

Chan, T. M., Sherbino, J., & Mercuri, M. (2017). Nuance and noise: Lessons learned from longitudinal aggregated assessment data. *J Grad Med Educ, 9*(6), 724–729. https://doi.org/10.4300/JGME-D-17-00086.1

Chary, M., Parikh, S., Manini, A. F., Boyer, E. W., & Radeos, M. (2019). A review of natural language processing in medical education. *West J Emerg Med, 20*(1), 78–86. https://doi.org/10.5811/westjem.2018.11.39725

Cheung, W. J., Wagner, N., Frank, J. R., Oswald, A., Van Melle, E., Skutovich, A., Dalseg, T. R., Cooke, L. J., & Hall, A. K. (2022). Implementation of competence committees during the transition to CBME in Canada: A national fidelity-focused evaluation. *Med Teach, 44*(7), 781–789. https://doi.org/10.1080/0142159X.2022.2041191

Cleland, J., Blitz, J., Cleutjens, K., Oude Egbrink, M. G. A., Schreurs, S., & Patterson, F. (2023). Robust, defensible, and fair: The AMEE guide to selection into medical school: AMEE Guide No. 153. *Med Teach*, 1–14. https://doi.org/10.1080/01421 59x.2023.2168529

Croft, H., Gilligan, C., Rasiah, R., Levett-Jones, T., & Schneider, J. (2020). Developing a validity argument for a simulation-based model of entrustment in dispensing skills assessment framework. *Curr Pharm Teach Learn*, *12*(9), 1081–1092. https://doi.org/10.1016/j.cptl.2020.04.028

Dagnone, J. D., Bandiera, G., & Harris, K. (2021). Re-examining the value proposition for competency-based medical education. *Can Med Educ J*, *12*(3), 155–158. https://doi.org/10.36834/cmej.68245

David, V., Walsh, M., Lockyer, J., & Mintz, M. (2021). Entrustable professional activities: An analysis of faculty time, trainee perspectives and actionability. *Can J Gen Intern Med*, *16*(1), 8–13. https://doi.org/10.22374/cjgim.v16i1.415

Dong, T., Saguil, A., Artino, A. R., Jr., Gilliland, W. R., Waechter, D. M., Lopreaito, J., Flanagan, A., & Durning, S. J. (2012). Relationship between OSCE scores and other typical medical school performance indicators: A 5-year cohort study. *Mil Med*, *177*(9 Suppl), 44–46. http://ovidsp.ovid.com/ovidweb.cgi?T=JS&PAGE=refere nce&D=medl&NEWS=N&AN=23029860

Echeverria, V., Martinez-Maldonado, R., & Shum, S. B. (2019). Towards collaboration translucence: Giving meaning to multimodal group data. Proceedings of the 2019 CHI Conference on Human Factors in Computing Systems, Glasgow, Scotland UK. https://doi.org/10.1145/3290605.3300269

Epstein, R. M. (2007). Assessment in medical education. *N Engl J Med*, *356*(4), 387–396. https://doi.org/10.1056/NEJMra054784

Fong, S., Yain-Whar, S., & Biuk-Aghai, R. P. (2009). Applying a hybrid model of neural network and decision tree classifier for predicting university admission. In *2009 7th International Conference on Information, Communications and Signal Processing (ICICS)* (pp. 1–5). New York: IEEE.

Frank, J., Snell, L., & Sherbino, J. (2017). *CanMEDS 2015 Physician Competency Framework*. Ottawa: Royal College of Physicians and Surgeons of Canada; 2015. *Google Scholar*.

Gingerich, A., Kogan, J., Yeates, P., Govaerts, M., & Holmboe, E. (2014). Seeing the 'black box' differently: Assessor cognition from three research perspectives. *Med Educ*, *48*(11), 1055–1068. https://doi.org/10.1111/medu.12546

Goldhamer, M. E. J., Martinez-Lage, M., Black-Schaffer, W. S., Huang, J. T., Co, J. P. T., Weinstein, D. F., & Pusic, M. V. (2022). Reimagining the clinical competency committee to enhance education and prepare for competency-based time-variable advancement. *J Gen Intern Med*, *37*(9), 2280–2290. https://doi.org/10.1007/s11 606-022-07515-3

Gordon, J. (2022). Harvard Macy Institute Podcast. In The Harvard Macy Institute Podcast S3 E6: The Learning Hospital with Jim Gordon. https://harvardmacy.org/blog/the-harvard-macy-institute-podcast-s3-e6

Grierson, L., Kulasegaram, K., Button, B., Lee-Krueger, R., McNeill, K., Youssef, A., & Cavanagh, A. (2022). Data-Sharing in Canadian Medical Education Research: Consensus Recommendations and Principles for Governance. Available from: www.dataconnection.ca

Hall, A. K., Schumacher, D. J., Thoma, B., Caretta-Weyer, H., Kinnear, B., Gruppen, L., Cooke, L. J., Frank, J. R., Van Melle, E., & Collaborators, I. (2021). Outcomes of competency-based medical education: A taxonomy for shared language. *Med Teach*, *43*(7), 788–793. https://doi.org/10.1080/0142159X.2021.1925643

Hennus, M. P., van Dam, M., Gauthier, S., Taylor, D. R., & ten Cate, O. (2022). The logic behind entrustable professional activity frameworks: A scoping review of the literature. Med Educ. https://doi.org/10.1111/medu.14806

Hodges, B. (2013). Assessment in the post-psychometric era: Learning to love the subjective and collective. *Med Teach, 35*(7), 564–568. https://doi.org/10.3109/0142159X.2013.789134

Holmboe, E. S., Sherbino, J., Long, D. M., Swing, S. R., & Frank, J. R. (2010). The role of assessment in competency-based medical education. *Med Teach, 32*(8), 676–682. https://doi.org/10.3109/0142159X.2010.500704

Hsu, T., De Angelis, F., Al-Asaaed, S., Basi, S. K., Tomiak, A., Grenier, D., Hammad, N., Henning, J. W., Berry, S., Song, X., & Mukherjee, S. D. (2021). Ten ways to get a grip on designing and implementing a competency-based medical education training program. *Can Med Educ J, 12*(2), e81–e87. https://doi.org/10.36834/cmej.70723

Hunt, T., Carter, R., Zhang, L., & Yang, S. (2019). Micro-credentials: The potential of personalized professional development. *Dev Learn Organ, 34*(2), 33–35. https://doi.org/10.1108/dlo-09-2019-0215

James, C. A., Wheelock, K. M., & Woolliscroft, J. O. (2021). Machine learning: The next Paradigm Shift in Medical Education. *Acad Med, 96*(7), 954–957. https://doi.org/10.1097/ACM.0000000000003943

Jeyalingam, T., Walsh, C. M., Tavares, W., Mylopoulos, M., Hodwitz, K., Liu, L. W. C., Heitman, S. J., & Brydges, R. (2022). Variable or fixed? Exploring entrustment decision making in workplace–and simulation-based assessments. *Acad Med, 97*(7), 1057–1064. https://doi.org/10.1097/acm.0000000000004661

Joy, T. R. (2022). Strategies for enhancing equity, diversity, and inclusion in medical school admissions – A Canadian medical school's journey. *Front Public Health, 10,* 879173. https://doi.org/10.3389/fpubh.2022.879173

Kamhawy, R., Chan, T. M., & Mondoux, S. (2021). Enabling positive practice improvement through data-driven feedback: A model for understanding how data and self-perception lead to practice change. *J Eval Clin Pract, 27*(4), 915–925. https://doi.org/https://doi.org/10.1111/jep.13504

Kinnear, B., Kelleher, M., Sall, D., Schauer, D. P., Warm, E. J., Kachelmeyer, A., Martini, A., & Schumacher, D. J. (2021). Development of resident-sensitive quality measures for inpatient general internal medicine. *J Gen Intern Med, 36*(5), 1271–1278. https://doi.org/10.1007/s11606-020-06320-0

Knight, S., & Buckingham Shum, S. (2017). Theory and learning analytics. In Lang, C., Siemens, G., Wise, A. F., & Gaševic, D. (eds.) *The Handbook of Learning Analytics* (1 ed., pp. 17–22). Society for Learning Analytics Research (SoLAR). http://solaresearch.org/hla-17/hla17-chapter1

Kogan, J. R., Conforti, L., Bernabeo, E., Iobst, W., & Holmboe, E. (2011). Opening the black box of clinical skills assessment via observation: A conceptual model. *Med Educ, 45*(10), 1048–1060. https://doi.org/10.1111/j.1365-2923.2011.04025.x

Li, S. A., Acai, A., Sherbino, J., & Chan, T. M. (2021). The teacher, the assessor, and the patient protector: A conceptual model describing how context interfaces with the supervisory roles of academic emergency physicians. *AEM Educ Train, 5*(1), 52–62. https://doi.org/10.1002/aet2.10431

Lockyer, J., Carraccio, C., Chan, M.-K., Hart, D., Smee, S., Touchie, C., Holmboe, E. S., & Frank, J. R. (2017). Core principles of assessment in competency-based medical education. *Med Teach, 39*(6), 609–616. https://doi.org/10.1080/0142159X.2017.1315082

Lockyer, L., Heathcote, E., & Dawson, S. (2013). Informing pedagogical action: aligning learning analytics with learning design. *Am Behav Sci, 57*(10), 1439–1459. https://doi.org/10.1177/0002764213479367

LoGiudice, A. B., Sibbald, M., Monteiro, S., Sherbino, J., Keuhl, A., Norman, G. R., & Chan, T. M. (2022). Intrinsic or invisible? An audit of CanMEDS roles in entrustable professional activities. Acad Med. https://doi.org/10.1097/ACM.0000000000004731

Ma, T. (2024). Considerations for implementation of a competency-based education program for preclerkship courses. In Schoenherr, J. R. & McConnell, M. M. (eds.) *Fundamentals and Frontiers in Medical Education and Decision-Making: Innovation, Implementation, and Translational Research*. Routledge.

Martinez-Maldonado, R., Gašević, D., Echeverria, V., Fernandez Nieto, G., Swiecki, Z., & Buckingham Shum, S. (2021). What do you mean by collaboration analytics? A conceptual model. *J Learn Anal, 8*(1), 126–153. https://doi.org/10.18608/jla.2021.7227

Marty, A. P., Linsenmeyer, M., George, B., Young, J. Q., Breckwoldt, J., & ten Cate, O. (2023). Mobile technologies to support workplace-based assessment for entrustment decisions: guidelines for programs and educators: AMEE Guide No. 154. *Med Teach*, 1–11. https://doi.org/10.1080/0142159X.2023.2168527

Miller, S., Caretta-Weyer, H., & Chan, T. (2022). Beyond competence: Rethinking continuing professional development in the age of competence-based medical education. *Can J Emerg Med, 24*(6), 563–565. https://doi.org/10.1007/s43678-022-00372-3

Oladokun, V. O., Adebanjo, A., & Charles-Owaba, O. E. (2008). Predicting students' academic performance using artificial neural network: a case study of an engineering course. *The Pacific Journal of Science & Technology, 9*(1), 72–79.

Ott, M. C., Pack, R., Cristancho, S., Chin, M., Van Koughnett, J. A., & Ott, M. (2022). "The Most Crushing Thing": Understanding resident assessment burden in a competency-based curriculum. *J Grad Med Educ, 14*(5), 583–592. https://doi.org/10.4300/JGME-D-22-00050.1

Peppler-Beechey, L., & Weingarten, H. P. (2021). Micro-credentials in the Applied Health Sciences: A Cautionary Tale about Quality (A Report from the School of Applied Health Sciences at the Michener Institute of Education at UHN for eCampusOntario, Issue.

Petosa, J. J., Jr., Martini, A., Klein, M., & Schumacher, D. (2021). Resident sensitive quality measures for general pediatrics: Alignment with existing care recommendations. *Acad Pediatr, 21*(6), 943–947. https://doi.org/10.1016/j.acap.2021.04.011

Prieto-Alvarez, C. G., Martinez-Maldonado, R., & Buckingham Shum, S. (2018). Mapping learner-data journeys. Proceedings of the 30th Australian Conference on Computer-Human Interaction.

Saqr, M., Fors, U., & Tedre, M. (2017). How learning analytics can early predict underachieving students in a blended medical education course. *Med Teach, 39*(7), 757–767. https://doi.org/10.1080/0142159X.2017.1309376

Schiff, K., Williams, D. J., Pardhan, A., Preyra, I., Li, S. A., & Chan, T. (2017). Resident development via progress testing and test-marking: An innovation and program evaluation. *Cureus, 9*(1), e992. https://doi.org/10.7759/cureus.992

Schoenherr, J. R., & Hamstra, S. J. (2016). Psychometrics and its discontents: An historical perspective on the discourse of the measurement tradition. *Adv Health Sci Educ Theory Pract, 21*(3), 719–729. https://doi.org/10.1007/s10459-015-9623-z

Schoenherr, J. R., & Hamstra, S. J. (2024). Validity in health professions education: From assessment instruments to program innovation and evaluation. In Schoenherr, J. R. & McConnell, M. M. (eds.) *Fundamentals and Frontiers in Medical Education and Decision-Making*. Routledge.

Schoenherr, J. R., Mahias-Ito, Y., & Li, X. Y. (2024). Collective competence and social learning in the health professions: Learning, thinking, and deciding in groups. In Schoenherr, J. R. (ed.), *Fundamentals and Frontiers in Medical Education and Decision-Making: Innovation, Implementation, and Translational Research*. Routledge.

Schoenherr, J. R., & Michael, K. (2024). AI-based technologies in the healthcare ecosystem: Applications in medical education and decision-making. In Schoenherr, J. R. (ed.), *Fundamentals and Frontiers in Medical Education and Decision-Making: Innovation, Implementation, and Translational Research*. Routledge.

Schumacher, D. J., Holmboe, E., Carraccio, C., Martini, A., van der Vleuten, C., Busari, J., Sobolewski, B., & Byczkowski, T. L. (2020). Resident-sensitive quality measures in the pediatric emergency department: Exploring relationships with supervisor entrustment and patient acuity and complexity. *Acad Med*, *95*(8), 1256–1264. https://doi.org/10.1097/acm.0000000000003242

Schumacher, D. J., Martini, A., Holmboe, E., Carraccio, C., van der Vleuten, C., Sobolewski, B., Busari, J., & Byczkowski, T. L. (2020). Initial implementation of resident-sensitive quality measures in the pediatric emergency department: A wide range of performance. *Acad Med*, *95*(8), 1248–1255. https://doi.org/10.1097/acm.0000000000003147

Schumacher, D. J., Martini, A., Holmboe, E., Varadarajan, K., Busari, J., van der Vleuten, C., & Carraccio, C. (2019). Developing resident-sensitive quality measures: Engaging stakeholders to inform next steps. *Acad Pediatr*, *19*(2), 177–185. https://doi.org/10.1016/j.acap.2018.09.013

Schumacher, D. J., Martini, A., Sobolewski, B., Carraccio, C., Holmboe, E., Busari, J., Poynter, S., van der Vleuten, C., & Lingard, L. (2020). Use of resident-sensitive quality measure data in entrustment decision making: A qualitative study of clinical competency committee members at one pediatric residency. *Acad Med*, *95*(11), 1726–1735. https://doi.org/10.1097/acm.0000000000003435

Sebok-Syer, S. S., Lingard, L., Panza, M., Van Hooren, T. A., & Rassbach, C. E. (2023). Supportive and collaborative interdependence: Distinguishing residents' contributions within health care teams. *Med Educ*. https://doi.org/10.1111/medu.15064

Sebok-Syer, S. S., Pack, R., Shepherd, L., McConnell, A., Dukelow, A. M., Sedran, R., & Lingard, L. (2020). Elucidating system-level interdependence in electronic health record data: What are the ramifications for trainee assessment? *Med Educ*, *54*(8), 738–747. https://doi.org/10.1111/medu.14147

Selwyn, N., & Gašević, D. (2020). The datafication of higher education: Discussing the promises and problems. *Teach High Educ*, *25*(4), 527–540. https://doi.org/10.1080/13562517.2019.1689388

Sherbino, J., Regehr, G., Dore, K., & Ginsburg, S. (2021). Tensions in describing competency-based medical education: A study of Canadian key opinion leaders. *Adv Health Sci Educ Theory Pract*, *26*(4), 1277–1289. https://doi.org/10.1007/s10459-021-10049-8

Smirnova, A., Chahine, S., Milani, C., Schuh, A., Sebok-Syer, S. S., Swartz, J. L., Wilhite, J. A., Kalet, A., Durning, S. J., Lombarts, K., van der Vleuten, C. P. M., & Schumacher, D. J. (2023). Using resident-sensitive quality measures derived from electronic health record data to assess residents' performance in pediatric emergency medicine. *Acad Med, 98*(3), 367–375. https://doi.org/10.1097/acm.0000000000005084

ten Cate, O., Carraccio, C., Damodaran, A., Gofton, W., Hamstra, S. J., Hart, D. E., Richardson, D., Ross, S., Schultz, K., Warm, E. J., Whelan, A. J., & Schumacher, D. J. (2021). Entrustment decision making: Extending Miller's Pyramid. *Acad Med, 96*(2), 199–204. https://doi.org/10.1097/ACM.0000000000003800

ten Cate, O., & Scheele, F. (2007). Competency-based postgraduate training: Can we bridge the gap between theory and clinical practice? *Acad Med, 82*(6), 542–547. https://doi.org/10.1097/ACM.0b013e31805559c7

ten Cate, O., & Schumacher, D. J. (2022). Entrustable professional activities versus competencies and skills: Exploring why different concepts are often conflated. *Adv Health Sci Educ Theory Pract, 27*(2), 491–499. https://doi.org/10.1007/s10459-022-10098-7

ten Cate, O., Schwartz, A., & Chen, H. C. (2020). Assessing trainees and making entrustment decisions: On the nature and use of entrustment-supervision scales. *Acad Med, 95*(11), 1662–1669. https://doi.org/10.1097/ACM.0000000000003427

Thai, K. P., Craig, S., Goodell, J., Lis, J., Schoenherr, J. R., & Kolodner, J. (2022). Learning Engineering Is Human-Centered. In (pp. 83–123). https://doi.org/10.4324/9781003276579-7

Thoma, B., Bandi, V., Carey, R., Mondal, D., Woods, R., Martin, L., & Chan, T. (2020). Developing a dashboard to meet Competence Committee needs: A design-based research project. *Can Med Educ J, 11*(1), e16–e34. https://doi.org/10.36834/cmej.68903

Thoma, B., Caretta-Weyer, H., Schumacher, D. J., Warm, E., Hall, A. K., Hamstra, S. J., Cavalcanti, R., & Chan, T. M. (2021). Becoming a deliberately developmental organization: Using competency based assessment data for organizational development. *Med Teach, 43*(7), 801–809. https://doi.org/https://doi.org/10.1080/0142159X.2021.1925100

Thoma, B., Ellaway, R. H., & Chan, T. M. (2021). From utopia through dystopia: Charting a course for learning analytics in competency-based medical education. *Acad Med, 96*(7S), 89–95. https://doi.org/https://doi.org/10.1097/ACM.0000000000004092

Thoma, B., Hall, A. K., Clark, K., Meshkat, N., Cheung, W. J., Desaulniers, P., Ffrench, C., Meiwald, A., Meyers, C., Patocka, C., Beatty, L., & Chan, T. M. (2020). Evaluation of a national competency-based assessment system in emergency medicine: A CanDREAM study. *J Grad Med Educ, 12*(4), 425–434. https://doi.org/10.4300/JGME-D-19-00803.1

Thoma, B., Monteiro, S., Pardhan, A., Waters, H., & Chan, T. (2022). Replacing high-stakes summative examinations with graduated medical licensure in Canada. *Can Med Assoc J (CMAJ), 194*(5), E168–E170. https://doi.org/https://doi.org/10.1503/cmaj.211816

Tolsgaard, M. G., Pusic, M. V., Sebok-Syer, S. S., Gin, B., Svendsen, M. B., Syer, M. D., Brydges, R., Cuddy, M. M., & Boscardin, C. K. (2023). The fundamentals of artificial intelligence in medical education research: AMEE guide no. 156. *Med Teach*, 1–9. https://doi.org/10.1080/0142159X.2023.2180340

Touchie, C., & ten Cate, O. (2016). The promise, perils, problems and progress of competency-based medical education. *Med Educ, 50*(1), 93–100. https://doi.org/10.1111/medu.12839

Van Melle, E., Frank, J. R., Holmboe, E. S., Dagnone, D., Stockley, D., Sherbino, J., & International Competency-based Medical Education, C. (2019). A core components framework for evaluating implementation of competency-based medical education programs. *Acad Med, 94*(7), 1002–1009. https://doi.org/10.1097/ACM.0000000000002743

Winkler-Schwartz, A., Bissonnette, V., Mirchi, N., Ponnudurai, N., Yilmaz, R., Ledwos, N., Siyar, S., Azarnoush, H., Karlik, B., & Del Maestro, R. F. (2019). Artificial intelligence in medical education: Best practices using machine learning to assess surgical expertise in virtual reality simulation. *J Surg Educ, 76*(6), 1681–1690. https://doi.org/10.1016/j.jsurg.2019.05.015

Witheridge, A., Ferns, G., & Scott-Smith, W. (2019). Revisiting Miller's pyramid in medical education: The gap between traditional assessment and diagnostic reasoning. *Int J Med Educ, 10*, 191–192. https://doi.org/10.5116/ijme.5d9b.0c37

Woods, R., Singh, S., Thoma, B., Patocka, C., Cheung, W., Monteiro, S., Chan, T. M., & Qu, A. L. V. c. (2022). Validity evidence for the quality of assessment for learning score: A quality metric for supervisor comments in competency based medical education. *Can Med Educ J, 13*(6), 19–35. https://doi.org/10.36834/cmej.74860

Yilmaz, Y., Carey, R., Chan, T. M., Bandi, V., Wang, S., Woods, R. A., Mondal, D., & Thoma, B. (2021). Developing a dashboard for faculty development in competency-based training programs: A design-based research project. *Can Med Educ J, 12*(4), 48–64. https://doi.org/10.36834/cmej.72067

Yilmaz, Y., Carey, R., Chan, T. M., Bandi, V., Wang, S., Woods, R. A., Mondal, D., & Thoma, B. (2022). Developing a dashboard for program evaluation in competency-based training programs: A design-based research project. *Can Med Educ J, 13*(5), 14–27. https://doi.org/10.36834/cmej.73554

Yilmaz, Y., Chan, M. K., Richardson, D., Atkinson, A., Bassilious, E., Snell, L., Chan, T. M., & Collaborators, I. (2023). Defining new roles and competencies for administrative staff and faculty in the age of competency-based medical education. *Med Teach, 45*(4), 395–403. https://doi.org/10.1080/0142159X.2022.2136517

Yilmaz, Y., Jurado Nunez, A., Ariaeinejad, A., Lee, M., Sherbino, J., & Chan, T. M. (2022). Harnessing natural language processing to support decisions around workplace-based assessment: Machine learning study of competency-based medical education. *JMIR Med Educ, 8*(2), e30537. https://doi.org/10.2196/30537

SECTION 2
Decision-Making

5

EMOTIONS AND CLINICAL DECISION-MAKING

Meghan M. McConnell

Introduction

Clinical reasoning is central to clinical practice. Clinical reasoning and decision-making encompass a range of cognitive processes required to observe, collect, and evaluate clinical information in order to generate differential diagnoses, initiate treatment plans, and organize necessary follow ups (Higgs, Jensen, Loftus, & Christensen, 2018; Schoenherr & McConnell, 2024). Much research has focused on understanding factors that influence clinical reasoning and decision-making, with the ultimate goal being to improve patient safety and reduce diagnostic errors (Bowes et al., 2020; Nendaz & Perrier, 2012; Norman & Eva, 2010). Such research has focused primarily on the cognitive processes involved in diagnostic reasoning, and other than a few exceptions (Estrada, Isen, & Young, 1997; Isbell, Bourdeaux, et al., 2020; Isbell, Tager, Beals, & Liu, 2020; Kozlowski et al., 2017; Liu, Chimowitz, & Isbell, 2022), the impact of emotions on clinical reasoning and decision-making has been largely overlooked. This is somewhat surprising given the affectively ladened nature of healthcare practices. Clinical decisions are frequently made in time-pressured, emotionally charged environments, and healthcare professionals are expected to manage their own and others' emotions throughout the medical care and treatment process (Kozlowski et al., 2017). It seems reasonable to expect emotions to influence clinical judgments. As Dr. Danielle Ofri writes,

> The emotional layers in medicine are far more nuanced and pervasive than we may like to believe. In fact, they can often be the dominant players in medical decision-making, handily overshadowing evidence-based

DOI: 10.4324/9781003316091-7

medicine, clinical algorithms, quality-control measures, even medical experience. And this can occur without anyone's conscious awareness.

(Ofri, 2013, p. 3)

The health professions community would benefit from a more thorough examination of the impact of emotions on clinical reasoning and decision-making.

Research within cognitive psychology has long acknowledged that emotions have a substantial impact on cognition and performance across a broad range of contexts. Emotion has been shown to influence cognitive processes such as perception, attention, learning, memory, judgment, reasoning, and problem-solving (for reviews, see Gasper & Spencer, 2018; Lemaire, 2022; Okon-Singer, Hendler, Pessoa, & Shackman, 2015; Pessoa, 2008). Understanding the relationship between cognition and emotion can provide new insights into clinical reasoning and decision-making and might ultimately improve the quality of patient care. The primary goal of this chapter is to use research within cognitive psychology to (a) highlight some of the theoretical approaches used to explain how emotions modulate cognition, (b) summarize cognitive research describing the interplay between emotions and various cognitive processes, and (c) describe recent research examining the influence of emotions on clinical reasoning and decision-making.

What Is an Emotion?

Perhaps due to the ubiquitous nature of emotions, there is substantial diversity in how emotions are defined and conceptualized across the various disciplines that study the phenomenon (Mulligan & Scherer, 2012). Much of this confusion is attributable to the semantic overlap of different affective constructs, such as *affect, emotion, mood,* and *feeling*. The use of inconsistent terminology creates ambiguity and confusion and reduces the quality, persuasiveness, and overall impact of a program of research (Ekkekakis, 2013).

In cognitive psychology, affect refers to a neurophysiological state that is interpreted as a simple, non-reflective experience (Russell, 2003). People are continuously in an affective state, although its nature and intensity vary over time. Affect is an umbrella term that encompasses a broad range of affective experiences, including temperament, attitude, emotion, and mood.

Of the affective constructs, moods and emotions are the most studied phenomena. Moods refer to low-intensity affective states that can last for hours, days, or weeks and are not associated with a specific object or event (Frijda, 2009). For this reason, the cause of a given mood might not be easily identifiable. A clinician might wake up in a frustrated mood, and this mood may subsequently impact the healthcare professional's judgment in clinical contexts.

While moods are characterized by a certain "diffuseness" – that is, they are not associated to a particular object or event (Frijda, 2009) – emotions are temporally linked to a specific event or moment, real or imagined, that can take place in the past, present, or future (Ekkekakis, 2013). Keltner and Gross (Keltner & Gross, 1999) defined emotions as "episodic, relatively short term, biologically based patterns of perception, experience, action, and communication that occur in response to specific physical and social challenges and opportunities" (p. 468). Examples of emotions include being proud about successfully diagnosing a difficult clinical problem, frustrated with a problematic, non-compliant patient, or nervous about performing an unfamiliar procedure. In most cases, emotions are accompanied by a variety of psychophysiological changes, such as behavioral responses (e.g., actions such as approach or avoidance), expressive reactions (e.g., facial and/or vocal expressions), physiological changes (e.g., neuronal or hormonal), and cognitive appraisals (e.g., subjective evaluations of the situation) (Frijda & Scherer, 2009).

Constructing Emotions: Scientific Taxonomies of Emotions

Given the wide range of moods and emotions, much debate has centered around how to best classify affective constructs (Hamann, 2012; Harmon-Jones, Harmon-Jones, & Summerell, 2017; Keltner, 2019). Researchers have proposed a variety of taxonomies to define the structure and function of affect, two of which are particularly relevant when examining the impact of moods and emotions on decision-making and reasoning.

Dimensional vs. Discrete Emotions

One major dispute in the literature concerns whether emotions are best conceptualized along shared dimensions or as discrete entities. Researchers espousing *dimensional approaches* argue that emotions comprise combinations of underlying dimensions. As an analogy, while individual labels can be applied to different colors, the spectrum of colors can be characterized using various dimensions, such as brightness, hue, and saturation (Fontaine, Scherer, Roesche, & Ellsworth, 2007). When applied to emotions, this approach maintains that seemingly distinct emotional labels can be ordered along a continuum of underlying dimensions. While there is some debate regarding the number of dimensions, most researchers agree that two fundamental dimensions characterize all emotions: valence (degree of pleasantness or unpleasantness) and arousal (strength or intensity) (Posner, Russell, & Peterson, 2005; Russell, 1980). According to this two-dimensional model, valence and arousal are orthogonal, bipolar dimensions that enable one to quantify different emotional states as a combination of these two dimensions. Emotions that are similar to one another (e.g., terror, fear) represent similar levels of valence and arousal, while those that are dissimilar to one another (e.g., excited, depressed) represent different levels of valence and/or arousal.

Some researchers argue that too much information is lost by trying to identify a set of underlying dimensions that transcend affective categories (Remington, Fabrigar, & Visser, 2000). Consequently, a growing number of researchers have endorsed a *discrete states approach*, which argues that each emotion is associated with unique behavioral and cognitive manifestations, somatic and visceral symptoms, expressive behaviors (e.g., facial, postural, vocal expressions), coping responses, and so forth (Fontaine et al., 2007; Siemer, Mauss, & Gross, 2007). For example, anxiety is triggered by the presence of "uncertain, existential threat" (R. Lazarus, 1991) and is associated with unique attention- and action-related biases, such as limited attention to peripheral details and avoidance strategies (Berman, Wheaton, McGrath, & Abramowitz, 2010; Eysenck, Derakshan, Santos, & Calvo, 2007), specific physiological symptoms, such as increases in respiratory rate, heart rate, and cardiovascular output (Kreibig, 2010; Levenson, 2009), and tense facial, postural, and vocal expressions (Banse & Scherer, 1996). Indeed, a discrete state account can also accommodate cross-cultural studies that have argued for cultural-specific emotions (Mesquita, De Leersnyder, & Boiger, 2016; Russell, 1991).

Incidental vs. Integral Emotions

Healthcare professions must often move rapidly between different contexts. By shifting from one situation to another, cognitive and emotional processes that were active in one situation might be carried over into another. When studying the impact of emotions on clinical decision-making, it is important to differentiate between incidental and integral emotions (Blanchette & Richards, 2010; Ferrer & Ellis, 2021; Västfjäll et al., 2016). *Incidental* emotions are affective states that arise from factors that are unrelated to the task at hand. For example, a physician might arrive at the clinic feeling frustrated after another driver cut her off on her way to work. *Integral* emotions, on the other hand, are those that arise directly from the task itself, such as feeling frustrated when interacting with a confrontational patient. An accumulating body of research suggests that the impact of emotions on various cognitive processes depends on whether the emotion is related (i.e., integral) or unrelated (i.e., incidental) to the task (Ferrer & Ellis, 2021; Västfjäll et al., 2016). In a review of the literature on the relationship between stress and clinical performance, LeBlanc (2009) argued that when a clinician's stress is integrally related to the task being performed (e.g., resuscitating a patient), attention will be focused toward the task itself, and performance might be enhanced. Alternatively, when the source of stress is incidental to the task (e.g., loud noises, disruptive team members), attention will be directed away from the task and toward the source of the stress, which will have detrimental effects on performance. Differentiating between incidental and integral affect can help explain why emotions can be both detrimental and beneficial, depending on the source of the emotion.

Theoretical Approaches

Researchers have developed a host of theoretical frameworks to explain the interplay between emotions and cognition. One such framework is the affect-as-information (AAI) model (Clore et al., 2001; Storbeck & Clore, 2008; Zadra & Clore, 2011). According to the AAI model, affect provides information about the overall value (e.g., pleasant vs. unpleasant, desirable vs. undesirable) and importance (e.g., urgent vs. not urgent, important vs. unimportant) of a situation; this information then guides subsequent thought processes and behaviors. Proponents of AAI approach argue that negative emotions signal that a situation is problematic, and as a result, individuals are more inclined to process information in a careful, systematic manner to solve the problem. In contrast, positive emotions signal that the situation is safe and benign and facilitates reliance on dominant, accessible processing styles, which have served them well in the past (Isbell, Lair, & Rovenpor, 2013). For example, consider a physician treating a critically injured child. In such a case, feelings of anxiety signify that the stakes are high, that the child's well-being is at risk, and that time is of the essence (LeBlanc, McConnell, & Monteiro, 2015). The AAI model argues that emotions influence decision-making and reasoning by prioritizing certain information and problem-solving strategies within the clinical environment.

Another common framework used to explore the relationship between cognition and emotion is the appraisal tendency framework (ATF; Lerner & Keltner, 2000). The key assumption of ATF is that emotions are adaptive reactions based on how individuals interpret, or *appraise*, a given event or situation (Moors, Ellsworth, & Fridja, 2013). Appraisal theorists argue that emotions are not triggered by the situation, *per se*, but arise from an individual's interpretation and appraisal of the situation (Stein & Hernandex, 2007). For this reason, the same situation can produce different emotions in different people based on their appraisal of the situation. For example, consider a scenario where a pediatrician is treating an infant, while dealing with a difficult mother who is constantly questioning the doctor's competence. According to ATF, the physician's emotions will depend on how he interprets the situation. He might feel angry if he interprets the mothers' behavior as unfair and ultimately obstructing his ability to treat the child. Or he might feel compassion if he believes that the mother is afraid and worried for her child's well-being. Appraisals are important in clinical settings because they mediate the impact of situational factors and can be targeted by interventions intended to improve clinical decision-making.

Emotion and Cognition

Emotions impact a wide range of cognitive processes necessary for clinical decision-making and reasoning. The following section summarizes relevant empirical findings on the impact of emotions on what we attend to, what we remember, and how we make decisions and reason about the world around us.

Attention. Human beings are presented with an endless stream of information from their environment, and only a subset of this information is relevant at any given moment. Performing complex tasks requires individuals to monitor, detect, and process useful information and inhibit irrelevant or distracting information (Carretié, 2014). Attention is critical for all these cognitive processes. A wealth of literature has shown that emotions impact a variety of attentional processes, such as selective attention and the breadth of attention.

Selective attention. Selective attention has been described as a spotlight that illuminates specific features of the environment, ensuring prioritized processing of these features. There is abundant evidence that emotions strongly influence selective attention, whereby people pay more attention to emotional relative to non-emotional stimuli (for reviews, see Carretié, 2014; Yiend, 2010). This prioritization of attentional resources can facilitate or impair performance, depending on whether the emotional content is relevant to the task at hand. When emotional content is relevant to task (e.g., identifying emotional stimuli from an array), emotions can improve attention and subsequent task performance (Anderson, 2005; Keil & Ihssen, 2004). On the other hand, emotions can disrupt performance when the emotional content is not relevant to the task. In such instances, emotional content captures and sustains our attention. Additional attentional resources must be deployed to inhibit the processing of emotional (i.e., irrelevant) information, and as a result, task performance is hindered (Dresler, Meriau, Heekeren, & van der Meer, 2009; Sebastian, McCrory, De Brito, & Viding, 2017). Therefore, whether emotion hinders or facilitates performance depends on whether the task requires focusing attention on emotional or non-emotional content.

In addition to being impacted by the emotional content in the environment, selective attention is also influenced by internal emotions and moods (Becker & Leinenger, 2011). Internal affective states have been shown to direct attention toward specific types of information in our environment. For example, individuals in negative affective states, such as anxiety, fear, and worry, are more likely to pay attention to negative or threatening stimuli compared to neutral or positive stimuli (Macatee, Albanese, Schmidt, & Cougle, 2017; Sänger et al., 2014). Similarly, when in positive affective states, people are more likely to focus on rewarding or positive stimuli (Pool, Brosch, Delplanque, & Sander, 2016; Tamir & Robinson, 2007). These findings demonstrate that temporary moods and emotions can influence attentional processing, such that attention is biased toward stimuli that are congruent with an individual's current affective state.

This selective processing of emotional content might impact clinical reasoning and decision-making by biasing attention on certain clinical features, and away from others. Research has shown that doctors attach importance to different information and gather different information when diagnosing a patient, and as a result, different doctors make different decisions about the same patient (Kostopoulou & Wildman, 2004). While a variety of individual, institutional, and environmental factors have been identified to explain, and ideally reduce, variability in medical decision-making, the influence of emotions as a potential contributor of this variability has been largely overlooked. More research is needed to examine if, and to what extent, emotions impact how clinicians select and process clinical information during the treatment process.

Scope of attention. Emotions not only influence what people attend to but also modulate the scope of attention. More specifically, emotions are capable of broadening or narrowing the attentional spotlight. Individuals in positive moods have a broader attentional focus, meaning they are more likely to focus on information at the global level and view the scene as a whole; individuals in negative moods have a more narrow attentional focus, resulting in their attention being focused on individual details of the scene (Huntsinger, 2013). The influence of emotions on the scope of attention has been studied using interference paradigms such as the flanker task (Eriksen, 1995). In such studies, participants are required to identify a centrally presented target that is surrounded by distractors that are either congruent (e.g., FFF) or incongruent (e.g., FTF) with the target. Generally speaking, individuals in positive moods are slower to identify targets that are surrounded by incongruent distractors, compared to individuals in negative moods (Rowe, Hirsh, & Anderson, 2007; Wadlinger & Isaacowitz, 2006; Wegbreit, Franconeri, & Beeman, 2015). This slowed response time to incongruent versus congruent trials (e.g., "flanker interference") is attributed to the broadened scope of attention associated with positive affective states. This increase in attentional scope facilitates processing of irrelevant flanking distractors, thereby impairing performance. In contrast, individuals in negative moods have a narrowed scope of attention, which allows them to focus on the target and pay less attention to the distracting flankers.

The impact of emotions on the scope of attention might impact clinical reasoning and decision-making by regulating the types of information that are attended to in clinical settings. For example, in a recent study examining failures to identify and respond to clinical deterioration, Jones and Johnstone (2017) describe a case where a patient presented with postoperative hypotension following a laparoscopic cholecystectomy. Both the nurse and anesthetist recognized and treated the hypotension but failed to recognize that the hypotension was unusual following a laparoscopic procedure. Shortly after being transferred to the ward, the patient had a hypotensive cardiac arrest, and it was subsequently determined that the cause of the hypotension was internal bleeding. The staff's failure to attribute the patient's hypotension as a sign of clinical deterioration was thought to occur because the staff "focused on the individual signs at the expense of thinking about the 'big picture' and why the patient was hypotensive" (p. 222). It is possible that negative emotions experienced by members of the healthcare team might have contributed to their inattention to the patient's clinical deterioration, although this was outside the scope of this study. Future research is needed to examine whether the relationship between emotions and the scope of attention impacts clinical reasoning and decision-making.

Memory. Moods and emotions also have a substantial impact on what we remember. Converging evidence from cognition and neuroimaging studies shows that emotional events are remembered disproportionately better than non-emotional events, a phenomenon referred to as *emotional memory enhancement* (Kensinger & Schacter, 2016; Levine & Pizarro, 2005). Moreover, when comparing memory for positive and negative experiences, negative information is more likely to be remembered, and with greater detail, than positive information (Kensinger, 2009; Mickley Steinmetz, Addis, & Kensinger, 2010; Williamson et al., 2019). While the cognitive mechanisms behind the memorial advantage for negative emotions are still debated in the literature, the effect has been replicated across a variety of different stimuli and domains, suggesting that (Alves, Koch, & Unkelbach, 2017; Bowen, Kark, & Kensinger, 2018; Lazarus, 2021).

While emotional events, particularly negative ones, tend to be remembered better than neutral events, emotions do not enhance memory for all aspects of a scene but rather produce selective memory benefits. Specifically, emotions are associated with *memory narrowing effects*, whereby memory is enhanced for central or core features of an emotional event (e.g., details central to the appearance or meaning of the emotional stimuli) and impaired for peripheral or background features (for review, see Kensinger, 2009; Levine & Edelstein, 2009). Memory narrowing has been demonstrated across a range of studies using both simple emotional stimuli (Kensinger, Garoff-Eaton, & Schacter, 2007; MacKay & Ahmetzanov, 2005) and more complex simulated or real-world settings (Alexander et al., 2005; Congleton & Berntsen, 2020; Sotgiu & Galati, 2007). The detrimental effect of emotion on memory for peripheral details has been attributed to attentional mechanisms. Because attention is automatically directed toward emotional information, such information receives prioritized processing, which leaves fewer cognitive resources available to process peripheral details. Emotional content "benefits from privileged processing, resulting in the typical pattern of enhanced memory for core features of emotional events and poorer memory for peripheral features" (Levine & Edelstein, 2009, p. 844).

Interestingly, not all studies show memory narrowing effects. For example, Laney et al. (2004) had participants listen to a story about either a date rape (emotional story) or a successful first date (neutral story) and then tested participants memories for the stories. No evidence of memory narrowing was found for the emotional stories. Rather, participants who listened to the emotional story had better memory for both central and peripheral details relative to those who heard the neutral story. Other studies have found that emotions can actually impair memory for information that could be considered central (Morgan et al., 2004; Morgan et al., 2013). For instance, Morgan et al. (Morgan et al., 2004) assessed memory in over 500 military personnel who underwent interrogation as part of a military survival training program. Researchers interviewed participants and found that soldiers who were exposed to extremely stressful interrogation tactics (e.g., food and sleep deprivation, physical confrontation) were less likely to recognize their interrogator compared to soldiers who underwent a less stressful interrogation. These findings indicate that emotions do not always enhance memory for central details. Practitioners and educators must be mindful of these results. For example, learners who are exposed to excessive negative environment (e.g., yelling, time-pressure) during a clinical simulation in an attempt to replicate a real-world scenario may not retain specific details of the scenario, thereby impairing learning.

Observations that emotions can either enhance or disrupt memory for central details raise the question of what determines whether a given detail should be classified as central or peripheral. Levine and Pizzaro (2005) argue that the types of information that are considered central will vary across different emotional states. Building on the ATF of emotions, these researchers argue that different emotions will trigger selective encoding and retrieval of motivationally relevant information. For example, if fear motivates people to avoid threats, frightened people will selectively remember information associated with threats and ways of avoiding them. If anger motivates people to overcome obstacles to their goals, angry people will selectively remember information associated with goals and the objects obstructing the achievement of such goals. Therefore, a frightened person will have better memory for sources of threats and means of avoiding them, while an angry person will have better memory for objects obstructing their goals and means of removing them. The motivations associated with discrete emotions might play an important role in determining what types of information are more likely to be remembered.

While the research discussed so far has provided convincing evidence that emotional events, especially negative ones, are associated with enhanced memory compared to non-emotional events, it is important to acknowledge that emotional memories are fallible. There is empirical evidence that memories for emotional events are susceptible to distortion. For example, memories for positive experiences are associated with a greater number of inconsistencies and memory errors, despite the fact that people are more confident in the accuracy of their positive memories relative to negative ones (Bohn & Berntsen, 2007; Levine & Bluck, 2004). Furthermore, acute stress has been shown to impair various memory processes (Kuhlmann, Piel, & Wolf, 2005; Morgan et al., 2006; Oei et al., 2006; Talmi, Lohnas, & Daw, 2019). Kuhlmann et al. (2005) found that individuals who were exposed to an acute stressor prior to learning had poorer memory for materials than those who were not exposed to a stressor. Lastly, emotion can impair memory when people engage in emotional regulation strategies (Bonanno et al., 2004; Raes, Hermans, Williams, & Eelen, 2006; Richards & Gross, 2006). For example, memory for emotional experiences is impaired when individuals suppress behavioral displays of emotion, relative to those who did not attempt to regulate their emotions (Bonanno et al., 2004). This finding might be particularly relevant in clinical contexts, where healthcare professionals are expected to control their emotions during their interactions with patients and colleagues. The tendency for clinicians to regulate, and at times even stifle or ignore, their emotions requires a substantial proportion of their mental resources, and as a result, fewer cognitive resources are available to solve the problem, and clinical performance is impaired.

Judgment, Decision-Making, and Reasoning. High-level cognitive abilities include judgment, decision-making, and reasoning (metacognition and communication are covered elsewhere, see Gago et al., this 2024; Schoenherr & Le-Bouar, 2024; Schoenherr et al., 2024). Historically, researchers focused on rational, deliberate, reason-based processes underlying these higher order cognitive abilities. This approach assumes that moods and emotions interfere with judgment, decision-making, and reasoning. During the past three decades, a growing body of literature has illustrated that moods and emotions exert wide-ranging influences on judgment, decision-making, and reasoning (for reviews, see Angie, Connelly, Waples, & Kligyte, 2011; Blanchette & Richards, 2010; George & Dane, 2016; Lerner, Li, Valdesolo, & Kassam, 2015), which additionally highlight the integral nature of emotions to decision-making (e.g., Damasio, 1994).

Judgment. Judgment is the ability to infer, estimate, and predict events (Hastie & Dawes, 2009). Individuals in positive moods tend to overestimate the likelihood of positive events relative to individuals in negative moods, while those in negative moods overestimate the likelihood of negative events. In a seminal study, Wright and Bower (1992) found that happy participants judged positive events to be more likely and negative events to be less likely, while sad participants judged negative events as more likely and positive events as less likely, relative to participants in a control condition. Such mood congruence effects on likelihood estimates have been documented in both laboratory (Bhanji & Beer, 2012; Maner & Gerend, 2007; Quraishi & Oaksford, 2013; Wright & Bower, 1992) and real-world contexts (Cohen-Charash, Scherbaum, Kammeyer-Mueller, & Staw, 2013; Danvers, Hu, & O'Neil, 2018).

Complementary findings have been found regarding the influence of emotions on individuals' perception of risk, whereby people in negative moods are more likely to judge events as being risker than people in positive moods (Hogarth, Portell, Cuxart, & Kolev, 2011; Slovic & Peters, 2006; Tompkins, Bjälkebring, & Peters, 2018). For example, Hu et al. (2013) induced positive, negative, and neutral moods and then had participants rate the probability of different types of traffic accidents. The results showed that individuals in negative moods believed they were more likely to be involved in traffic accidents (e.g., greater risk perception) than those in positive or neutral moods. Such findings suggest that people in negative moods will judge the same event as being riskier than people in positive moods.

Interestingly, not all negative emotions appear to have the same effects on judgments of risk. For example, fear and anger can differentially impact risk perceptions (Angie et al., 2011; Jeon, Yim, & Walker, 2011; Lu, Xie, & Zhang, 2013; She, Eimontaite, Zhang, & Sun, 2017). Across a series of studies, Lerner and collaborators (Fischhoff, Gonzalez, Lerner, & Small, 2005; Lerner, Gonzalez, Small, & Fischhoff, 2003) examined how fear and anger affected perceived risks of terrorism following the September 11 terrorist attacks (from a few days to a year later). Participants were induced to feel either fear or anger and were then asked to estimate risks related to future terrorist attacks. The study showed that fear and anger had opposite effects on risk perceptions – fearful participants reported greater risk estimates than did angry participants, who reported lower risk estimates. These findings illustrate that specific negative emotions can have divergent effects on risk estimates, suggesting it is important to consider discrete emotions, as opposed to more global dimensions, when examining the relationship between affect and risk perception.

Together, these findings suggest that clinicians' affective states may influence their judgments about a patient's susceptibility to (or risk of) a given disease, as well as the probability that the patient may benefit from interventions. Such perceptions of risk could have significant implications for the use of preventative health services and highlight the importance of considering the influence of affective states on practitioners' perceptions and estimates of risk factors when making clinical judgments, as well as patients' responses to the recommendations of healthcare professionals.

Decision-making. While studies on judgment examine how people estimate the likelihood of different events, research on decision-making investigates how people choose among these different options (Blanchette & Richards, 2010). Early research adopted a valence-based approach, focusing on the impact of negative and/or positive emotional states on decision-making. This valence-based perspective suggests that people tend to make less risky decisions when they are in positive moods than when they are in negative moods (Chuang & Kung, 2005; Isen & Geva, 1987; Isen, Nygren, & Ashby, 1988). However, several researchers have criticized these valence-based approaches, arguing that it is important to distinguish between specific emotions when examining the impact of emotions on decision-making and risk-taking (DeSteno, Petty, Wegner, & Rucker, 2000; Raghunathan & Pham, 1999; Yang, Zhou, Gu, & Wu, 2020). This perspective is based on findings that discrete emotions within the same valence can have contrasting effects on decision-making (Raghunathan & Pham, 1999; Yang et al., 2018, 2020). For example, Ragunathan and Phan (1999) compared risk preferences among participants who were induced into sad, anxious, or neutral affective states. Following the mood induction, participants were asked to choose between two jobs, one with a high salary but low job security (riskier option) and another with an average salary but high job security (safer option). The results revealed that sad individuals were more likely to select the risker option, while anxious individuals selected the safer option. More recently, Yang et al. (2020) induced anger, fear, and happiness and had participants choose between two gambling options, where there was a tradeoff between risk and reward. Fearful participants made fewer risky decisions than angry or happy participants, while there was no difference in risk preferences between angry and happy individuals. Such findings suggest that affective valence in and of itself cannot fully explain the complex relationship between emotions and decision-making, as same-valence emotions can impact decision-making in different ways.

The relationship between affective states and risk-taking has implications for clinical reasoning and decision-making. Consider a situation where a physician needs to decide between two treatment options: one "safer" option that presents fewer risks to the patient but also leads to less optimal care and one "risky" option that presents significant risks to a patient but also has a greater possibility of resolving the clinical problem at hand. Based on the findings described above, the emotion of the physician could impact which option is chosen – an anxious physician would be more likely to select the safer option, while an angry physician would be more likely to choose the riskier option. More research is needed to understand how emotions shape clinical decisions and if (and when) they are beneficial or harmful to patient care.

In addition to influencing decision-making and risk-taking, affective states also influence the types of strategies individuals use to make decisions. More specifically, emotions modulate decision-making strategies by influencing how deeply individuals process information (for review, see Huntsinger, Isbell, & Clore, 2014; Huntsinger & Ray, 2016). People in positive affective states are more likely to engage in top-down, abstract, heuristic processing styles when making decisions, while people in negative states are more likely to use bottom-up, detailed-oriented, analytic processing styles. These different processing styles can impact how individuals make decisions. For example, relative to negative or neutral affective states, individuals in positive moods are more likely to use stereotypes when forming judgments and making decisions about others (Bodenhausen, 1993; Curtis, 2013). Conversely, people in negative moods are more likely to use systematic processing strategies when making decisions, processing information in a careful, detail-oriented manner (Li et al., 2022; Li et al., 2020; Moons & Mackie, 2007).

This tendency to adopt more top-down, heuristic processing strategies while in positive moods has been associated with greater propensity for cognitive errors. For example, individuals in positive moods are less likely to rely on logical decision rules when making decisions compared to those in negative moods (de Vries et al., 2012). Positive moods are also associated with increased susceptibility to weak persuasive arguments relative to negative moods (Burger & Bless, 2016; Griskevicius, Shiota, & Neufeld, 2010; Hullett, 2005). For example, people in positive mood are persuaded more by superficial features of an argument as opposed to quality; those in negative moods are persuaded more by the quality of argument and are more persuaded by strong as opposed to weak arguments (Hullett, 2005; DM Mackie & Worth, 1989). The extent to which such findings generalize to clinical errors is unknown. More research is needed to examine the role of physicians' emotions on diagnostic errors, as refining our understanding of this relationship will help improve diagnostic performance and patient safety.

While positive moods have been associated with greater cognitive errors, this is not to say that positive affective states do not have any beneficial effects on decision-making. There has been a wealth of research showing that relative to negative affective states, positive states are associated with greater cognitive flexibility, the "ability to organize ideas in multiple ways and to access alternative cognitive perspectives" (Ashby, Isen, & Turken, 1999, p 530; for reviews, see Bolte & Goschke, 2010; Isen, 2008). As a result of this increased cognitive flexibility, people experiencing positive emotions are more likely to think of alternative strategies and solutions (De Dreu, Baas, & Nijstad, 2008; Gasper, 2003), consider multiple sources of information (Dreisbach & Goschke, 2004; Lin, Tsai, Lin, & Chen, 2014), be more open to information (Djamasbi, 2007), and explore new ideas (Fredrickson, 2003; Fredrickson & Branigan, 2005) relative to those experiencing negative affective states. Positive affect has also been associated with increased creativity and problem-solving (Chen, Hu, & Plucker, 2016; Davis, 2009). Together, these findings suggest that positive affect might enhance clinical reasoning and decision-making by facilitating integration of clinical information, promoting the consideration of alternative diagnoses, and allowing for more creative solutions to clinical problems.

Reasoning. Reasoning is the process of constructing arguments to justify conclusions (Ball & Thompson, 2018). Early research has shown that emotions have deleterious effects on reasoning skills (for review, see Clore, 2011; Pham, 2007). For example, Oaksford et al. (1996) induced either positive, negative, or neutral moods and then had participants complete a deductive reasoning task. The results showed that participants in positive and negative moods had poorer performance on the reasoning task relative to those in neutral moods. These effects have since been replicated using a variety of reasoning tasks (Causse et al., 2012; Cianci & Bierstaker, 2009; Oaksford, Carlile, & Moore, 2004), illustrating that both positive and negative affective states can impair reasoning. Similar effects have been found when examining the impact of emotional materials on reasoning skills. Across different reasoning tasks, individuals are less likely to draw valid inferences and are more prone to logical errors when reasoning about emotional content compared to non-emotional content (Blanchette & Leese, 2010; Blanchette & Richards, 2004). Together, these findings indicate that both experimentally induced affective states and emotional materials can deleteriously impact reasoning skills.

Not all studies, however, have found that emotions impair reasoning abilities. Several studies have shown that emotions improve reasoning in circumstances where emotional contents are personally relevant to individuals (Blanchette & Campbell, 2012; Blanchette, Gavigan, & Johnston, 2014; Blanchette, Richards, Melnyk, & Lavda, 2007; Caparos & Blanchette, 2017). For example, following the 2005 terrorist attacks in London, Blanchette et al. (2007) examined whether emotions related to the bombings impacted individuals' reasoning skills for content related to the attacks. They found that participants from London, UK provided more correct responses on a reasoning task containing terrorist-related content compared to participants from Canada. Similar effects have been found with victims of sexual abuse, who reasoned more logically about topics related to sexual abuse (Caparos & Blanchette, 2017), and war veterans, who showed superior reasoning about combat-related contents (Blanchette & Campbell, 2012). Such findings illustrate that emotional content that is personally relevant to an individual can enhance reasoning skills.

Reasoning within clinical contexts inevitably involves a range of emotions, which can arise from within the physician (e.g., anxiety over a challenging clinical case or sadness over a patient's deterioration) and from external sources (e.g., troublesome behaviors from patients or colleagues). The question that needs to be addressed, then, is what makes an emotion relevant to a given clinical reasoning task. One could argue that emotions linked to key features of a clinical presentation will facilitate diagnostic reasoning. For example, a physician's frustration in response to an agitated and disruptive elderly patient may facilitate identification of a urinary tract infection as the presumption cause of the patient's disruptive behavior. However, even if such emotions are relevant to the clinical diagnosis, physicians traditionally do not pay much attention to their emotions and often believe that they must suppress their emotions to provide optimal care to their patients. This emotional suppression might inevitably lead to all emotional states and content being interpreted as being irrelevant to the clinical task, thereby impeding diagnostic performance.

Emotion and Clinical Decision-Making

The extensive literature reviewed here clearly illustrates that emotions influence a variety of cognitive processes, including attention, memory, judgment, decision-making, and reasoning. Building on these findings, researchers have started to acknowledge that healthcare providers' emotions can impact clinical decision-making and reasoning. Healthcare professionals and educators must ensure that they account for these influences in their practice.

Stress is arguably the most studied negative affective state in healthcare. This is not surprising given that clinicians face myriad stressors in their work environment. Stress has been shown to impair clinical performance across a range of healthcare professionals, settings, and clinical tasks (Groombridge, Kim, Maini, & Fitzgerald, 2019; LeBlanc et al., 2005; LeBlanc, Regehr, Shlonsky, & Bogo, 2012; Piquette et al., 2014; Williams, Manwell, Konrad, & Linzer, 2007). For example, paramedics' drug dose calculations have been shown to be less accurate during high-stress scenarios relative to low-stress scenarios (LeBlanc et al., 2005). Within medicine, feelings of stress have been linked to self-reported suboptimal clinical care and medical errors (Williams et al., 2007). Stress is thought to impair clinical reasoning by narrowing individuals' information processing scope. Pottier et al. (2013) randomly assigned senior medical students to either a high-stress or low-stress simulated ambulatory consultation and assessed students' decision-making and communication skills. While stress did not have an impact on students' diagnostic accuracy or communication skills, students in the high-stress condition were less likely

Meghan M. McConnell

to report signs of differential diagnosis. The authors suggested that stress might restrict individuals' reasoning scope when establishing a differential diagnosis, consequently leading to premature closure – the tendency to stop considering other alternatives after the initial diagnosis is made.

Stress has also been shown to influence healthcare professionals' assessments of risk. In a study examining the effects of stress on child protection workers' assessment of children at risk of abuse and neglect, researchers presented workers with two simulated scenarios – one non-confrontational and one confrontational – and asked them to conduct a 15-minute interview with a mother who was played by a specially trained actor. Child protection workers had greater stress responses during confrontational scenarios and rated the overall risk to the child as being greater in the confrontational than non-confrontational scenarios (LeBlanc et al., 2012).

One way that negative affect impacts diagnostic processes is by reducing the quality of physician-patient interactions. For example, Kushnir, Kushnir, Sarel, Cohen (2011) found that when in negative moods, family physicians reported spending less time talking to their patients, prescribing more medications, ordering more laboratory and diagnostic tests, and making more referrals to specialists. The opposite was true for positive moods – respondents believed they talked more, prescribed fewer medications, and made fewer referrals for tests and specialists. These findings suggest that negative moods can impact diagnostic behaviors, which subsequently affects the quality of physician-patient interactions.

During doctor-patient interactions, there are times that the patients themselves elicit strong emotions in healthcare providers. A number of studies have shown that some patients are more likely than others to evoke strong emotional responses in healthcare providers, such as demanding, disrespectful, or demeaning patients, those who are aggressive or arrogant toward the provider, those with unrealistic expectations, non-compliant patients or those who ignore the practitioner's advice, and patients with either difficult-to-diagnose or mental health problems (Jackson & Kroenke, 1999; Sharpe et al., 1994; Smith & Zimny, 1988). A small body of literature has shown that clinicians' emotional responses to these patients can negatively impact diagnostic decisions (Isbell, Bourdeaux, et al., 2020; Isbell, Tager, et al., 2020; Mamede et al., 2017; Schmidt et al., 2017). A recent qualitative study explored emotional experiences of emergency department physicians and nurses and the perceived effects of these emotions on clinical decision-making and patient safety (Isbell, Bourdeaux, et al., 2020). The majority of providers interviewed believed that negative emotions, particularly frustration and anger, adversely impacted patient care. For example, providers reported spending less time with patients who elicited negative emotions and ordering tests that allowed for quicker discharge to minimize time with patients who elicited negative emotions. Some providers acknowledged that this decrease in face time could result in suboptimal care and may increase the likelihood of diagnostic errors.

Other research has examined the influence of difficult patient behaviors on diagnostic accuracy (Mamede et al., 2017; Schmidt et al., 2017). For example, Mamede et al. (2017) presented internal medicine residents with eight clinical vignettes, half of which described "difficult" patients and the other half described "neutral" patients. After reading each vignette, residents were asked to provide a diagnosis and to recall the patient's clinical findings and behaviors. When diagnosing difficult patients, residents made more diagnostic errors, recalled fewer clinical findings, and recollected more patient behaviors compared to diagnosing neutral patient vignettes. The authors argued that difficult patients induced negative emotions in healthcare providers, and as a result, providers must divert cognitive resources to process these behaviors, which impedes processing of clinical findings and reduces diagnostic accuracy.

Working in multidisciplinary clinical teams can also elicit emotions that can affect clinical decision-making and reasoning. Several studies have shown that teams characterized by rudeness or incivility can adversely impact both individual and collective clinical judgments (Johnson et al., 2020; Riskin et al., 2015, 2017). For example, using a simulation-based randomized controlled study, Riskin et al. (2015) examined the impact of colleague-based rudeness on patient outcomes in a neonatal intensive care unit context. The study found that exposure to rudeness negatively impacted diagnostic accuracy and clinical performance of individual team members. Rudeness also negatively affected information-sharing and help-seeking behaviors, suggesting that rudeness can detrimentally influence team-level processes (Riskin et al., 2015). A follow-up study confirmed these findings, demonstrating that rudeness not only disrupted diagnostic performance of individual team members but also had adverse effects on team dynamics (e.g., information and workload sharing, helping behaviors, and communication) (Riskin et al., 2017). These findings illustrate that the deleterious effects of negative emotions are not limited to individual healthcare professionals but also extend to team performance.

While studies show that negative affect can hinder clinical performance, research suggests that positive affect can facilitate clinical reasoning and decision-making (Crane et al., 2017; Estrada et al., 1997; Isen, Rosenzweig, & Young, 1991). For example, Isen et al. (1991) examined the impact of positive affect on diagnostic reasoning in third year medical students. After being induced into a positive or neutral mood state, students were presented with six hypothetical patients and were asked to decide which patient was most likely to have lung cancer. Participants were asked to verbalize their clinical reasoning as they assessed the patients. While the positive and neutral emotion groups did not differ in their diagnostic accuracy, participants in the positive affect group made their decisions more quickly than those in the neutral group. Furthermore, relative to the control group, those in positive affective states were more likely to go beyond the task at hand and considered potential diagnoses of the other hypothetical patients. Positive moods were also associated with greater integration of information from different diagnostic dimensions (e.g., age, occupation, smoking status), which the authors interpreted as being indicative of more holistic and integrative styles of problem-solving. In a subsequent study, Estrada et al. (1997) used a similar procedure to investigate the influence of positive moods on diagnostic reasoning among practicing physicians. Following a mood induction, internists were provided with a written vignette describing a 45-year-old woman who presented with a six-month history of arthralgias, fatigue, dark urine, and "red spots" on both legs, along with additional clinical information (e.g., laboratory results and medical history). Physicians were asked to verbalize their reasoning as they diagnosed the patient (with chronic active hepatitis). The results showed that physicians in positive moods considered liver disease as a potential diagnosis earlier than those in neutral moods. The authors suggested that positive affect facilitated processing of clinical information, which consequently improved diagnostic reasoning. Furthermore, compared to the neutral group, those in the positive affect group showed less evidence of anchoring (e.g., ignoring or discounting of non-supportive or disconfirming evidence) in their reasoning, suggesting that emotions modulate not only the integration of information but also the ability to adjust one's hypothesis based on disconfirming evidence. Together, the results of these studies suggest that positive moods are associated with a more flexible processing style, allowing practitioners to consider multiple sources of information when formulating a diagnosis or generating a clinical judgment.

Building on these findings, a recent simulation-based study examined the relationship between positive and negative affect and fixation errors among practicing anesthetists (Crane et al., 2017). Fixation errors occur when a provider focuses on a single aspect of a case and excludes other more relevant aspects (Fioratou, Flin, & Glavin, 2010). Practicing anesthesiologists rated how frequently they experienced positive and negative moods during the three days prior to the study. The anesthetists then participated in a high-fidelity simulated scenario as part of their continuing professional development. Prior to beginning the simulation, the practitioners were provided with a case history and an anesthetic assessment of a simulated patient, who was a 48-year-old man who was bitten by a dog on his left hand two days prior. The anesthetists' task was to provide a general anesthetic to allow wound debridement. Shortly after the simulation began, the patient began to deteriorate rapidly into a "can't intubate, can't ventilate" scenario, and the anesthetists were observed for their degree of fixation. The study found that anesthesiologists who reported more frequent positive moods showed less fixation, were quicker to identify a decline in patient oxygen saturation, and initiated the airway management intervention more quickly. Collectively, these findings illustrate that positive affect is associated with a more flexible thinking, allowing practitioners to integrate multiple sources of information, consider alternative solutions, and promote more efficient decision-making.

The research described in this section suggests that positive and negative affective states improve or impair clinical reasoning and decision-making, respectively. However, such conclusions run the risk of oversimplifying what is undoubtedly a complex relationship between emotions and clinical judgment. Moreover, the limited research that has examined the impact of emotions on clinical reasoning and decision-making has adopted primarily a valence-based approach. As reviewed in earlier sections, emotions with similar valence and arousal can have contrasting effects on cognitive processing. More research is needed to further our understanding of how emotions shape clinical thinking and determine when they are beneficial and when they can be harmful to patient care.

Conclusion

Emotions permeate medical practice, and yet, the influence of emotions on clinical reasoning and decision-making has been largely ignored. The goal of this chapter was to review evidence from cognitive psychology showing that emotions deeply influence a wide range of cognitive processes involved in clinical judgments. In reviewing research of affect and cognition, this chapter demonstrates that emotional states and emotional content can strongly influence key cognitive processes involved in clinical reasoning and decision-making. Recent research within the medical field confirms that emotions can have substantial impact on healthcare professionals' judgments and behaviors in clinical settings. Emotions should be better incorporated into theories and frameworks of clinical reasoning and decision-making. Addressing the positive and negative impacts of emotions on doctor-patient interactions will ultimately lead to better medical care and will enhance outcomes for patients, healthcare professionals, and healthcare organizations.

Recommendations. Research in psychological science can provide valuable insight into the design and implementation of medical education (Schoenherr & McConnell, 2024). Based on the research reviewed here, several recommendations can be created to inform medical education and clinical practice. These recommendations see the identification of, and responses to, emotions as a core competency that must be developed in practitioners and educators.

Emotion and Mood are Ubiquitous Features of a Situation and Should be Accepted. Clinicians and educators must acknowledge the role that emotions can play in clinical practice. Encouraging healthcare professionals to be aware of their affective states and how their emotions may influence their perceptions, interpretations, and behaviors will have important implications for patient safety. As Borrell-Carrió and Epstein state, "emotional self-awareness and self-regulation of attention can be consciously cultivated as habits to help physicians function better in clinical situations" (Borrell-Carrió & Epstein, 2004, p. 310). More research is needed to examine what factors facilitate or impeded healthcare professionals' ability to accurately identify and reflect on their own emotions during clinical practice.

Educational Activities Should be Designed to Address Emotion in a Principled Manner. Educators should not simply assume that "high fidelity" simulation that involves "stress" in any way addresses the nuances of affective states on learning and decision-making. As the review here illustrates, multiple emotional responses are possible and are shaped by learners' and clinicians' experiences. Emotions tend to be heightened during early clinical experiences (Ofri, 2013). As McNaughton (2013) eloquently states, "under great pressure to prove themselves worthy of entering the profession, students are afraid to admit that they have uncomfortable feelings about patients or procedures and hide these feelings behind a cloak of competence" (p. 75). Medical educators may be able to train physicians to be aware of their emotional states and understand how emotions may influence clinical decision-making and reasoning.

References

Alexander, K., Quas, J., Goodman, G., Ghetti, S., Edelstein, R., Redlich, A., ... & Jones, D. (2005). Traumatic impact predicts long-term memory for documented child sexual abuse. *Psychological Science, 16*(1), 33–40.

Alves, H., Koch, A., & Unkelbach, C. (2017). Why good is more alike than bad: Processing implications. *Trends in Cognitive Sciences, 21*(2), 69–79.

Anderson, A. (2005). Affective influences on the attentional dynamics supporting awareness. *Journal of Experimental Psychology: General, 134*(2), 258–281.

Angie, A., Connelly, S., Waples, E., & Kligyte, V. (2011). The influence of discrete emotions on judgement and decision-making: A meta-analytic review. *Cognition and Emotion, 25*(8), 1393–1422.

Ashby, F., Isen, A., & Turken, A. (1999). A neuropsychological theory of positive affect and its influence on cognition. *Psychological Review, 106*, 529–550.

Ball, L., & Thompson, V. (2018). *The Routledge International Handbook of Thinking and Reasoning.* New York: Psychology Press.

Banse, R., & Scherer, K. (1996). Acoustic profiles in vocal emotion expression. *Journal of Personality and Social Psychology, 70*, 614–636.

Becker, M., & Leinenger, M. (2011). Attentional selection is biased toward mood-congruent stimuli. *Emotion, 11*(5), 1248–1254.

Berman, N., Wheaton, M., McGrath, P., & Abramowitz, J. (2010). Predicting anxiety: The role of experiential avoidance and anxiety sensitivity. *Journal of Anxiety Disorders, 24*, 109–113.

Bhanji, J., & Beer, J. (2012). Unpacking the neural associations of emotion and judgment in emotion-congruent judgment. *Social Cognitive and Affective Neuroscience, 7*(3), 348–356.

Blanchette, I., & Campbell, M. (2012). Reasoning about highly emotional topics: Syllogistic reasoning in a group of war veterans. *Journal of Cognitive Psychology, 24*(2), 157–164.

Blanchette, I., Gavigan, S., & Johnston, K. (2014). Does emotion help or hinder reasoning? The moderating role of relevance. *Journal of Experimental Psychology: General, 143*, 1049–1064.

Blanchette, I., & Leese, J. (2010). The effect of negative emotion on deductive reasoning. *Experimental Psychology, 58*(3), 235–246.

Blanchette, I., & Richards, A. (2004). Reasoning about emotional and neutral materials. Is logic affected by emotion? *Psychological Science, 15*, 745–752.

Blanchette, I., & Richards, A. (2010). The influence of affect on higher level cognition: A review of research on interpretation, judgement, decision making and reasoning. *Cognition & Emotion, 24*, 561–596.

Blanchette, I., Richards, A., Melnyk, L., & Lavda, A. (2007). Reasoning about emotional contents following shocking terrorist attacks: A tale of three cities. *Journal of Experimental Psychology. Applied, 13*(1), 47–56. https://doi.org/10.1037/1076-898X.13.1.47

Bodenhausen, G. (1993). Emotions, arousal, and stereotypic judgments: A heuristic model of affect and stereotyping. In D Mackie & D. Hamilton (Eds.), *Affect, Cognition, and Stereotyping: Interactive Processes in Intergroup Perception* (pp. 13–37). San Diego, CA: Academic Press.

Bohn, A., & Berntsen, D. (2007). Pleasantness bias in flashbulb memories: Positive and negative flashbulb memories of the fall of the Berlin Wall among East and West Germans. *Memory and Cognition, 35*, 565–577.

Bolte, A., & Goschke, T. (2010). Thinking and emotion: Affective modulation of cognitive processing modes. In B. Glatzeder, V. Goel, & A. Müller (Eds.), *Towards a Theory of Thinking: Building Blocks for a Conceptual Framework* (pp. 261–277). Berlin: Springer-Verlag.

Bonanno, G., Papa, A., Lalande, K., Westphal, A., & Coifman, K. (2004). The importance of being flexible: The ability to both enhance and suppress emotional expression predicts long-term adjustment. *Psychological Science, 10*, 482–487.

Borrell-Carrió, F., & Epstein, R. (2004). Preventing errors in clinical practice: A call for self-awareness. *Annals of Family Medicine, 2*, 310–316.

Bowen, H., Kark, S., & Kensinger, E. (2018). NEVER forget: Negative emotional valence enhances recapitulation. *Psychonomic Bulletin & Review, 25*, 870–891.

Bowes, S., Ammirati, R., Costello, T., Basterfield, C., & Lilienfeld, S. (2020). Cognitive biases, heuristics, and logical fallacies in clinical practice: A brief field guide for practicing clinicians and supervisors. *Professional Psychology: Research and Practice, 51*, 435–445.

Burger, A., & Bless, H. (2016). Affect and the weight of idealistic versus pragmatic concerns in decision situations. *European Journal of Social Psychology, 46,* 323–340.

Caparos, S., & Blanchette, I. (2017). Independent effects of relevance and arousal on deductive reasoning. *Cognition and Emotion, 31*(5), 1012–1022.

Carretié, L. (2014). Exogenous (automatic) attention to emotional stimuli: A review. *Cognitive, Affective, & Behavioral Neuroscience, 14*(4), 1228–1258.

Causse, M., Pavard, B., Senard, J., Démonet, J., & Pastor, J. (2012). Positive and negative emotion induction through avatars and its impact on reasoning performance: Cardiovascular and pupillary correlates. *Studia Psychologica, 54,* 37–51.

Chen, B., Hu, W., & Plucker, J. (2016). The effect of mood on problem finding in scientific creativity. *Journal of Creative Behavior, 50,* 308–320.

Chuang, S., & Kung, C. (2005). The effects of emotions on risk-taking. *Journal of American Academy of Business, 6*(2), 113–117.

Cianci, A., & Bierstaker, J. (2009). The impact of positive and negative mood on the hypothesis generation and ethical judgments of auditors. *Auditing: A Journal of Practice & Theory, 28,* 119–144.

Clore, G. (2011). Psychology and the rationality of emotion. *Modern Theology, 27,* 325–338.

Clore, G., Wyer, R., Dienes, B., Gasper, K., Gohm, C., & Isbell, L. (2001). Affective feelings as feedback: Some cognitive consequences. In L. Martin & G. Clore (Eds.), *Theories of Mood and Cognition: A User's Handbook* (pp. 27–62). Mahwah, NJ: Erlbaum.

Cohen-Charash, Y., Scherbaum, C., Kammeyer-Mueller, J., & Staw, B. (2013). Mood and the market: Can press reports of investors' mood predict stock prices? *PLoS One, 8*(8), 72031.

Congleton, A., & Berntsen, D. (2020). The devil is in the details: Investigating the influence of emotion on event memory using a simulated event. *Psychological Research, 84,* 2339–2353.

Crane, M., Brouwers, S., Forrest, K., Tan, S., Loveday, T., Wiggins, M., ... & David, L. (2017). Positive affect is associated with reduced fixation in a realistic medical simulation. *Human Factors: The Journal of the Human Factors and Ergonomics Society, 59,* 821–832.

Curtis, G. (2013). Don't be happy, worry: Positive mood, but not anxiety, increases stereotyping in a mock-juror decision-making task. *Psychiatry, Psychology and Law, 20,* 686–699.

Damasio, A. R. (1994). *Descartes' Error: Emotion, Reason, and the Human Brain.* New York, NY: Avon Books.

Danvers, A., Hu, J., & O'Neil, M. (2018). Emotional congruence and judgments of honesty and bias. *Collabra: Psychology, 4*(1), 1–7.

Davis, M. (2009). Understanding the relationship between mood and creativity: A meta-analysis. *Organization Behavior and Human Decision Processes, 108,* 25–38.

De Dreu, C., Baas, M., & Nijstad, B. (2008). Hedonic tone and activation level in the mood creativity link: Toward a dual pathway to creativity model. *Journal of Personality and Social Psychology, 94,* 739–756.

DeSteno, D., Petty, R., Wegner, D., & Rucker, D. (2000). Beyond valence in the perception of likelihood: The role of emotion specificity. *Journal of Personality and Social Psychology, 78,* 387–416.

de Vries, M., Holland, R., Corneille, O., Rondeel, E., & Witteman, C. (2012). Mood effects on dominated choices: Positive mood induces departures from logical rules. *Journal of Behavioral Decision Making, 25,* 74–81.

Djamasbi, S. (2007). Does positive affect influence the effective usage of a decision support system? *Decision Support Systems, 43,* 1707–1717.

Dreisbach, G., & Goschke, T. (2004). How positive affect modulates cognitive control: Reduced perseveration at the cost of increased distractibility. *Journal of Experimental Psychology: Learning, Memory, and Cognition, 30,* 343–353.

Dresler, T., Meriau, K., Heekeren, H., & van der Meer, E. (2009). Emotional stroop task: Effect of word arousal and subject anxiety on emotional interference. *Psychological Research, 73,* 364–371.

Ekkekakis, P. (2013). *The Measurement of Affect, Mood, and Emotion: A Guide for Health-Behavioral Research.* New York, NY: Cambridge University Press.

Eriksen, C. (1995). The flankers task and response competition: A useful tool for investigating a variety of cognitive problems. *Visual Cognition, 2,* 101–118.

Estrada, C. A., Isen, A. M., & Young, M. J. (1997). Positive affect facilitates integration of information and decreases anchoring in reasoning among physicians. *Organizational Behavior and Human Decision Processes, 72*(1), 117–135.

Eysenck, M., Derakshan, N., Santos, R., & Calvo, M. (2007). Anxiety and cognitive performance: Attentional control theory. *Emotion, 7,* 336–353.

Ferrer, R., & Ellis, E. (2021). Preliminary evidence for differential effects of integral and incidental emotions on risk perception and behavioral intentions: A meta-analysis of eight experiments. *Journal of Behavioral Decision Making, 34*(2), 275–289.

Fioratou, E., Flin, R., & Glavin, R. (2010). No simple fix for fixation errors: Cognitive processes and their clinical applications. *Anesthesia, 65,* 61–69.

Fischhoff, B., Gonzalez, J., Lerner, J., & Small, D. (2005). Evolving judgments of terror risks: Foresight, hindsight, and emotion. *Journal of Experimental Psychology: Applied, 11,* 124–139.

Fontaine, J., Scherer, K., Roesche, E., & Ellsworth, P. (2007). The world of emotions is not two-dimensional. *Psychological Science, 18,* 1050–1057.

Fredrickson, B. (2003). The value of positive emotions: The emerging science of positive psychology is coming to understand why it's good to feel good. *American Science, 91,* 330–335.

Fredrickson, B., & Branigan, C. (2005). Positive emotions broaden the scope of attention and thought-action repertoires. *Cognition and Emotion, 19,* 313–332.

Frijda, N. (2009). Mood. In D. Sander & K. Scherer (Eds.), *The Oxford Companion to Emotion and the Affective Sciences* (pp. 258–259). New York, NY: Oxford University Press.

Frijda, N., & Scherer, K. (2009). Emotion definitions (psychological perspectives). In D. Sander & K. Scherer (Eds.), *The Oxford Companion to Emotion and the Affective Sciences* (2nd ed., pp. 142–144). Oxford: Oxford University Press.

Gago, F., Echagüe, C. L., & Lázaro, M. (2024). Reflection as a core skill in bioethics education: Application to the scientific and healthcare professions. In J. R. Schoenherr & M. M. McConnell (Eds.), *Fundamentals and Frontiers in Medical Education and Decision-Making.* New York: Routledge.

Gasper, K. (2003). When necessity is the mother of invention: Mood and problem solving. *Journal of Experimental Social Psychology, 39,* 248–262.

Gasper, K., & Spencer, L. (2018). Affective ingredients: Recipes for understanding how affective states alter cognitive outcomes. In E. Diener, S. Oishi, & L. Tay (Eds.), *Handbook of Well-Being*. Salt Lake City, UT: DEF Publishers.

George, J., & Dane, E. (2016). Affect, emotion, and decision making. *Organizational Behavior and Human Decision Processes, 136*, 47–55.

Griskevicius, V., Shiota, M., & Neufeld, S. (2010). Influence of different positive emotions on persuasion processing: A functional evolutionary approach. *Emotion, 10*(2), 190–206.

Groombridge, C., Kim, Y., Maini, A., & Fitzgerald, M. (2019). Stress and decision-making in resuscitation: A systematic review. *Resuscitation, 144*, 115–122.

Hamann, S. (2012). Mapping discrete and dimensional emotions onto the brain: Controversies and consensus. *Trends in Cognitive Sciences, 16*(9), 458–466.

Harmon-Jones, E., Harmon-Jones, C., & Summerell, E. (2017). On the importance of both dimensional and discrete models of emotion. *Behavioral Sciences, 7*(4), 66–82.

Hastie, R., & Dawes, R. (2009). *Rational Choice in an Uncertain World: The Psychology of Judgment and Decision Making*. New York, NY: Sage Publications.

Higgs, J., Jensen, G., Loftus, S., & Christensen, N. (2018). *Clinical Reasoning in the Health Professions*. Edinburgh: Elsevier Health Sciences.

Hogarth, R., Portell, M., Cuxart, A., & Kolev, G. (2011). Emotion and reason in everyday risk perception. *Journal of Behavioral Decision Making, 24*(2), 202–222.

Hu, T., Xie, X., & Li, J. (2013). Negative or positive? The effect of emotion and mood on risky driving. *Transportation Research Part F: Traffic Psychology and Behaviour, 16*, 29–40.

Hullett, C. (2005). The impact of mood on persuasion: A meta-analysis. *Communication Research, 32*, 423–442.

Huntsinger, J. (2013). Does emotion directly tune the scope of attention? *Current Directions in Psychological Science, 22*, 265–270.

Huntsinger, J., Isbell, L., & Clore, G. (2014). The affective control of thought: Malleable, not fixed. *Psychological Review, 121*(4), 600–618.

Huntsinger, J., & Ray, C. (2016). A flexible influence of affective feelings on creative and analytic performance. *Emotion, 16*, 826–838.

Isbell, L., Bourdeaux, E., Chimowitz, H., Liu, G., Cyr, E., & Kimball, E. (2020). What do emergency department physicians and nurses feel? A qualitative study of emotions, triggers, regulation strategies, and effects on patient care. *BMJ Quality & Safety, 29*, 1–2.

Isbell, L., Lair, E., & Rovenpor, D. (2013). Affect-as-information about processing styles: A cognitive malleability approach. *Social and Personality Psychology Compass, 7*(2), 93–114.

Isbell, L., Tager, J., Beals, K., & Liu, G. (2020). Emotionally evocative patients in the emergency department: A mixed methods investigation of providers' reported emotions and implications for patient safety. *BMJ Quality & Safety, 29*(10), 1–12.

Isen, A. (2008). Some ways in which positive affect influences decision-making and problem-solving. In M. Lewis & J. Haviland-Jones (Eds.), *Handbook of Emotions* (pp. 548–573). New York, NY: Guilford Press.

Isen, A., & Geva, N. (1987). The influence of positive affect on acceptable level of risk: The person with a large canoe has a large worry. *Organization Behavior and Human Decision Processes, 39*, 145–154.

Isen, A., Nygren, T., & Ashby, F. (1988). Influence of positive affect on the subjective utility of gains and losses: It is just not worth the risk. *Journal of Personality and Social Psychology, 55,* 710–717.

Isen, A., Rosenzweig, A., & Young, M. (1991). The influence of positive affect on clinical problem solving. *Medical Decision Making, 11*(3), 221–227.

Jackson, J., & Kroenke, K. (1999). Difficult patient encounters in the ambulatory clinic: Clinical predictors and outcomes. *Archives of Internal Medicine, 159,* 1069–1075.

Jeon, M., Yim, J., & Walker, B. (2011). An angry driver is not the same as a fearful driver: Effects of specific negative emotions on risk perception, driving performance, and workload. *In Proceedings of the 3rd International Conference on Automotive User Interfaces and Interactive Vehicular Applications,* 137–142.

Johnson, S., Haerling, K., Yuwen, W., Huynh, V., & Le, C. (2020). Incivility and clinical performance, teamwork, and emotions: A randomized controlled trial. *Journal of Nursing Care Quality, 35,* 70–76.

Jones, A., & Johnstone, M. (2017). Inattentional blindness and failures to rescue the deteriorating patient in critical care, emergency and perioperative settings: Four case scenarios. *Australian Critical Care, 30,* 219–223.

Keil, A., & Ihssen, N. (2004). Identification facilitation for emotionally arousing verbs during the attentional blink. *Emotion, 4*(1), 23–35.

Keltner, D. (2019). Toward a consensual taxonomy of emotions. *Cognition and Emotion, 33*(1), 14–19.

Keltner, D., & Gross, J. (1999). Functional accounts of emotions. *Emotion and Cognition, 13*(5), 467–480.

Kensinger, E. (2009). Remembering the details: Effects of emotion. *Emotion Review, 1,* 99–113.

Kensinger, E., Garoff-Eaton, R., & Schacter, D. (2007). Effects of emotion on memory specificity: Memory trade-offs elicited by negative visually arousing stimuli. *Journal of Memory and Language, 56,* 575–591.

Kensinger, E., & Schacter, D. (2016). Memory and emotion. In L. Feldman Barrett, M. Lewis, & J. Haviland-Jones (Eds.), *Handbook of Emotions* (4th ed., pp. 564–578). New York, NY: Guilford Press.

Kostopoulou, O., & Wildman, M. (2004). Sources of variability in uncertain medical decisions in the ICU: A process tracing study. *BMJ Quality & Safety, 13,* 272–280.

Kozlowski, D., Hutchinson, M., Hurley, J., Rowley, J., & Sutherland, J. (2017). The role of emotion in clinical decision making: An integrative literature review. *BMC Medical Education, 17,* 1–13.

Kreibig, S. (2010). Autonomic system activity in emotion: A review. *Biological Psychology, 84,* 394–421.

Kuhlmann, S., Piel, M., & Wolf, O. (2005). Impaired memory retrieval after psychosocial stress in healthy young men. *Journal of Neuroscience, 25,* 2977–2982.

Kushnir, T., Kushnir, J., Sarel, A., & Cohen, A. (2011). Exploring physician perceptions of the impact of emotions on behaviour during interactions with patients. *Family Practice, 28,* 75–81.

Laney, C., Campbell, H., Heuer, F., & Reisberg, D. (2004). Memory for thematically arousing events. *Memory and Cognition, 32,* 1149–1159.

Lazarus, J. (2021). Negativity bias: An evolutionary hypothesis and an empirical programme. *Learning and Motivation, 75,* 1–13.

Lazarus, R. (1991). *Emotion and Adaptation*. Oxford: Oxford University Press.

LeBlanc, V., MacDonald, R., McArthur, B., King, K., & Lepine, T. (2005). Paramedic performance in calculating drug dosages following stressful scenarios in a human patient simulator. *Prehospital Emergency Care, 9*, 439–444.

LeBlanc, V., Regehr, C., Shlonsky, A., & Bogo, M. (2012). Stress responses and decision making in child protection workers faced with high conflict situations. *Child Abuse and Neglect, 36*, 404–412.

LeBlanc, V. R. (2009). The effects of acute stress on performance: Implications for health professions education. *Academic Medicine, 84*, S25–S33.

LeBlanc, V. R., McConnell, M. M., & Monteiro, S. D. (2015). Predictable chaos: A review of the effects of emotions on attention, memory and decision making. *Advances in Health Sciences Education: Theory and Practice, 20*(1). https://doi.org/10.1007/s10459-014-9516-6

Lemaire, P. (2022). *Emotion and Cognition: An Introduction*. New York, NY: Routledge.

Lerner, J., Gonzalez, R., Small, D., & Fischhoff, B. (2003). Effects of fear and anger on perceived risks of terrorism: A national field experiment. *Psychological Science, 14*, 144–150.

Lerner, J., & Keltner, D. (2000). Beyond valence: Toward a model of emotion-specific influences on judgment and choice. *Cognition and Emotion, 14*, 473–493.

Lerner, J., Li, Y., Valdesolo, P., & Kassam, K. (2015). Emotion and decision making. *Annual Review of Psychology, 66*, 799–823.

Levenson, R. (2009). Autonomic specificity and emotion. In R. Davidson, K. Scherer, & H. Goldsmith (Eds.), *Handbook of Affective Science* (pp. 212–224). Oxford: Oxford University Press.

Levine, L., & Bluck, S. (2004). Painting with broad strokes: Happiness and the malleability of event memory. *Cognition and Emotion, 18*, 559–574.

Levine, L., & Edelstein, R. (2009). Emotion and memory narrowing: A review and goal-relevance approach. *Cognition and Emotion, 23*(5), 833–875.

Levine, L., & Pizarro, D. (2005). Emotion and memory research: A grumpy overview. *Social Cognition, 22*, 530–554.

Li, X., Li, Y., Wang, X., Bai, H., & Hu, W. (2022). Affective valence moderates the influence of thinking style on insight problem solving: Electrophysiological evidence. *Biological Psychology, 170*, 108317.

Li, X., Li, Y., Wang, X., Fan, X., Tong, W., & Hu, W. (2020). The effects of emotional valence on insight problem solving in global-local processing: An ERP study. *International Journal of Psychophysiology, 155*, 194–203.

Lin, W., Tsai, P., Lin, H., & Chen, H. (2014). How does emotion influence different creative performances? The mediating role of cognitive flexibility. *Cognition and Emotion, 28*, 834–844.

Liu, Chimowitz, H., & Isbell, L. (2022). Affective influences on clinical reasoning and diagnosis: Insights from social psychology and new research opportunities. *Diagnosis, 9*(3), 295–305.

Lu, J., Xie, X., & Zhang, R. (2013). Focusing on appraisals: How and why anger and fear influence driving risk perception. *Journal of Safety Research, 45*, 65–73.

Macatee, R., Albanese, B., Schmidt, N., & Cougle, J. (2017). Attention bias towards negative emotional information and its relationship with daily worry in the context of acute stress: An eye-tracking study. *Behaviour Research and Therapy, 90*, 96–110.

MacKay, D., & Ahmetzanov, M. (2005). Emotion, memory, and attention in the taboo Stroop paradigm: An experimental analogue of flashbulb memories. *Psychological Science*, *16*(1), 25–32.

Mackie, D. M., & Worth, L. (1989). Processing deficits and the mediation of positive affect in persuasion. *Journal of Personality and Social Psychology*, *57*, 27–40.

Mamede, S., Van Go, T., Schuit, S., Van den Berge, K., Van Daele, P., Bueving, H., ... & Schmidt, H. (2017). Why patients' disruptive behaviours impair doctors' diagnostic reasoning: A randomized experiment. *BMJ Quality & Safety*, *26*, 13–18.

Maner, J., & Gerend, M. (2007). Motivationally selective risk judgments: Do fear and curiosity boost the boons or the banes? *Organization Behavior and Human Decision Processes*, *103*, 256–267.

McNaughton, N. (2013). Discourse(s) of emotion within medical education: The ever-present absence. *Medical Education*, *47*, 71–79.

Mesquita, B., De Leersnyder, J., & Boiger, M. (2016). The cultural psychology of emotions. In L. Feldman Barrett, M. Lewis, & J. Haviland-Jones (Eds.), *Handbook of Emotions* (pp. 393–411). New York, NY: Guilford Press.

Mickley Steinmetz, K., Addis, D., & Kensinger, E. (2010). The effect of arousal on the emotional memory network depends on valence. *NeuroImage*, *53*(1), 318–324.

Moons, W., & Mackie, D. (2007). Thinking straight while seeing red: The influence of anger on information processing. *Personality and Social Psychology Bulletin*, *33*, 706–720.

Moors, A., Ellsworth, P., & Fridja, N. (2013). Appraisal theories of emotion: State of the art and future development. *Emotion Review*, *5*(2), 119–124.

Morgan, C., Doran, A., Steffian, G., Hazlett, G., & Southwick, S. (2006). Stress-induced deficits in working memory and visuo-constructive abilities in special operations soldiers. *Biological Psychology*, *60*, 722–729.

Morgan, C., Hazlett, G., Doran, A., Garrett, S., Hoyt, G., & Thomas, P. (2004). Accuracy of eyewitness memory for persons encountered during exposure to highly intense stress. *International Journal of Law and Psychiatry*, *27*, 265–279.

Morgan, C., Southwick, S., Steffian, G., Hazlett, G., & Loftus, E. (2013). Misinformation can influence memory for recently experienced, highly stressful events. *International Journal of Law and Psychiatry*, *36*, 11–17.

Mulligan, K., & Scherer, K. (2012). Toward a working definition of emotion. *Emotion Review*, *4*(4), 345–357.

Nendaz, M., & Perrier, A. (2012). Diagnostic errors and flaws in clinical reasoning: Mechanisms and prevention in practice. *Swiss Medical Weekly*, *142*, 1–9.

Norman, G. R., & Eva, K. W. (2010). Diagnostic error and clinical reasoning. *Medical Education*, *44*(1), 94–100.

Oaksford, M., Carlile, J., & Moore, S. (2004). The effects of reasoning, prior mood, and personality on emotion. *Psychologia*, *47*, 250–263.

Oaksford, M., Morris, F., Grainger, B., & Williams, J. (1996). Mood, reasoning, and central executive processes. *Journal of Experimental Psychology: Learning, Memory, and Cognition*, *22*, 476–492.

Oei, N., Everaerd, W., Elzinga, B., van Well, S., & Bermond, B. (2006). Psychosocial stress impairs working memory at high loads: An association with cortisol levels and memory retrieval. *The International Journal on the Biology of Stress*, *9*, 131–144.

Ofri, D. (2013). *What Doctors Feel: How Emotions Affect the Practice of Medicine.* Boston: Beacon Press.

Okon-Singer, H., Hendler, T., Pessoa, L., & Shackman, A. (2015). The neurobiology of emotion – Cognition interactions: Fundamental questions and strategies for future research. *Frontiers in Human Neuroscience, 9,* 1–14.

Pessoa, L. (2008). On the relationship between emotion and cognition. *Nature Reviews Neuroscience, 9*(2), 148–158.

Pham, M. T. (2007). Emotion and rationality: A critical review and interpretation of empirical evidence. *Review of General Psychology, 11*(2), 155–178. https://doi.org/10.1037/1089-2680.11.2.155

Piquette, D., Tarshis, J., Sinuff, T., Fowler, R., Pinto, R., & Leblanc, V. R. (2014). Impact of acute stress on resident performance during simulated resuscitation episodes: A prospective randomized cross-over study. *Teaching and Learning in Medicine, 26,* 9–16.

Pool, E., Brosch, T., Delplanque, S., & Sander, D. (2016). Attentional bias for positive emotional stimuli: A meta-analytic investigation. *Psychological Bulletin, 142,* 79–106.

Posner, J., Russell, J., & Peterson, B. (2005). The circumplex model of affect: An integrative approach to affective neuroscience, cognitive development, and psychopathology. *Development and Psychopathology, 17,* 715–734.

Pottier, P., Dejoie, T., Hardouin, J., Le Loupp, A., Planchon, B., Bonnaud, A., & Leblanc, V. (2013). Effect of stress on clinical reasoning during simulated ambulatory consultations. *Medical Teacher, 35,* 472–480.

Quraishi, S., & Oaksford, M. (2013). Emotion as an argumentative strategy: How induced mood affects the evaluation of neutral and inflammatory slippery slope arguments. In I. Blanchette (Ed.), *Emotion and Reasoning* (pp. 95–118). London: Psychology Press.

Raes, F., Hermans, D., Williams, J., & Eelen, P. (2006). Reduced autobiographical memory specificity and affect regulation. *Emotion and Cognition, 20,* 402–429.

Raghunathan, R., & Pham, M. (1999). All negative moods are not equal: Motivational influences of anxiety and sadness on decision making. *Organization Behavior and Human Decision Processes, 79*(1), 56–77.

Remington, N., Fabrigar, L., & Visser, P. (2000). Reexamining the circumplex model of affect. *Journal of Personality and Social Psychology, 79,* 286–300.

Richards, J., & Gross, J. (2006). Personality and emotional memory: How regulating emotion impairs memory for emotional events. *Journal of Research in Personality, 40,* 631–651.

Riskin, A., Erez, A., Foulk, T., Kugelman, A., Gover, A., Shoris, I., ... & Bamberger, P. (2015). The impact of rudeness on medical team performance: a randomized trial. *Pediatrics, 136,* 487–495.

Riskin, A., Erez, A., Foulk, T., Riskin-Geuz, K., Ziv, A., Sela, R., ... & Bamberger, P. (2017). Rudeness and medical team performance. *Pediatrics, 139,* 1–11.

Rowe, H., Hirsh, J., & Anderson, A. (2007). Positive affect increases the breadth of attentional selection. *Proceedings of the National Academy of Sciences, 104,* 383–388.

Russell, J. (1980). A circumplex model of affect. *Journal of Personality and Social Psychology, 39,* 1161.

Russell, J. (1991). Culture and the categorization of emotions. *Psychological Bulletin, 110,* 426–450.

Russell, J. (2003). Core affect and the psychological construction of emotion. *Psychological Review, 110*, 145–172

Sänger, J., Bechtold, L., Schoofs, D., Blaszkewicz, M., & Wascher, E. (2014). The influence of acute stress on attention mechanisms and its electrophysiological correlates. *Frontiers in Behavioral Neuroscience, 8*, 1–13.

Schmidt, H., van Gog, T., Schuit, S., Van den Berge, K., Van Daele, P., Bueving, H., ... & Mamede, S. (2017). Do patients' disruptive behaviours influence the accuracy of a doctor's diagnosis? A randomised experiment. *BMJ Quality & Safety, 26*, 19–23.

Schoenherr, J. R., & Le-Bouar, C. (2024). Fundamentals of persuasive health communication: Representing, communicating, and distributing health information. In J. R. Schoenherr & M. M. McConnell (Eds.), *Fundamentals and Frontiers in Medical Education and Decision-Making*. New York: Routledge.

Schoenherr, J. R., Waechter, J., & Lee, C. H. (2024). Quantifying expertise in the healthcare professions: Cognitive efficiency and metacognitive calibration. In J. R. Schoenherr & M. M. McConnell (Eds.), *Fundamentals and Frontiers in Medical Education and Decision-Making*. New York: Routledge.

Schoenherr, J. R. & McConnell, M. M. (2024). Human-centered design in health professions education: Informing competency-based education with psychological science. In J. R. Schoenherr & M. M. McConnell (Eds.), *Fundamentals and Frontiers in Medical Education and Decision-Making*. New York: Routledge

Sebastian, C., McCrory, E., De Brito, S., & Viding, E. (2017). Modulation of amygdala response to task-irrelevant emotion. *Social Cognitive and Affective Neuroscience, 12*(4), 643–650.

Sharpe, M., Mayou, R., Seacroatt, V., Surawy, C., Warwick, H., Bulstrode, C., ... & Lane, D. (1994). Why do doctors find some patients difficult to help? *QJM: An International Journal of Medicine, 87*, 187–193.

She, S., Eimontaite, I., Zhang, D., & Sun, Y. (2017). Fear, anger, and risk preference reversals: An experimental study on a Chinese sample. *Frontiers in Psychology, 8*, 1371.

Siemer, M., Mauss, I., & Gross, J. (2007). Same situation–different emotions: How appraisals shape our emotions. *Emotion, 7*, 592–600.

Slovic, P., & Peters, E. (2006). Risk perception and affect. *Current Directions in Psychological Science, 15*(6), 322–325.

Smith, R., & Zimny, G. (1988). Physicians emotional reactions to patients. *Psychosomatics, 29*, 392–397.

Sotgiu, I., & Galati, D. (2007). Long-term memory for traumatic events: Experiences and emotional reactions during the 2000 flood in Italy. *Journal of Psychology, 141*, 91–108.

Stein, N., & Hernandex, M. (2007). Assessing understanding and appraisals during emotional experience. In J. Coan & J. Allen (Eds.), *Handbook of Emotion Elicitation and Assessment* (pp. 298–317). Oxford: Oxford University Press.

Storbeck, J., & Clore, G. (2008). Affective arousal as information: How affective arousal influences judgments, leaning, and memory. *Social and Personality Psychology Compass, 2*, 1824–1843.

Talmi, D., Lohnas, L., & Daw, N. (2019). A retrieved context model of the emotional modulation of memory. *Psychological Review, 126*(4), 455–485.

Tamir, M., & Robinson, M. (2007). The happy spotlight: Positive mood and selective attention to rewarding information. *Personality and Social Psychology Bulletin, 33*(8), 1124–1136.

Tompkins, M., Bjälkebring, P., & Peters, E. (2018). Emotional aspects of risk perceptions. In M. Raue, E. Lermer, & B. Streicher (Eds.), *Psychological Perspectives on Risk and Risk Analysis: Theory, Models, and Applications* (pp. 109–130). Cham, Switzerland: Springer.

Västfjäll, D., Slovic, P., Burns, W., Erlandsson, A., Koppel, L., Asutay, E., & Tinghög, G. (2016). The arithmetic of emotion: Integration of incidental and integral affect in judgments and decisions. *Frontiers in Psychology, 7*(325), 1–10.

Wadlinger, H., & Isaacowitz, D. (2006). Positive mood broadens visual attention to positive stimuli. *Motivation and Emotion, 30*, 87–99.

Wegbreit, E., Franconeri, S., & Beeman, M. (2015). Anxious mood narrows attention in feature space. *Cognition and Emotion, 29*(4), 668–677.

Williams, E., Manwell, L., Konrad, T., & Linzer, M. (2007). The relationship of organizational culture, stress, satisfaction, and burnout with physician-reported error and suboptimal patient care: Results from the MEMO study. *Health Care Management Review, 32*, 203–212.

Williamson, J., Drago, V., Harciarek, M., Falchook, A., Wargovich, B., & Heilman, K. (2019). Chronological effects of emotional valence on the self-selected retrieval of autobiographical memories. *Cognitive and Behavioral Neurology, 32*, 11–15.

Wright, W., & Bower, G. (1992). Mood effects on subjective probability assessment. *Organizational Behavior and Human Decision Processes, 52*, 276–291.

Yang, Q., Zhao, D., Wu, Y., Tang, P., Gu, R., & Luo, Y. (2018). Differentiating the influence of incidental anger and fear on risk decision-making. *Physiology and Behavior, 184*, 179–188.

Yang, Q., Zhou, S., Gu, R., & Wu, Y. (2020). How do different kinds of incidental emotions influence risk decision making? *Biological Psychology, 154*, 107920.

Yiend, J. (2010). The effects of emotion on attention: A review of attentional processing of emotional information. *Cognition and Emotion, 24*(1), 3–47.

Zadra, J., & Clore, G. (2011). Emotion and perception: The role of affective information. *Wiley Interdisciplinary Reviews. Cognitive Science, 2*(6), 676–685.

6

SEPARATING THE NOISE FROM THE SIGNAL

The Role of Familiarity and Pattern Recognition in the Development of Clinical Expertise

Sandra Monteiro, Alice Cavanagh, Bapujee Biswabandan, and Matthew Sibbald

6.1 Introduction

Expert clinical decision-making skills are central to effective healthcare (Kligler et al., 2004). At its core, decision-making is a cognitive process triggered by the identification of a goal (Edwards, 1954). Medical expertise is distinctive in that it is defined by others, in contrast to experts in competitive domains like chess, or golf, who are identified by number of wins and trophies (Wahls & Futz, 2000). Expert clinicians are notable because of their perceived efficient analysis of a situation and their ability to identify effective solutions as well (Schoenherr et al., 2024). Novices, such as undergraduate medical learners, who might have mastered the acquisition of medical facts and clinical guidelines, typically struggle to make clinical decisions. For most learners, simply identifying the most immediate and pertinent goal is the primary challenge given the complex interplay between their medical knowledge, professional role, commitment to provide care, and responsibility to honor the patient's request. For example, a medical student might struggle to summarize the primary concerns of a patient, who was referred to a cardiologist's office, but now reports that his pain goes away quickly after he starts exercising, while his adult daughter, who accompanied him to the appointment, insists there is a serious issue. The medical student must address the patient's expectations of the encounter, the family member's concern, but also read into the family physicians' referral of the testing, and long-term management of risk factors that is hoped for through the consultation. Somewhere buried in this clinical interaction is the need to rule coronary disease in or out and determine if the disease is life-threatening and should be addressed regardless of the patient's

DOI: 10.4324/9781003316091-8

BOX 6.1 LEARNING TO SORT THE NOISE CREATES SIGNAL

I know you want me to be seeing what you're seeing, but right now I just don't: we're looking at the same printed cardiotocograph (CTG) – hearing the same insistent alarm – but I'm confused when the resident I'm trailing decides her patient should continue labouring and silences the beeping. Just three hours earlier, looking at a seemingly identical read out, some sign in the tangled lines mapping fetal and maternal heart rate and uterine contractions, were grounds to call for an emergent caesarean section. In these early days of my first obstetrics observership it feels as though I am watching everyone and everything but seeing nothing. It makes me feel very anxious.

A few days later, a patient nurse offers me a framework for interpretation: start with the baseline fetal heart rate – what is it over ten minutes (and how does that compare with what we might expect)? Next look for variability – how much does the fetal heart rate change peak to trough? Finally, look for accelerations and decelerations – where do these dips and rises come relative to uterine contractions, and how long do they take to wane? With these rules of thumb in mind, my classroom learning about acidosis and alkalosis comes into sharper focus: fetal heart rate is a proxy for fetal oxygenation and therefore fetal distress. I cling to the electronic fetal monitoring like a life raft, glad to finally understand one aspect of what is going on.

Still, these first principles only take me so far: the seasoned senses of the midwives, nurses and physicians working around me find layers of meaning in the delivery suite that evade me. Although I can see if there is trouble from the instruments used to mediate labour, its severities and subtleties still elude me and my suggestions for treatment and monitoring, when I'm asked, are almost always too reactive. Moreover, my field of vision has narrowed: I'm glued so closely to the CTG that I'm surprised when a resident informs me that she prefers to attend births that progress without electronic fetal monitoring. What does she use to monitor progress or to know when contractions are coming? The patient answers for her, when she informs us with a groan that another contraction is building. With the patient's permission, the resident places my hands on her belly and I feel the wave of hardness passing. Soon it is time to push.

Beyond the labour ward, learning medicine is as much about learning how to see as it is about learning bone names or how to calculate the anion gap. Some medical educators give students practice with this task, by asking them to categorize patients into a simple binary, based on appearance: sick or not sick? Then, how sick? These broad-stroke exercises help us to develop the clinical sense that corresponds to our growing classroom physiology – what to look for and which signs, symptoms or lab results portend trouble ahead. Reflecting on this, it feels like learning medicine is about learning what is important, and then tuning the rest out.

I worry, though, about what this process of honing my vision might lead me to miss: before learning to read the tocograph, I talked to patients – what else could I do? – about their pregnancies, their lives, and their previous medical histories. These conversations meandered, and more than once, I was able to present a patient to my attending with a relevant, but obscure, detail that a more experienced clinician had missed. More than that, though, it's still not clear to me how to manage the principle of patient-centred care when medical values (physicians' perceptions of safety, evidence-based practice) come into conflict with the values and epistemologies that underpin patients' decisions; after all, what we choose to see and evaluate as important is inherently a process of values. Birth plans are a site of common conflict on this theme in the labour ward.

symptom burden which could involve balancing the benefits and risks of an invasive angiogram.

6.1.1   The Role of Diagnosis in Clinical Decision-Making

Correct diagnoses can inform good decisions about treatment as many diagnoses are linked to evidence-based therapeutic recommendations. Conversely, thoughtful decisions can create the right context to identify the correct diagnosis. For example, while it is necessary that a clinician makes the decision to admit a patient clearly in active labor, this hinges on first confirming that the patient is in active labor – straightforward assessment – in which case there is an obvious next step. Instead, if we return to the patient indifferent to his chest pain, there are multiple considerations regarding the patient's concerns, the underlying diagnosis, and appropriate therapy. Direct imaging of the coronary arteries with an angiogram carries some procedural risk but the greatest diagnostic clarity. Perhaps his family would like to see this happen, even if he is unclear about taking this risk. The alternative of stress testing might clarify how much risk his chest pain poses but might induce a delay in appropriate intervention if his pain reflects life-threatening coronary disease and carry some reduced sensitivity and specificity to identify the disease. Given his demographics and pain pattern, the pretest likelihood of disease may be sufficient alone to make a clinical diagnosis and justify medical therapy. Typically, the processes involved in diagnosis conclude in assigning a label to a pattern of symptoms. A diagnostic label can provide an anchoring point to guide further clinical decision-making and considerations – such as, what are the potential outcomes, risks, and benefits related to the diagnosis? Are there viable treatments? What information is relevant to ensure the patient is comfortable with the decision? What supports are needed to help the patient?

In this chapter, we explore the process of gaining clinical efficiency through the acquisition of knowledge and experience. We begin with a brief explanation of the *neuroscience of learning* throughout the lifespan. Building on this understanding of learning, we evaluate two dominant *theories of clinical decision-making* and their implications for teaching and learning strategies. We then offer a *synthesis of research on decision-making* and elaborate on three interrelated concepts, specifically recognition-primed decision-making (RPD), situational awareness, and metacognition. We conclude the chapter with a *knowledge translation of theories* into practice to help guide training on clinical decision-making.

6.2 Neuroscience of Learning

Expectations that learners will engage in self-directed learning are often justified by the fast pace of innovation and knowledge creation in the healthcare professions (Murad et al., 2010; Schoenherr et al., 2024). However, capacity for self-directed learning is experience dependent, and novice learners (i.e. learners who are inexperienced at learning in a given context) will be least effective at directing their own learning. We argue that a novice learner, such as a first-year medical student, will benefit most from a blend of instructor-directed and self-directed learning. A medical student is inexperienced at both learning in a complex clinical environment and engaging with clinical decision-making. Early in training, medical students initiate an experience-dependent developmental path, analogous to that of early child development (de Bruin et al., 2018). Indeed, the model of experience-dependent learning and neuroplasticity that describes early childhood development can also be applied to adults learning a new skill, or in the case of medical education, developing a new professional identity (Lövdén et al., 2013).

As newborns, we experience much of the world as random noise, with fuzzy islands of signals. In these early developmental years, many important neural events tune our system to the world we live in and sharpen these signals (Vida et al., 2012). In this way, we begin to recognize faces, language, and shapes, yet the significance or meaning of the things we see, hear, or feel continues to evolve throughout our life. Neuroscience research has confirmed that neuroplasticity of the brain, that is, the capacity for neural networks to alter in response to changing environmental and experiential events, is present throughout the lifespan (Lövdén et al., 2013; Vida et al., 2012). The implication is that engaging in skill development in adulthood contributes to neural adaptation. Through this process, medical learners increase their perceptual sensitivity for distinguishing between relevant sights, sounds,

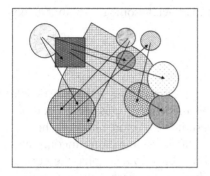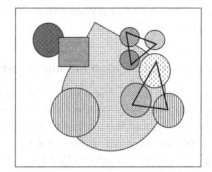

FIGURE 6.1   Abstract representation of different processes performed by novice learners and experienced clinicians. Learners serially scan all available information (left), whereas experienced healthcare professionals use prior knowledge to organize information (triangles, right). Learners might also struggle to differentiate relevant or related information from "background noise".

smells, and touch. Figure 6.1 depicts an abstract representation of different processes performed by novice learners and experienced clinicians.

When learners enter a novel environment, such as medical school, they are immersed in what might feel like random noise. Yet, to the experienced health professionals, the signals are loud and clear. Without sufficient prior experience, a medical student attempting to interpret novel stimuli (e.g., cardiotocograph [CTG] or radiographs) is essentially trying to make sense of random *noise*. While novices can certainly perceive the waveforms on a CTG, they cannot yet detect the subtle differences between waveforms that signal an emergency caesarean and those that call for continued laboring. Novices have not had enough experience to detect patterns or recognize structures that can provide meaning. However, as learners gain experience with CTGs from different patients, they can focus attention on familiar patterns and build on them. Managing this sense-making by complete reliance on self-directed learning is more time consuming and uncertain than instructor-directed learning in a supportive environment (de Bruin et al., 2018; Vida et al., 2012).

Consider a representative narrative (Box 6.1). In the narrative, a medical student reflects on their experience in a labor ward. The learner is not struggling with seeing or hearing a fetal heart monitor over the background noise of the labor ward – instead they are struggling with interpreting and prioritizing the input in ways that acknowledge the nuances of tone and sound from both machine and patient. The narrative emphasizes the *feeling* of not knowing how to interpret the perceptions. A brief focused exposure to multiple examples of CTGs, with guided training by an instructor on the relevance of the most common patterns, can alleviate some of the uncertainty experienced by a novice.

6.3 Clinical Decision-Making Theories

The literature on effective and accurate decision-making reflects a debate between two sets of theorists. One set of theorists propose that decision-making requires the evaluation of multiple strategies, before choosing the best option. Another set of theorists propose that decision-making incorporates prior experience and so clinicians would first have to recognize the current situation as similar to a problem they solved in the past and then apply a similar solution (Edwards, 1954).

Within the first account, decision-making starts with an analysis of the goal, reviewing what is required to achieve it, what options for solutions are available, and an analysis of the risks and benefits associated with each option before deciding on one best path forward (Kahneman, 2003). According to this account, decision-making involves weighing the risks and benefits of multiple options and selecting the one that best meets the goal or solves the problem.

The implications are significant; according to the first account, clinical decision-making strategies are similar for novices and experts. Critically, the difference in efficiency and effectiveness of decisions can be explained by the improper application of the analytic process. An example of this process in action is reflected by the Situation, Background, Assessment, Recommendation (SBAR) (Shahid & Thomas, 2018) acronym which highlights the importance of first defining the *Situation* or clinical context and then clarifying the *Background* or evidence that demonstrates understanding of the situation.

The next step in the process is an *Assessment* of the available options to address the situation. Wrapping up with a single, best *Recommendation* based on an evaluation of the strengths and weaknesses of the various options. Similar tools have been developed to help clinicians organize the relevant information for the purpose of communicating with colleagues, particularly at the point of handover (Farhan et al., 2012). While these tools can improve efficiency and clarity of communication between experienced clinicians, they are not an accurate representation of real-time cognitive processing but instead embody a retrospective description of the decision-making process.

The second set of theorists draw on models of memory processes, which are believed to operate in parallel (Newell & Bröder, 2008). Rather than having to calculate risks and benefits in real time, decision-making is the application of prior solutions based on recognizing a familiar pattern in the current situation. As an expert clinician is likely to have encountered numerous similar situations, with similar goals, their ability to quickly retrieve an effective solution from memory distinguishes them from a novice. The only difference between an expert and a novice then is the number and variety of experiences. While novices might initially find a tool like SBAR useful for organizing their thoughts, the discrete stages of the SBAR communication tool do not ensure effective decisions. Without an understanding of the situation or the evidence, learners might not have appropriate insights for assessing the situation, let alone what recommendations to offer to the patient or their supervisor. Without the requisite experience to draw from, a learner might be restricted to relying on guidelines, algorithms, and any cues they glean from experts around them.

The narrative in Box 6.1 highlights the potential for increasing complexity and confusion for learners regarding which cues to respond to and how to prioritize actions. In the complex context of healthcare, both theories are correct, as a situation might warrant both an analytic and an experience-based solution. In considering how best to support clinicians' advancement from novice to expert, it is critical that we pay attention to our natural learning processes and use caution when interpreting these processes retrospectively (Banning, 2008; Monteiro & Norman, 2013).

6.3.1   Clinical Decision-Making Research

The cognitive processes related to decision-making have been researched for decades (Banning, 2008), yet the focus has been different across disciplines and time. Early research in psychology focused on understanding how people evaluate a limited set of *given* options, to better predict human behavior in similar situations (Edwards, 1954). A typical study design presented participants with realistic scenarios, requiring a decision to solve a problem. Researchers then rated the quality of participants' decisions. The main outcome measured was accuracy as each scenario could be solved with a single best decision. Often certain details of the scenarios were controlled to determine their impact on the accuracy of the decision. For example, the way information is presented about risk can bias participants toward the correct or incorrect response (Kahneman, 2003; Kahneman, 2011; Tversky & Kahneman, n.d.). Because there are many examples of classic psychology studies demonstrating how participants can be influenced to select the incorrect response, some medical education research drawing on this subset of psychology characterizes humans as irrational and prone to emotion and bias (Kahneman, 2003; Graber, 2020). The framing of this research fits within the definition of *decision-making as a process of consciously weighing multiple options.* Other work that fits in this perspective has examined the alignment to Bayes' theorem (Ashby & Smith, 2000), influence of epidemiological evidence (Ashby & Smith, 2000; Elstein, 2004; Hasselblad & McCrory, 1995) (i.e., prevalence and incidence rates) and modeling of algorithmic clinical decision-making (Arocha et al., 2005).

Within many early research paradigms designed to observe the decision making process, participants were not selected for expertise in the context of the scenario – for example, people with no medical training being asked to analyze a clinical problem and select an appropriate therapeutic to treat a disease. Evidence from these research paradigms showed that participants made qualitatively better decisions when they followed an algorithm or used logical decision-making rules (Larrick & Feiler, 2015). In contrast, evidence from research paradigms that accounted for participants' expertise and matched participants' training to the context of the scenarios, the impact of various factors and the pattern of results tended to be very different (Klein, 2008; Salas et al., 2010); expertise facilitated accurate decision-making far better than algorithms. This finding fits within the proposal that *decision-making incorporates prior experience*; experienced individuals efficiently pick the most likely solution because they have already solved a similar problem before (Klein, 1993, chapter 6).

Recognition-Primed Decision-Making

The RPD model, which is associated with a naturalistic decision-making framework, is often integrated into research in domains characterized by uncertainty and risk, like medicine (Elstein, 2001; Lavoie et al., 2022). The RPD model was developed based on observations that taking the time to develop and consider multiple options increased risks and reduced safety in time-sensitive contexts. Critically, the actions and self-reports of experts did not indicate a slower analytic approach (Klein et al., 2010). Klein proposed that familiar situations prime a decision or strategy, which might be altered with additional evaluation, such as mentally simulating the outcome. There might also be a need to align the primed decision with current professional practice guidelines and safety protocols. Therefore, the model allows for some analysis at various points during the event.

RPD also highlights the importance of assessing the situation to retrieve an effective solution more accurately, which is different from assessing viable options. In time-sensitive contexts, experts assess the situation through a more efficient recognition process. Therefore, in contrast to a popular conception of decision-making as a process of identifying and then evaluating the risks and benefits of various options, RPD involves the recognition of cues, expectations, goals, and actions (Lavoie et al., 2022). From this perspective, experts are better able to detect cues, signaling what kind of problem or situation needs to be addressed, and possibly also which situation must be prioritized (Chan et al., 2020). Also, because of their prior experience, experts are better able to evaluate expectations, goals, and actions.

If we consider the environment of a novice in medicine, it seems reasonable that they have not had time to understand, let alone identify important cues. The learner in the narrative concludes that "… learning medicine is about learning what is important, and then tuning the rest out". Indeed, experts are far more efficient at tuning out the noise. Given their vast experience in the same clinical context, a labor ward, for example, they can also develop more accurate expectations, whereas the learner in the narrative realizes that "subtleties still elude [them] and [their] suggestions for treatment and monitoring, when … asked, are almost always too reactive".

Situational Awareness

The concept of situational awareness might seem an intuitive one, but the literature on human cognition and behavior contains multiple definitions, theories, and models of this concept. Stanton et al. (2010) synthesized these multiple perspectives into three epistemological approaches: cognitive psychology, computing/engineering, and human factors/behavioral psychology/sociology. The most popular conceptualization of situational awareness comes from cognitive psychology, described as an individual's momentary perception and comprehension of their current environment and how it might influence their immediate future. Within the context of computing and engineering, situational awareness is often discussed by systems designers or operators referring to the accuracy and timeliness of technology-supported data displays (Stanton et al., 2010). From a human factor or sociological perspective, situational awareness refers to the ways in which information, or access to information, brings technology, culture, and people together (Levin et al., 2012; Stanton et al., 2010). Stanton describes these three perspectives simply as in-mind, in-world, and in-interaction. If we consider the feelings and observations of the learner in the narrative, we might appreciate their challenge with situational awareness as they cannot manage awareness of in-world and in-interaction very well. The learner recognizes that they are unable to keep up with the more experienced clinicians, from the moment they examine a diagnostic image.

Metacognition

The concept of metacognition has produced rich programs of research that span decades (Gago et al., 2024; Schoenherr et al., 2024; Nelson, 1996). A basic definition of metacognition is awareness of one's own mental processes (*Definition of METACOGNITION*, 2023), i.e., "thinking about thinking" (*Definition of METACOGNITION*, 2023). Here we consider two kinds of metacognition proposed in the literature (Regehr & Eva, 2006): self-monitoring and self-regulation (Nelson & Narens) (Nelson, 1996). As a topic of research, metacognition has been studied as an evaluation of knowledge and as an evaluation of reasoning. The metacognition of knowledge is like an analytic process, or System 2, while the metacognition of reasoning is considered similar to a non-analytic process, or System 1 (Evans, 2008) (see Schoenherr & McConnell, 2024; Schoenherr et al., 2024). When novices engage in evaluating their knowledge, they might be able to determine what they know, but may not understand everything they do not know. This evaluation is an analytic process as novices must consciously compare the current situation to the knowledge they can recall. When novices engage in evaluating their performance, they might also be considering their affective responses (McConnell, 2024), or their cognitive uncertainty in their knowledge (e.g., Burleigh & Schoenherr, 2015; Schoenherr & Burleigh, 2020; Schoenherr & Lacroix, 2020)).

Our understanding of metacognition is often linked back to the work of Vygotsky (Yardley et al., 2012). Vygotsky's theory of cognitive development emphasizes the role of social interactions in the development of metacognitive skills. Specifically, Vygotsky's theory suggests that children (or novices) learn to regulate their own thinking and behavior through interactions with more knowledgeable others. This process of other-regulation eventually leads to self-regulation, which is a key aspect of metacognition. This aspect is key, as educators are critical for supporting the self-regulation process. Vygotsky's theory highlights the importance of verbalized self-observation, or introspection, in the development of metacognitive skills. This means that novices *learn to perceive* their own cognitive processes as meaningful and develop knowledge about their own thinking and learning strategies. For emphasis, in contrast to the implications of concepts like self-monitoring, self-assessment, and self-regulation, scaffolding is critical for helping novices complete a task, while *gradually* reducing that support as the novice becomes more capable. Given the fast pace of medicine and healthcare in general, it may have escaped most clinicians that appropriate gradual reduction in scaffolding will be different for each learner and for each domain they must master.

In the narrative, the trainee's initial confusion while interpreting CTGs reflects their difficulty regulating their own thinking and decision-making in the complex context of fetal heart monitoring. The nurse's guidance on interpreting the CTG data, a form of social interaction, provides a scaffold for verbalized self-observation or introspection. This interaction helps the trainee perceive their own cognitive processes as meaningful, leading to the development of knowledge about interpreting the patterns and making clinical decisions. As the narrative progresses, the trainee moves from a state of confusion and limited understanding to a more nuanced comprehension of fetal heart monitoring. This growth is guided by interactions with more experienced medical professionals. The trainee's progress aligns with

Vygotsky's emphasis on the role of social interactions and guidance in cognitive development.

Synthesis

Overall research on decision-making processes often suggests a slightly adversarial relationship between analytic and non-analytic models. One line of research contrasts conscious exploration of multiple options with experience-dependent recognition of solutions. However, in a complex environment like healthcare, competence in both forms of decision-making is required. Similarly, the three different forms of situational awareness are valued within different contexts in the literature; the complexities of healthcare education contain multiple contexts and so require clinician educators to consider which perspective to apply when teaching. Metacognitive processes have also been described as analytic when focused on knowledge and non-analytic when focused on reasoning; clearly both are required.

The first sentence of the narrative (Box 6.1) describes the confusion and uncertainty of a medical student who examines something they believe to be objective, or visually undeniable, like a diagnostic image through visual perception, but does not *understand* the meaning or urgency indicated by the image pattern. When more experienced clinicians see and understand how seemingly similar images inform very distinct management plans, we might assume that a student is not looking closely or analytically enough, or the student might assume that. This assumption can leave educators and trainees frustrated and confused about next steps toward developing clinical competence. For example, a clinician sees the obvious lack of lung markings on a chest X-ray, spanning a substantial portion of the lung apex and intuits that a chest tube is needed. The same finding is appreciated by the student – decreased lung markings – but is not salient, does not prime any actions, or provide a clear diagnosis for the patient's sudden chest pain and shortness of breath. Instead, the student might only manage slowly constructing and evaluating a differential based on the clinical symptoms.

The shifts between analytic and non-analytic reasoning and decision-making have been studied for decades, but typically as separate processes. Some cognitive psychology has explored these concepts to better understand how the mind works (Klein, 1993) and some cognitive psychology, economics, and education psychology have extended this research to describe some of the factors that limit human performance (Tversky & Kahneman, n.d.). Additionally, applied psychologists have cautioned against focusing only on one process (Monteiro et al., 2020; Monteiro & Norman, 2013). Certainly, learners do not benefit from trying to evaluate or categorize their reasoning process. Importantly, for the purpose of designing education, distinguishing between processes is not the primary goal. As demonstrated by the narrative, explained by recognition decision-making research, and supported by theories of situational awareness and metacognition, the process, or metrics that we deem to represent the process, reflects the clinician's level of expertise and comfort with the context. The process does not drive performance, and it is not possible to control the process in a way that affects performance in a positive way (Monteiro et al., 2020; Monteiro et al., 2020). The last section is dedicated to translating theories into teaching strategies that support learners to identify the signals they will need to practice independently.

6.4 Decision Tuning Strategies for Novices

Clinical teaching is not as simple as pointing directly to the *signal* to help students "see" or "hear". Instead, we must think of medical students as learning to read, interpret, and communicate in a new language (Schoenherr & LeBouar, 2024). Like musicians, they must not only learn musical notes but also entire musicals. Initially, the novice does not see what the expert sees; they perceive the same information through their senses, but they do not yet understand the structure (Schoenherr, 2024). This lack of understanding creates uncertainty, frustration, and emotions that can misdirect attention and attempts to learn (McConnell, 2024). Experts can easily make these distinctions based on previous experience. For example, evidence from eye-tracking studies (Al-Moteri et al., 2017; Fox & Faulkner-Jones, 2017) demonstrate that novices and experts employ different search strategies when scanning diagnostic images. These search strategies have been used to distinguish between holistic processing that is often supported by prior experience and analytic processing that is indicative of exploring individual elements and details.

Decision-making research indicates that an expert clinician rapidly and simultaneously (1) recruits prior experience relevant to the context, creating a focused lens to interpret new information, and (2) interprets the familiarity of new information and consequently their confidence in making decisions. However, these classic studies have offered limited understanding about novice's metacognition, the ways in which novices evaluate their own knowledge, and where they might judge the learning gap to be.

What experiential learning opportunities can we provide trainees who are consistently pushed from uncertainty to recognition and back in again? Can we prepare trainees and educators to accept/predict these transitions (Chorley et al., 2021)? Table 6.1 provides some strategies for matching instructional design to the learner's learning stage.

TABLE 6.1 Translations of Developmental Stages into Approaches that Can Be Used by Instructors and Learners

Strategy and Level of Learner	Developmental Stage	What Can the Teacher Do to Help the Learner?	What Can the Learner Do to Help the Teacher?
Pre-clinical learner	Naïve novice little or no book knowledge	Frame book knowledge within a clinical context to help learners build perspective around how clinical decision-making draws from basic science	Share with clinical educators stage of training and knowledge base to date
New clinical learner	Relative novice with good book knowledge little or no clinical experience	Model clinical reasoning and approaches to interactions. Make explicit thought process. Focus on key clinical variables that inform decisions	Create conversation spaces around expectations for engagement. Balance active engagement with observation. Prioritize and highlight areas of focus for active learning that are small and manageable
Intermediate to senior clinical learner	Experienced clinical learner without understanding of YOUR clinical environment (e.g., new to rotation but not new to clerkship)	Orient learners around expectations in participating in the workplace environment. Highlight goals that must be integrated in clinical reasoning	Focus on the organization of written and oral communication to facilitate sharing mental models of clinical reasoning details. Attend to differences in the way teachers frame clinical reasoning problems and remain curious around them

(Continued)

TABLE 6.1 (Continued)

Strategy and Level of Learner	Developmental Stage	What Can the Teacher Do to Help the Learner?	What Can the Learner Do to Help the Teacher?
New medical resident	Working clinical and book knowledge without robust experience to confidently manage situations	Signal where situations are typical and clear from where situations are complex and require more engagement in clinical reasoning Provide opportunities for learners to see multiple exemplars where management should be clear but learners are uncertain	Identify areas of low confidence, and ask for templates around information collection and management
Intermediate to senior medical resident	Experience to back clinical and book knowledge with gaps encountering unusual or rare situations	Provide the learner opportunity to share their mental model. Identify areas of nuance of uncertainty and distinguish from clearly established pathways for clinical decision-making	Learn from different teachers

6.5 Conclusion

Whether by a novice or expert, perceiving and making meaning of an observed event is relative. Many scholars in health professions education acknowledge this by referencing "different lenses", which often refers to individual differences in lived experiences. This relativity of perception extends beyond research paradigms and philosophies; what we perceive through all our senses is relative. Not only can there be variations in how individual learners process or attend to the same stimuli (e.g., sound or image), but also the meaning or significance assigned to a stimulus can vary. This also implies that it is not possible to transfer the set of patterns that one clinician recognizes to another clinician; each clinician's knowledge base and pattern structures will be quite unique in the same way that their experiences are.

References

Al-Moteri, M. O., Symmons, M., Plummer, V., & Cooper, S. (2017). Eye tracking to investigate cue processing in medical decision making: A scoping review. *Computers in Human Behavior*, 66, 52–66. https://doi.org/10.1016/j.chb.2016.09.022

Arocha, J. F., Wang, D., & Patel, V. L. (2005). Identifying reasoning strategies in medical decision making: A methodological guide. *Journal of Biomedical Informatics*, 38(2), 154–171. https://doi.org/10.1016/j.jbi.2005.02.001

Ashby, D., & Smith, A. F. M. (2000). Evidence-based medicine as Bayesian decision making. *Statistics in Medicine*, 19(23), 3291–3305. https://doi.org/10.1002/1097-0258(20001215)19:23

Banning, M. (2008). A review of clinical decision making: Models and current research. *Journal of Clinical Nursing*, 17(2), 187–195. https://doi.org/10.1111/j.1365-2702.2006.01791.x

Burleigh, T. J., & Schoenherr, J. R. (2015). A reappraisal of the uncanny valley: Categorical perception or frequency-based sensitization? *Frontiers in Psychology*, 5. www.frontiersin.org/articles/10.3389/fpsyg.2014.01488

Chan, T. M., Mercuri, M., Turcotte, M., Gardiner, E., Sherbino, J., & de Wit, K. (2020). Making decisions in the era of the clinical decision rule: How emergency physicians use clinical decision rules. *Academic Medicine*, 95(8), 1230–1237. https://doi.org/10.1097/ACM.0000000000003098

Chorley, A., Welsher, A., Pardhan, A., & Chan, T. M. (2021). Faculty-lead opinions on workplace-based methods for graduated managerial teaching (FLOW MGMT): A national cross-sectional survey of Canadian emergency medicine lead educators. *AEM Education and Training*, 5(1), 19–27. https://doi.org/10.1002/aet2.10429

de Bruin, A. B., Sibbald, M., & Monteiro, S. (2018). 3. The science of learning. In *Understanding Medical Education: Evidence, Theory, and Practice* (23–36). Wiley.

Definition of METACOGNITION. (2023, July 14). www.merriam-webster.com/dictionary/metacognition

Edwards, W. (1954). The theory of decision making. *Psychological Bulletin*, 51(4), 380–417.

Elstein, A. S. (2001). Naturalistic decision making and clinical judgment. *Journal of Behavioral Decision Making*, 14(5), 363.

Elstein, A. S. (2004). On the origins and development of evidence-based medicine and medical decision making. *Inflammation Research*, 53, S184–S189. https://doi.org/10.1007/s00011-004-0357-2

Evans, J. S. B. T. (2008). Dual-processing accounts of reasoning, judgment, and social cognition. *Annual Psychological Review, 59*, 255–278.

Farhan, M., Brown, R., Woloshynowych, M., & Vincent, C. (2012). The ABC of handover: A qualitative study to develop a new tool for handover in the emergency department. *Emergency Medicine Journal, 29*(12), 941–946. https://doi.org/10.1136/emermed-2011-200199

Fox, S. E., & Faulkner-Jones, B. E. (2017). Eye-tracking in the study of visual expertise: Methodology and approaches in medicine. *Frontline Learning Research, 5*(3), 43–54. https://doi.org/10.14786/flr.v5i3.258

Gago, F., Echagüe, C. L., & Lázaro, M. (2024). Reflection as a core skill in bioethics education: Application to the scientific and healthcare professions. In J. R. Schoenherr & M. M. McConnell (Eds.), *Fundamentals and Frontiers in Medical Education and Decision-Making: Educational Theory and Psychological Practice.* Routledge.

Graber, M. (2020). Progress understanding diagnosis and diagnostic errors: thoughts at year 10. *Diagnosis, 7*(3), 151–159. https://doi.org/10.1515/dx-2020-0055

Hasselblad, V., & McCrory, D. C. (1995). Meta-analytic tools for medical decision making: A practical guide. *Medical Decision Making, 15*(1), 81–96. https://doi.org/10.1177/0272989X9501500112.

Kahneman, D. (2003). A perspective on judgment and choice: Mapping bounded rationality. *American Psychologist, 58*(9), 697–720. https://doi.org/10.1037/0003-066X.58.9.697

Kahneman, D. (2011). *Thinking, Fast and Slow.* Macmillan.

Klein, G. (Ed.). (1993). *Decision Making in Action: Models and Methods.* Ablex Pub.

Klein, G. (2008). Naturalistic decision making. *Human Factors, 50*(3), 456–460.

Klein, G., Calderwood, R., & Clinton-Cirocco, A. (2010). Rapid decision making on the fire ground: The original study plus a postscript. *Journal of Cognitive Engineering and Decision Making, 4*(3), 186–209. https://doi.org/10.1518/155534310X12844000801203

Kligler, B., Maizes, V., Schachter, S., Park, C. M., Gaudet, T., Benn, R., Lee, R., & Remen, R. N. (2004). Core competencies in integrative medicine for medical school curricula: A proposal. *Academic Medicine, 79*(6), 521.

Larrick, R. P., & Feiler, D. C. (2015). Expertise in decision making. In *The Wiley Blackwell Handbook of Judgment and Decision Making* (pp. 696–721). John Wiley & Sons, Ltd. https://doi.org/10.1002/9781118468333.ch24

Lavoie, P., Deschênes, M.-F., Maheu-Cadotte, M.-A., Lapierre, A., Mailhot, T., Rodriguez, D., & Desforges, J. (2022). Nursing students' decision making regarding postpartum hemorrhage: An exploration using the recognition-primed decision model. *Nurse Education in Practice, 64*, 103448. https://doi.org/10.1016/j.nepr.2022.103448

Levin, S., Sauer, L., Kelen, G., Kirsch, T., Pham, J., Desai, S., & France, D. (2012). Situation awareness in emergency medicine. *IIE Transactions on Healthcare Systems Engineering, 2*(2), 172–180. https://doi.org/10.1080/19488300.2012.684739

Lövdén, M., Wenger, E., Mårtensson, J., Lindenberger, U., & Bäckman, L. (2013). Structural brain plasticity in adult learning and development. *Neuroscience & Biobehavioral Reviews, 37*(9, Part B), 2296–2310. https://doi.org/10.1016/j.neubiorev.2013.02.014

Monteiro, S., Sherbino, J., Sibbald, M., & Norman, G. (2020). Critical thinking, biases and dual processing: The enduring myth of generalisable skills. *Medical Education, 54*(1), 66–73. https://doi.org/10.1111/medu.13872

Monteiro, S. D., Sherbino, J., Schmidt, H., Mamede, S., Ilgen, J., & Norman, G. (2020). It's the destination: Diagnostic accuracy and reasoning. *Advances in Health Sciences Education, 25*(1), 19–29. https://doi.org/10.1007/s10459-019-09903-7

Monteiro, S. M., & Norman, G. (2013). Diagnostic reasoning: Where we've been, where we're going. *Teaching and Learning in Medicine, 25*, S26–S32. https://doi.org/10.1080/10401334.2013.842911

Murad, M. H., Coto-Yglesias, F., Varkey, P., Prokop, L. J., & Murad, A. L. (2010). The effectiveness of self-directed learning in health professions education: A systematic review. *Medical Education, 44*(11), 1057–1068. https://doi.org/10.1111/j.1365-2923.2010.03750.x

Nelson, T. O. (1996). Consciousness and metacognition. *American Psychologist, 51*(2), 102–116. https://doi.org/10.1037//0003-066X.51.2.102

Newell, B. R., & Bröder, A. (2008). Cognitive processes, models and metaphors in decision research. *Judgment and Decision Making, 3*(3), 195–204. https://doi.org/10.1017/S1930297500002400

Regehr, G., & Eva, K. (2006). Self-assessment, self-direction, and the self-regulating professional. *Clinical Orthopaedics & Related Research, 449*, 34–38. https://doi.org/10.1097/01.blo.0000224027.85732.b2

Salas, E., Rosen, M. A., & DiazGranados, D. (2010). Expertise-based intuition and decision making in organizations. *Journal of Management, 36*(4), 941–973. https://doi.org/10.1177/0149206309350084

Schoenherr, J. R., & Burleigh, T. J. (2020). Dissociating affective and cognitive dimensions of uncertainty by altering regulatory focus. *Acta Psychologica, 205*, 103017. https://doi.org/10.1016/j.actpsy.2020.103017

Schoenherr, J. R., & Lacroix, G. L. (2020). Performance monitoring during categorization with and without prior knowledge: A comparison of confidence calibration indices with the certainty criterion. *Canadian Journal of Experimental Psychology/Revue canadienne de psychologie expérimentale, 74*(4), 302.

Schoenherr, J. R., Waechter, J., & Lee, C. H. (2024). Quantifying expertise in the healthcare professions: Cognitive efficiency and metacognitive calibration. In: Schoenherr, J. R. & McConnell, M. M. (eds.), *Fundamentals and Frontiers of Medical Education and Decision-Making: Educational Theory and Psychological Practice*. Routledge.

Shahid, S., & Thomas, S. (2018). Situation, background, assessment, recommendation (SBAR) communication tool for handoff in health care–A narrative review. *Safety in Health, 4*(1), 7. https://doi.org/10.1186/s40886-018-0073-1

Stanton, N. A., Salmon, P. M., Walker, G. H., & Jenkins, D. P. (2010). Is situation awareness all in the mind? *Theoretical Issues in Ergonomics Science, 11*(1–2), 29–40.

Tversky, A., & Kahneman, D. (1974). Judgment under uncertainty: Heuristics and biases. *Science, 185*(4157), 1124–1131.

Vida, M. D., Vingilis-Jaremko, L., Butler, B. E., Gibson, L. C., & Monteiro, S. (2012). The reorganized brain: How treatment strategies for stroke and amblyopia can inform our knowledge of plasticity throughout the lifespan. *Developmental Psychobiology, 54*(3), 357–368.

Wahls, T. L., & Futz, D. N. (2000). The master clinician project. *The Journal of Ambulatory Care Management, 23*(4), 9.

Yardley, S., Teunissen, P. W., & Dornan, T. (2012). Experiential learning: Transforming theory into practice. *Medical Teacher, 34*(2), 161–164. https://doi.org/10.3109/0142159X.2012.643264

7

OPTIMIZING PSYCHOMOTOR SKILLS ACQUISITION IN HEALTHCARE SIMULATION THROUGH KNOWLEDGE MOBILIZATION

Sandy Abdo, Leanne Elliott, Julia Micallef, Mithusa Sivanathan, and Adam Dubrowski

7.1 Simulation in Health Profession Education

A growing body of literature suggests that teaching technical clinical skills through simulation contributes to skill retention (Motola et al., 2013) and skill transfer to clinical settings (Doody & Condon, 2013). In the context of health professions education, simulation employs models, actors, animal parts, digital technologies, and supplementary materials and scripts to create an immersive, replicable, safe, and standardized learning environment without posing harm to patients (Barjis, 2011; Kothari et al., 2017). This is ideal for training technical clinical skills where healthcare professionals provide direct patient care that has a demonstrable impact on clinical outcomes (Chiniara et al., 2013; Tolsgaard, 2013). According to the literature, technical skills are types of psychomotor skills, and we will be using these terms interchangeably throughout this chapter (Dubrowski & Backestein, 2004; Grantcharov & Reznick, 2008; Kovacs, 1997).

For the effective teaching of technical clinical skills in simulation settings, simulationists need to understand the pedagogical frameworks, derived from the field of motor learning and control, that underpin and drive the process of learning (Peyre & Ashley, 2011). Nonverbal technical skills represent a unique challenge for competency-based medical education (Schoenherr & McConnel,2024; Schoenherr & Hamstra, 2024). The acquisition of technical skills involves (a) learning how to perform specific movements (procedural knowledge), (b) understanding why one should execute the procedure (scientific knowledge), and (c) understanding what the clinical results might imply (clinical reasoning; Martina et al., 2012).

DOI: 10.4324/9781003316091-9

Using psychomotor learning theory to guide the development of simulation training sessions has been shown to enhance technical skills learning among healthcare students and professionals (Perry et al., 2022). Fitts and Posner's (1967) widely cited model considers the general process of how a learner transitions from a novice to an expert in any given psychomotor skill (for a discussion of cognitive expertise development, see Montiero et al., 2024). This well-established theory suggests that it is possible to organize psychomotor skills training as a planned activity, with predetermined learning objectives (Feil et al., 1994; for issues in the translation of this model in medical education, see Schoenherr & McConnell, 2024).

To understand the implications of incorporating evidence-based design elements, one needs to understand in general how people acquire psychomotor skills. Therefore, we will highlight the stages of learning in Fitts and Posner's Three Stage Model of Learning.

7.2   Fitts and Posner Three Stage Model of Learning

Fitts and Posner (1967) introduced a structured model of psychomotor skills acquisition comprising three stages: cognitive, associative, and autonomous. In the cognitive stage, learners grasp the skill and its motor patterns through instruction, guidance, feedback, and trial and error. This stage witnesses significant performance improvement, though errors are common, and efficiency increases gradually. Transitioning to the associative stage, learners identify effective psychomotor patterns, making minor adjustments. This phase's duration varies with skill complexity and practice time. Focus narrows to skill details, transitions, and subtle adjustments, aiming for smooth execution. The autonomous stage, the final phase, signifies gradual performance improvement. Skills become automated, requiring minimal cognitive engagement. Ideally, this phase balances speed and accuracy, with fewer distractions impacting performance (Schoenherr et al., 2024).

Fitts and Posner's model aligns with the typical performance and learning curve, involving cognitive effort, rapid improvement, slow progress, and eventual plateau (Taylor & Ivry, 2012; Guadagnoli & Lee, 2004; Guadagnoli et al., 2012).

Despite its comprehensive view of learning stages, Fitts and Posner's model lacks insight into practice design elements crucial for psychomotor learning. This chapter's objective is to describe key practice design elements in the psychomotor domain, catering to simulationists with limited prior knowledge.

Table 7.1 summarizes the seven principles that will be discussed in this chapter that can be used to modify simulation-based practice to optimize its effectiveness.

However, some practice design elements may yield paradoxical effects during skill acquisition and transfer to clinical settings. A deep understanding

TABLE 7.1 Summary of the Conditions of Practice Depending on the Expertise Level of the Learner

Condition	Novice	Intermediate	Advanced
Motivation	Ensure the task is not very difficult and discouraging	Ensure the task is challenging but not too challenging	Ensure the task is challenging enough
Information	Enough information to guide the learner	Little to no information	Only if absolutely necessary
Observation	Very important	Less important	Not important
Distribution of Practice	Not a lot of time between practice sessions	Adequate amount of time between practice sessions	A lot of time between practice sessions
Variability	No variability	Few variability	A lot of variability
Contextual Interference	Blocked practice	Moving toward random practice	Random practice
Feedback	A lot of feedback	Some feedback	Little feedback

of the learning-performance distinction is essential for clinicians and simulationists to structure training programs promoting enduring learning. This ensures newly that acquired skills stand the test of time (retention) and transfer effectively to real clinical environments (Dubrowski, 2005).

7.3 Transfer Appropriate Processing

Behavioral research in cognitive psychology distinguishes between immediate performance changes during practice and lasting changes in performance over time (Kantak & Winstein, 2012). Learning implies relatively permanent, transferable changes, while performance denotes temporary, measurable changes during or immediately after practice (Guadagnoli & Lee, 2004). Notably, practice-induced performance improvements often do not translate into enduring learning, and learning can occur without immediate performance gains (Soderstrom & Bjork, 2015). Paradoxically, conditions leading to significant practice errors often facilitate substantial learning (Soderstrom & Bjork, 2015).

Assessing competencies indirectly is standard in simulation-based education (Schoenherr & Hamstra, 2024). Educators infer learning by examining performance changes using retention and transfer tests (Moulton et al., 2006). These tests gauge performance after a specific time interval following practice (Kantak & Winstein, 2012). While a 24-hour retention interval is common, it may not suit many real-world skill applications that require performance days, weeks, or months later. Thus, training sessions should promote robust learning. Aligning retention periods with local curricular activities, like weekly sessions for surgical residents, can be ideal (Dubrowski & MacRae, 2006).

Simulationists must also decide what kind of test to use. Two types are prevalent: retention and transfer tests. Retention tests evaluate the permanence of learned skills, replicating acquisition conditions after a delay. Transfer tests assess the adaptability and generalizability of learning by introducing variations or different conditions (Kantak & Winstein, 2012). Practice conditions can be tailored to manipulate the difficulty level, with the Challenge Point Framework (CPF) helping instructors adjust training difficulty based on learners' skill levels.

7.4 Challenge Point Framework

The CPF (Guadagnoli & Lee, 2004), is a model grounded in information theory and processing. It revolves around the idea that the level of learning is linked to the amount of interpretable information available during practice, which is perceived as a "challenge" by learners. Psychomotor tasks, like clinical procedures, vary in the challenge they pose to learners of different skill levels. According to the CPF, training sessions should tailor the challenge level to match the performers' skill level for optimal learning. To achieve this, clinicians should consider both nominal and functional task difficulty in simulation-based learning environments.

Nominal task difficulty represents the inherent challenge of a task, regardless of who performs it or the conditions it's done . It's based on the task's inherent perceptual and motor demands. For instance, a chest tube insertion on an adult mannequin may be perceived differently in difficulty by different individuals, but the nominal difficulty is determined solely by the task's characteristics, such as the procedure's complexity and simulator size.

Functional task difficulty, on the other hand, considers the challenge level in light of the performer's skill and the practice conditions. For example, a chest tube procedure would be less challenging for an experienced emergency medicine fellow compared to a medical resident with no prior experience. Changing the simulator to an infant mannequin or adding an observer/evaluator would increase functional difficulty, particularly for the resident.

The learner's processing capacity becomes overwhelmed when the challenge exceeds their abilities, hindering efficient information processing and learning. Conversely, if action-planning processes are not challenged enough during skill acquisition, learning suffers as well. The optimal challenge point (OPC) represents the point where learners experience maximal learning due to exposure to the right level of task difficulty for their skill level.

The CPF adheres to three fundamental corollaries:

1 Learning depends on the presence of information.
2 Too much or too little information impairs learning.
3 The optimal amount of information varies based on the learner's skill level and task difficulty.

In summary, psychomotor skill learning involves stages of learning, the learning-performance paradox, and the CPF. Fitts and Posner's (1967) model provides insight into learners' needs, instructions, guidance, feedback, and environmental interference, and how these evolve as proficiency grows. The learning-performance paradox emphasizes the impact of practice quality on learning outcomes. Lastly, the CPF offers a practical framework for educators to adjust functional task difficulty based on performer skill levels, optimizing the simulation environment for learning.

7.5 Conditions to Enhance Technical Skills Learning

In the remainder of the chapter, we will provide an overview of some of the key instructional design elements that can help with the adjustment of functional task difficulty, focusing on the procedural knowledge component of technical skills learning. We use suturing as the main example to explain the conditions of practice and how CPF plays a role in how the conditions of practice should be laid out according to the type of learner, whether novice or advanced. In the next section, we will introduce a few selected conditions (as outlined in Table 7.1) that may enhance simulation-based training (e.g., Guadagnoli & Lee, 2004).

7.5.1 Motivation – "Keep them interested"

Most learners in health professions will be highly intrinsically motivated to learn psychomotor skills. However, for some of the most fundamental skills, motivation might be limited as they might be unaware as to why the skill is needed and how it is used in the delivery of care (George & Doto, 2001). Learners' motivational influences are conditions that encourage learners to practice more (Lewthwaite & Wulf, 2010a). Research exploring the relationship between simulation-based learning and motivation shows that motivation is a key player in optimal learning and improved transfer of skills for healthcare learners (Arizo-Luque et al., 2022). For example, Escher et al. (2017), demonstrated that medical students felt more motivated to use simulations with the understanding that using this training tool could help improve patient safety.

Learners are motivated when they are in situations where expectations of their performance are enhanced or their desire for autonomy is supported. Learner expectancies of performance are proportional to their self-efficacy (i.e., confidence in one's ability to perform well). High self-efficacy in learners can occur when they receive positive social-comparative information, when a task is made to appear less difficult, or when learners' concerns about their abilities are reduced (Ávila et al., 2012; Wulf et al., 2012). Defining what success means for a set of performance criteria, highlighting the acquirability of a task, or structuring practice schedules with errorless practice at the beginning and gradually increasing difficulty can also raise one's self-efficacy (Dweck, 1999; Maxwell et al., 2001; Palmer et al., 2016).

Giving the learner control over a certain aspect of the practice (called self-controlled practice) has been shown to enhance motor learning as well (Sanli et al., 2013). Examples of choices include deciding when to receive feedback, using an assistive device, viewing a demonstration of the skill, deciding the order in which they want to practice different tasks, or even how much to practice (Brydges et al., 2010; Brydges et al. 2012; Sanli et al., 2013). These tactics could be added before and during simulation training to motivate the learner through the learning process (Schmidt et al., 2019).

Examples. Before practice, giving learners a general comment about their peer group's performance would make suturing less of a daunting skill and alleviate concern. For example, the instructor can say "in the past, students have been very fast at picking up how to hold the forceps correctly and mount the needle after a few tries." During practice, encouraging words can increase motivation though it is important that the message is delivered in a way that describes the performance as a function of practice rather than the result of inherent ability (Drews et al., 2013). Instead of commenting "you are a great surgeon!" while a student suture or has completed suturing, the trainer could say "you did a great job suturing!" to not diminish motivation if and when mistakes are made in future practice sessions, and to eliminate the association of the mistake with the profession (the belief that they are a bad surgeon). False-positive feedback has been shown to increase motivation; however, providing it in the context of suturing performance, a technical skill that will be performed on patients, would be ethically problematic (Schmidt et al., 2019) and might lead to overconfidence bias (Schoenherr et al., 2024). Giving the learners a choice about how often they receive feedback on their performance during practice (Nousiainen et al., 2008), how often they practice (Jowett et al., 2007), and how they view demonstrations of the suturing technique (Cheung et al., 2016), could increase their motivation to learn suturing as it might fulfill their need for autonomy. Specific to suturing, students could be given a choice of simulators and instruments to work with to give the feeling of being autonomous (Brydges et al., 2006).

Motivation is closely related to the level of difficulty. If we designed a suturing task that was too easy based on the learner's skill level (i.e., the OPC was not achieved), the lack of difficulty would hinder learning. On the other hand, if the practice tasks are too difficult and the learner starts feeling discouraged, these conditions would also hinder learning (Brydges et al., 2007). This highlights the importance of matching the level of difficulty of the practice with the skill level of the learner. A novice learner who perceives suturing as a challenging task will become overwhelmed if the instructor makes the task harder. In this case, the instructor should dial back the practice difficulty to match the skill level of the learner. An advanced learner with extensive suturing experience might not be as enthusiastic about practicing the easy version of the suturing task. Hence, the instructor must increase the difficulty enough to keep the advanced learner challenged.

One way to accomplish this is to start the training session with suturing models offering minimal difficulty so novice participants would be able to increase their confidence early on in practice, and then, as the training goes on, suturing models offering higher levels of difficulty could be introduced (Brydges et al., 2006). The confidence created in the beginning would support the learner as they encounter more difficult practice activities throughout the session. The conditions of practice that will be discussed in the remainder of the chapter could be used by the instructor to adjust the level of difficulty to enhance the learner's motivation. By regulating motivation, the learner will be more attentive and engaged to complete and acquire a particular task.

7.5.2 Instructions – "Communication is the key"

Communication is an essential competency in the health professions (Schoenherr & LeBouar, 2024). Verbal information is mainly used in healthcare simulation during pre-briefing in the form of instructions and during and after hands-on practice in the form of feedback. In the pre-brief, verbal information about the task has been found to improve learning and performance and promote critical thinking (Tyerman et al., 2016). Outlining objectives during pre-briefing is very important to learner success (Brackney & Priode, 2015). During and after simulation practice, feedback on participant performance is critical because it fosters long-lasting learning, enables students to reflect deeply on their work, and slows the loss of knowledge (Issenberg et al., 2005). Giving students oral feedback has allowed trainers to be more flexible in their questioning, allowing the students to respond right away, and provided clarification on any misunderstandings (Gardner, 2012).

Walker and Peyton's (1998) Four Step approach is the most popular and tested method of skills instruction. Instructions are delivered as follows:

Step 1. The teacher demonstrates the skill at a normal pace without any comments ("Demonstration")
Step 2. The teacher repeats the procedure, this time describing all necessary sub-steps ("Deconstruction")
Step 3. The learner has to explain each sub-step while the teacher follows the learner's instructions ("Comprehension")
Step 4. The learner performs the complete skill on his/her own ("Performance")

Giving learners clear instructions on how to perform a skill improves performance and learning. Unfortunately, many times instructors are unable to break down the steps of a skill as they have become proficient and the skill no longer requires that level of processing – that is, the instructors are in the autonomous stage and, as such, have difficulty verbalizing the steps necessary to execute the skill. Developing these steps ahead of time and preparing them in a format that is accessible to the learner and the instructor often takes significant effort; cognitive task analysis has been shown to be effective in simulation (Read & Baillie, 2013; Sullivan et al., 2014). For example, Axt et al. (2018) showed that breaking down the steps of a laparoscopy procedure into a limited number of essential key steps improved learning and internalization of the skill. Having a list of such steps not only helps with practice in the lab but also with mental rehearsal.

A frequently omitted element of instruction is errors. Instruction about the most common errors and how to avoid them improves the acquisition of psychomotor skills (Gardner et al., 2015). With error-focused training, learners experience common errors, how to correct them, and how to avoid them during training (Rogers et al., 2002). Encouraging or focusing on errors, in addition to flawless performances, during instructions can enhance learning and performance of psychomotor skills (Cheung et al., 2013; Cheung et al., 2016; Rojas et al., 2012).

Example. Verbal information can be provided in the form of learning materials, diagrams, books, online tools, and videos narrated by experts in simulation-based suturing training (Denadai et al., 2014). The skill can be broken down into steps that can benefit the learning process early on. Following Peyton's four steps, the instructor could first perform the suturing task from start to finish, then perform it a second time while verbally explaining each step as they go. After they have outlined each step in the skill, verbal information could be used to explain the rationale behind the steps. Next, the trainees could try the suturing skill for themselves while providing verbal information on the skill, just as the trainer did during their demonstration, narrating and explaining their every move. At this point the trainee will begin to internalize the steps, requiring less verbal information as they develop the skill over time. Once the trainee has performed the verbalization exercise, they should be encouraged to practice the skill independently without verbalizing each step.

According to the CPF, it is hard to learn complex psychomotor skills (e.g., intubation) without information. Verbal information needs to be provided in appropriate amounts according to the skill level of the learner, as learning might be impaired by insufficient or excessive amounts of verbal information. For instance, a novice learning how to intubate a simulated patient would benefit from more verbal information about the steps of the procedure compared to an advanced learner. Thus, the amount of verbal information provided by instructors should be reduced as the learner becomes more skilled (i.e., diminishing feedback schedule). Novices are concerned with learning the mechanics of the skill; hence, a lot of verbal information on this would be supportive during this stage of learning. Providing excessive details about the skill, however, might hinder the novice learner since details aside from how to do the skill can contribute to information overload. Therefore, limiting this kind of verbal information would be appropriate during this time. As the learner becomes more advanced, it is expected that they will have internalized the steps and no longer need this verbal information about procedural steps and mechanics. Instead, verbal information on details like the type of equipment required will offer the advanced learner something new and augment their performance.

7.5.3   Observation – "Imitation is the highest form of flattery"

Observational learning is learning by observing elements of action. It is a basic form of learning that has historically promoted the transmission of medical and therapeutic knowledge and skills across cultures (Schoenherr & Beaudoin, 2024). Asking learners in healthcare simulations to watch live or video-recorded demonstrations modeled by experts exemplifies observation learning (Ferrari, 1996; Maslovat et al., 2010; McCullagh & Weiss, 2001; Scully & Newell, 1985).

Similar to physical practice, observing others can enhance learning by generating or updating the motor schema, an organizational structure that allows for an internal mental representation of the action in the central nervous system (Cheung et al., 2016; Schmidt, 1975). Observational practice allows the learner to deduce cognitive and perceptual information by observing a particular skill. It is believed that a similar pattern of the generated action is produced inside the brain mirror neuron system modifying their own version of the action accordingly (Cheung et al., 2016).

There is a paucity of research that examines the role that observational learning plays in health professions education. A systematic review by O'Regan et al. (2016) found that observational learning can be just as effective as physically using the simulation for some, while others might prefer hands-on learning and will not benefit as much from observation. Observational learning has also been shown to be beneficial for novice healthcare learners to watch their peers go through the simulation to observe their errors and techniques (LeBel et al., 2018). This highlights the potential utility of non-expert demonstrations and links back to the idea that tremendous learning can occur by observing what not to do.

In addition, evidence suggests that observational learning might be a powerful way to prepare learners for simulation-based practice in an online environment (Cheung et al., 2016; Rojas et al., 2016; Dubrowski et al., 2021). Collectively, these studies demonstrate that providing video-based observational learning opportunities, especially ones where the learners need to interact with the videos, and ones that incorporate errors, serve as an ideal way to prepare the learners for upcoming hands-on practice, leading to more proficient first hands-on attempts, enhancing confidence and self-efficacy, and reducing of time spent in practice.

However, although observational learning in face-to-face and online preparation for practice is effective, currently no research seeks to understand if this effectiveness changes as a function of learners' level of proficiency in the skills learned. That is, one potential research avenue in this line of work should explore how observational practice can be integrated with CPF.

Example. An observational component of suturing training could be provided in the form of instructional videos conducted by a professional performing the skill, e.g., a simple suturing task. Prior to simulation training, the learner could be asked to watch a video where an expert is performing the suturing task with guided instructions on what they are doing. Cheung et al. (2016) found that those who participated in observational learning (receiving reading materials and web-based activities) one week prior to simulation training took significantly less time to perform the skill compared to those who simply read through the material before practice, i.e., the traditional approach. Cheung et al. (2016) called this phenomenon the "worked-example effect" where presenting working examples to the learners helps reduce learning task complexity, and the CPF by Guadagnoli and Lee (2004) also states that providing the learner with instructional information when the task is complex would enhance the learner's proficiency.

Conforming to the idea of joint attention (Schoenherr,2024), a demonstration of the suturing skill would offer novice and advanced learners the information needed for learning. A novice learner in suturing would benefit from observing an expert demonstrating every step being explained at a slow pace so that the information can be assimilated. A more experienced learner in suturing, on the other hand, would be better off seeing the skill in action by an expert at the expert's regular pace so that they know how the skill would be performed in a clinical setting. Whereas an advanced learner might not need to observe an expert perform a skill, they might still find observing another expert useful to reassess and reflect on their knowledge (Calvo-Merino et al., 2005). A novice learner should be shown simple sutures by an expert as they offer less complexity, allowing the learner to master the basics. As the learner advances in the suturing skill, they could be shown advanced sutures by an expert as they would offer greater complexity, allowing the learner to challenge themselves accordingly. A simulationist should consider the type of learner they are working with, either novice or advanced, in order to prepare the appropriate demonstration required according to CPF in relation to observational learning.

These observations raise the question of how best to assess the learner's current level of performance. One possibility is to employ an abbreviated version of the Objective Structured Assessments of Technical Skills (OSATS) proposed by Martin et al. (1997). Although typically OSATS are a 12-minute, minimum six-station test of technical skills scored by an expert through direct observations guided by a skill-specific checklist and global rating scales, some notable alternatives have been explored to improve the utility of this approach to quickly assess the learners. Here, a single station is set up during curricular activities. All learners rotate through the station and perform the skill to be learned once (Bann et al., 2005). The skill is scored to establish the learners' baseline.

7.5.4 Distribution of Practice – "Give the learners a break!"

Distribution of practice refers to practice periods for a particular task that are separated by periods of rest that can vary in frequency and duration (Ruch, 1928; Smith & Rothkopf, 1984). A practice schedule with no times of rest in between is known as a massed practice, whereas a practice schedule containing periods of rest is known as a distributed practice schedule (Bjerrum et al., 2016; Lee & Genovese, 1988; Schmidt et al., 2019).

Giving periods of rest to learners in between practice sessions is a viable way to diminish the cognitive overload of learners (Smith & Rothkopf, 1984). According to the American Psychological Association, cognitive overload signifies a greater demand on the working memory than what a person's mental ability is able to cope with. Having massed practice sessions can result in diminished learning as the learner can become tired and distracted throughout the session (Lee & Genovese, 1988; Smith & Rothkopf, 1984). Distributing the practice sessions provides learners with the chance to effectively recover in between sessions so they are less likely to lose attention and get tired, which results in more effective learning (Schmidt et al., 2019; Smith & Rothkopf, 1984). In addition to the immediate positives that distributing practice sessions can have on learners, there are also long-lasting benefits as it is said by Smith and Rothkopf (1984) that spaced-out practice sessions can improve memory recall, which ultimately improves retention (Moulton et al., 2006).

The scheduling of practice can provide flexible and feasible training methods through healthcare simulation. It has been shown to influence skills acquisition and retention in the psychomotor domain in varying ways (Cepeda et al., 2006). For example, Verdaasdonk et al. (2007) found that laparoscopic skills taught through a virtual reality simulator were more effective in terms of the speed of performance when done through a training schedule that was distributed over three consecutive days compared to a one-day distributed training schedule. Moulton et al. (2006) discovered that learners in the weekly distributed practice treatment performed microvascular anastomosis better on the retention test than those in the one-day distributed practice. Interestingly, in a study by Bjerrum et al. (2016), they found that there was no significant difference in skill acquisition for learning bronchoscopy skills on a simulator when comparing a daily versus weekly distribution schedule. Therefore, while there are no guidelines for the optimal practice-to-rest ratio, these studies suggest that distributed practice provides benefits to trainees, and the magnitude of its effect is dependent on the task type, task complexity, and the interval between practice sessions (Donovan & Radosevich, 1999). For a more physical task that is not very complex, such as suturing skills, a distributed practice schedule with more rest time in between might be more beneficial to the learner.

Despite the benefits of distributed practices, implementation must also be considered (Schoenherr & Hamstra, 2024). Distributed practice takes longer and requires more coordination from an administrative perspective when compared to mass practice. Unsurprisingly, a lack of time among trainees, instructors, and program facilitators has consistently been identified as a large barrier to the implementation of medical training programs (Bucklin et al., 2021; Krishnan et al., 2017; Price et al., 2010; Reis et al., 2022). When a one-day structured practice session is all that is feasible for a group of trainees, the window for facilitating true learning becomes more constrained, and the structure of said training session becomes that much more important. Considerations of training variables such as motivation, instructions, observation, variability, contextual interference, and feedback are crucial for the development of all simulation-training programs, especially when structured practice cannot be distributed, and the training program is confined to a single group session. In addition to the single group training session, program facilitators should consider including minimum time requirements for self-directed or peer-to-peer training in the simulation lab (or an alternative, suitable training space). For example, learners could be required to sign up for a 30-minute self-directed or peer-to-peer training session in the simulation lab once a week for four weeks following the group training day. This would allow trainees to accumulate practice in a distributed manner, while also minimizing additional administrative work for program facilitators. Program administrators would need to book blocks of time in the simulation lab and ensure the training equipment/learning objectives are available/clear for trainees, but the scheduling/management of individuals' training times within those blocks should be left up to the trainees to reduce administrative burden while also providing scheduling flexibility for busy trainees. An additional benefit of this format is that it does not require instructors to be onsite; the learners themselves and/or their training peers take on the role of the instructor during these additional sessions. To increase compliance, it should be made explicitly clear that self-directed or peer-to-peer training sessions are a mandatory component of the training program (Reis et al., 2022). A sign-in sheet could also be implemented in the training space for attendance tracking.

Example. Simulation-based education is an effective way to teach learners suturing skills (Emmanuel et al., 2021; Theodoulou et al., 2018), and specifically, with suturing, a distributed practice schedule is effective for knowledge retention (O'Connor et al., 1998; Theodoulou et al., 2018). To practice suturing using a simulator in a distributed fashion, educators can organize the teaching so that the learners are taught how to suture in various sessions spread out over some time so that there is a rest period in between. This will allow the learners to learn the skill during the practice session, then have time to reflect and understand what they just learned and be able to come back after rest and practice the skill again.

7.5.5   *Variability – "Repetition without repetition"*

Variability of practice is when multiple variations of a given skill are practiced (Schmidt, 1975; Schmidt et al., 2019; Shea & Kohl, 1990).

This practice condition is derived from Schmidt's (1975) schema theory of motor learning (Shea & Kohl, 1990). This theory explains that practicing psychomotor tasks that have no variability in them leads to the development of a single solution to achieve a specific motor outcome (Schmidt, 1975). Therefore, practicing a motor skill with a variety of versions leads to the development of a schema, which has many solutions to the same problem, so that the skill is effectively learned (Schmidt, 1975; Shea & Kohl, 1990). This is especially important for skill transfer and adaptability in clinical settings.

In a study by Brydges et al. (2006), the researchers assessed the effect of teaching learners how to perform one-handed knot-tying using a superficial (simple) and a deep (complex) knot-tying simulator. It was found that changing the context of the skill had an impact on both novice and experienced learners, indicating that different movement patterns had to be learned to tackle the same skill with different levels of difficulty (Brydges et al., 2006). While both contexts are essentially the same in the outcome, a new skill had to be learned to execute both scenarios, which ultimately increased the knowledge of the learners as they developed a more robust schema (Brydges et al., 2006; Schmidt, 1975).

Example. To explain this in relation to learning how to suture, if learners are given a simple superficial suture pad to learn suturing skills, they will only learn how to perform that skill under that condition. This is ideal for novice learners who are still learning the basics; however, variation is needed to increase task difficulty and optimize learning (Guadagnoli & Lee, 2004). To achieve this variation, educators can introduce different types of suturing simulators, such as deep suture pads, or perineal repair simulators, which still teach suturing, but in different ways. Another way to add variation and difficulty to suturing education is to alter the simulation environments. For example, educators can add oil onto the suture pad to simulate blood, so the learner has to accommodate for that interference, or even place the suture pad on a moving "patient" so that the learners need to account for movement. Each of these is an example of how variability can be added to simulation suture training. With these variations, the learners can learn not only how to execute a suture but also how to perform this skill in various scenarios. Increasing variability with skill level encourages the development of a rich schema (Schmidt, 1975). One question that relates to the notion of variability is how to select these variabilities. Haji et al. (2015) adopted a consensus-building methodology, specifically Delphi methods, to accomplish this. In their study, Haji and colleagues used the Delphi method to identify conditions impacting the variability of procedural skills for novice learners. They have recruited a panel of 16 advanced learners from six hospitals and universities to define and converge on a set of variations on lumbar puncture skills. This study demonstrated the feasibility of this approach and suggested that this method might be applied to the design of simulation training for other procedural and non-procedural skills, thereby advancing the agenda of theoretically based instruction design in health care simulation.

7.5.6 Contextual Interference – "Throw some curveballs"

Contextual interference is the interference that results from switching from one skill to another (e.g., suturing then intubating, i.e., between-skill variation) or changing the context in which a task is practiced from trial to trial (e.g., suturing different types of wounds or using different suturing techniques/equipment, i.e., within-skill variation) (Shea & Morgan, 1979). Practicing one task in a trial is called blocked practice and refers to a low degree of interference, whereas a high degree of interference happens when the learner practices different skills assigned at random in a trial (Guadagnoli et al., 2012).

Contextual interference consists of two types of practices, "blocked" and "random." In blocked practice, one skill is practiced multiple times before moving to a different skill. Whereas in random practice, multiple tasks are practiced in random order multiple times, the same task is not practiced in a row. Two hypotheses can help explain how contextual interference works. The first is called the "Action-plan hypothesis," which states that before performing a movement, an "action plan" is prepared in our minds. Although this plan is ready in blocked practice, in the long run, it loses effectiveness after it is retrieved from the working memory. On the other hand, random practice forces our minds to reconstruct the action plan every time we must use the skill, which results in prolonged retention of the skill (Rivard et al., 2015).

The second hypothesis called the *Elaboration-distinctiveness* approach suggests that in random practice, all of the skills remain in the working memory where the learner can compare and contrast each of the skills with one another, whereas in blocked practice, the tasks are separate and retrieved at different times putting the learner at a disadvantage since the higher processing that is happening in random practice, although more straining during practice, yields better results during retention (Rivard et al., 2015). In addition, task difficulty plays an important role in the type of contextual interference. Guadagnoli and Lee (2004) states that if the task is complex and high in difficulty, it is recommended to use blocked practice, whereas if the task is not challenging enough, then random practice can be used to elevate difficulty to a level more suitable to the skill level of the performer.

Numerous research literature used contextual interference in their studies to test its efficacy on surgical skills proficiency. Willis and colleagues (2013) used contextual interference under the name of "proactive interference" (PI) examining it when the medical students were taking a break from their main task (suturing) by subjecting them to five different learning conditions practice trials. Another study by Rivard et al. (2015) looked at whether blocked or random practice is better for skill acquisition and retention. These researchers also looked at suturing as the main skill and concluded that although acquisition in random practice is slower than in blocked practice, it was shown to allow for greater retention compared to blocked practice at the end of the study. Additionally, a study by Brydges and colleagues (2007) also looked at the effects of blocked and random practice for an orthopedic surgical task and found that blocked performance performed better than random practice on easier tasks in comparison to complex tasks. However, since orthopedic surgeries are composed of different skills that are associated with a cognitive effect, these skills should be practiced as a whole, and contextual interference was not recommended. It is important to consider the skill practiced when considering contextual interference (Brydges et al., 2007; Johnson et al., 2022).

Example. The extent to which contextual interference might improve suturing skill proficiency is dependent on how experienced the learner is in the skill. If the learner is a novice to suturing, it is best if they participate in a blocked structured practice where they only need to perform the suturing task (Guadagnoli & Lee, 2004). Since the task is very likely to be difficult for the learner who might easily get overwhelmed if they participate in multiple skills randomly assigned. Blocked practice will allow the learner to retrieve their acquired knowledge of the skill and practice it repeatedly to consolidate and improve the psychomotor skill. On the contrary, advanced learners who already know how to perform the task might find block practice very easy, and hence, a random practice might be a more ideal option (Guadagnoli & Lee, 2004). Random practice could be in the form of practicing multiple skills at random or variations of the same skill. Doing so will allow the advanced learner because it forces them to retrieve the knowledge about how to perform the skill each time they attempt to perform the skill before performing it. This coincides with the CPF that states that as the learner improves their execution of the skill, it is important for the practice to become more random to challenge the learner and enhance learning (Guadagnoli et al., 2012).

7.5.7 Feedback – "Another perspective"

Feedback, in the context of motor learning, can be defined as the information that is received during and after an action (Ende, 1983; Schmidt et al., 2019). It has been demonstrated that feedback is one of the most important features of learning psychomotor skills (Ende, 1983; Walsh et al., 2009). In the most basic form, feedback can be divided into inherent and augmented feedback. Inherent feedback is defined as the information that is naturally understood and gathered through our senses (Ende, 1983; Schmidt et al., 2019; Schoenmaker et al., 2022). Alternatively, augmented feedback supplements the inherent feedback by providing information about the movement sequence or outcome from another point of view (Ende, 1983; Schmidt et al., 2019; Schoenmaker et al., 2022). In this part of the chapter, we will focus on explaining different types of feedback and how they can be provided to learners.

Concurrent versus Terminal Feedback. When learning psychomotor skills using simulations, it is augmented feedback that is at the forefront. There are various dimensions of augmented feedback, and one important distinction is that when feedback is delivered during a simulation practice session, it is referred to as concurrent feedback (Ende, 1983; Walsh et al., 2009; Schmidt et al., 2019). While feedback is very important to learning psychomotor skills, there are instances where it can hinder the learning process (Walsh et al., 2009). This is especially true for concurrent feedback. While a learner is using a simulation to develop a psychomotor skill, they are focused on processing the inherent feedback. By providing augmented feedback at the same time, the learners' attention is disrupted, and they can no longer acquire the sensory information properly (Walsh et al., 2009). Under these conditions, the trainees do not learn at all, and they might begin to rely on the augmented feedback in order to perform the skill, rather than relying on their own procedural knowledge (Walsh et al., 2009). In other words, concurrent feedback imposes a cognitive overload on the learner so that they can no longer process their inherent feedback and will begin to rely on the augmented feedback which diminishes their overall learning experience (Walsh et al., 2009; Li et al., 2011). However, it has been found that concurrent feedback might be beneficial when dealing with novice learners who are still unfamiliar with the steps of performing a skill and need help interpreting their inherent feedback (Hadden, 1998). In these instances, concurrent feedback can improve practice performance; however, there are still implications with long-term knowledge retention suggesting that terminal feedback is a better solution (Hadden, 1998).

An alternative to concurrent feedback is terminal feedback, which is the information provided after a practice attempt (Salmoni et al., 1984; Schmidt et al., 2019). This type of feedback has been shown to positively impact knowledge retention and transfer (i.e., learning) (Walsh et al., 2009; Xeroulis et al., 2007). Terminal feedback contains two important categories: knowledge of results (KR) and knowledge of performance (KP). KR is the feedback that is given regarding the outcome of the action concerning the overall goal of the action (Salmoni et al., 1984; Schmidt et al., 2019). For example, if you think of a basketball player shooting a free throw, KR would be the coach telling the player that their throw resulted in the ball hitting the backboard too far to the right. KP is the feedback provided regarding the action movement that leads to the outcome (Ammons, 1956; Schmidt et al., 2019). Taking it back to the basketball example, when the player is shooting a free throw, their coach can comment on the angle of their arms or their stance to explain why their throw was too far to the right of the backboard. Research on terminal feedback in psychomotor skills training largely focuses on KR and not KP (Schmidt et al., 2019). This is because it is easier to measure the results of an action, compared to the performance itself, which usually requires a recording device to capture the movement (Schmidt et al., 2019). While it has been found that KP is more effective in knowledge acquisition of motor skills compared to KR, there are still some unknowns in relation to its role in simulation education (Sharma et al., 2016). This includes which type of feedback is more effective, if a combination of the two would work best, and if there are differences in the effectiveness of each type of feedback for different levels of learners (Oppici et al., 2021).

Feedback is one of the most critical components of skill acquisition. Normally, feedback is given by a knowledgeable other; these could be experts in a particular skill. These experts could be professional in the skill being learnt or other professionals (e.g., surgical skills and/or nurse educators). However, having a knowledgeable expert could be expensive and lack flexibility as these experts might not always be available, especially if the practice is being performed asynchronously at the learner's time. This leaves the need for other educational models such as dyad training, peer-assisted learning (PAL), and crowdsourcing of feedback.

Dyad training is an educational model that could replace the traditional feedback of the knowledgeable other. In dyad training, two learners partner up and take turns between practicing and observing (Shea et al., 1999). In dyad practice, partners communicate with each other and share tips and strategies, which not only help with skill acquisition but also build relationships and communication skills between partners (Granados & Wulf, 2007). Practicing in duo was shown to enhance the partners' skill retention and reduce the cost compared to individual practice (Shea et al., 1999; Granados & Wulf, 2007).

PAL is for peers who are neither professional instructors nor experts providing feedback to their other peers (Topping & Ehly, 2001). By providing feedback to their peers, learners are not only assisting others but also learning themselves. This strategy ensures that all learners get feedback in a timely and effective manner and develop teamwork skills and relationships with peers. Topping and Ehly (2001) found that PAL has similar efficiency as feedback given by a knowledgeable expert. Additionally, to be effective for skill acquisition, it is also cost-effective and provides flexibility in providing feedback when learners are learning the skill at their own time.

Crowdsourcing is another way learners could receive feedback by practicing in a large cohort of individuals. The individuals in the group do not need to be knowledgeable in all the topics, just by being part of a large cohort of individuals with different expertise, they will be able to add and acquire knowledge. Crowdsourcing was facilitated by the internet and brings a diversity of wisdom and flexibility to solve problems and acquire skills effectively (Dai et al., 2017). Dai et al. (2017) showed that crowdsourcing is cost-effective and efficient and provides quality feedback similar to expert feedback.

Feedback needs to be standardized to be an effective tool for skill acquisition. *How can feedback be structured?* The most effective way to provide feedback to learners in post-simulation environments is through OSATS (Faulkner et al. 1996; Martin et al., 1997; Reznick et al., 1997; MacRae et al., 2000). This model of testing utilizes global rating scales and skill-specific checklists to assess learners' ability to perform a skill and their knowledge retention (Faulkner et al., 1996; Martin et al., 1997; Reznick et al., 1997; MacRae et al., 2000). Other structured assessment tools are the Global Operative Assessment of Laparoscopic Skills (GOALS), and the Global Evaluative Assessment of Robotic Skills (GEARS) (Dai et al., 2017).

Example. The type and amount of feedback depend on how experienced the learner is in the skill and task difficulty. Since suturing is a complex skill with multiple steps, it is best to guide novice learners who are unfamiliar with the steps using concurrent feedback. Providing this type of feedback to novice learners will allow them to compare the practice to the feedback provided to enhance learning. However, as the learner becomes more advanced in suturing, delayed feedback should be used instead, with the amount of external feedback decreasing as expertise increases to provide the optimal level of challenge. This will allow the learners to count on their inherent feedback before obtaining any external feedback (Guadagnoli et al., 2012). Additionally, expert feedback might be preferred for novice learners, whereas more advanced learners might benefit more from other educational models such as dyad, PAL, and crowdsourcing. Having said that, it is worth noting that feedback is not recommended for easy tasks since learners might rely on the feedback rather than processing the information themselves. Instead, it is encouraged to be administered to complex tasks only (Guadagnoli et al., 2012).

7.6   Conclusion

This chapter provides a summary of the essential features required to provide training in technical skills that should be adopted by simulationists. Despite our focus on psychomotor skills, the majority of the features we have outlined (e.g., variability and distributed practice) are equally applicable to other kinds of learning. This primarily stems from the fact that the processes of automaticity and deliberation define all domains of health professions education (Gago et al., 2024; Montiero et al., 2024; Schoenherr et al., 2024) with feedback representing a form of communication that requires educators understanding the mental models of learners (Schoenherr & LeBouar, 2024).

While we have identified best practices in simulation-based education, it might not be feasible to implement these features in a specific programmatic context. Surgical skills learning engineers must therefore consider the implementation validity of their design. This requires understanding the resources (human, material, financial) and programmatic context (Schoenherr & Hamstra, 2024) and identifying when additional performance in a task will only provide minimal benefit (i.e., a performance asymptote; Schoenherr et al., 2024). Educators in the health professions must critically combine the knowledge from psychological science, neuroscience, and kinesiology in a principled manner that acknowledges and contextualizes the contributions from these fields to develop the most effective training approaches.

References

Ammons, R. B. (1956). Effects of knowledge of performance: A survey and tentative theoretical formulation. *The Journal of General Psychology*, 54(2), 279–299.

Arizo-Luque, V., Ramirez-Baena, L., Pujalte-Jesús, M. J., Rodríguez-Herrera, M. Á., Lozano-Molina, A., Arrogante, O., & Díaz-Agea, J. L. (2022). Does self-directed learning with simulation improve critical thinking and motivation of nursing students? A pre-post intervention study with the MAES© methodology. *Healthcare*, 10(5), 927. MDPI. https://doi.org/10.3390/healthcare10050927

Ávila, L. T. G., Chiviacowsky, S., Wulf, G., & Lewthwaite, R. (2012). Positive social-comparative feedback enhances motor learning in children. *Psychology of Sport and Exercise*, 13, 849–853.

Axt, S., Storz, P., Ehrenberg, C., Falch, C., Immenroth, M., Kirschniak, A., & Muller, S. (2018). Evaluation of self-educational training methods to learn laparoscopic skills–a randomized controlled trial. *BMC Medical Education*, 18(1), 85. https://doi.org/10.1186/s12909-018-1193-3

Bann, S., Khan, M., Datta, V., & Darzi, A. (2005). Surgical skill is predicted by the ability to detect errors. *The American Journal of Surgery*, 189(4), 412–415. https://doi.org/10.1016/j.amjsurg.2004.07.040. PMID: 15820451.

Barjis, J. (2011). Healthcare simulation and its potential areas and future trends. *SCS M&S Magazine*, 2(5), 1–6.

Bjerrum, A. S., Eika, B., Charles, P., & Hilberg, O. (2016). Distributed practice. The more the merrier? A randomised bronchoscopy simulation study. *Medical Education Online*, 21, 30517. https://doi.org/10.3402/meo.v21.30517

Brackney, K. D., & Priode, S. (2015). Creating context with prebriefing: A case example using simulation. *Journal of Nursing Education and Practice*, 5(1). https://libres.uncg.edu/ir/asu/f/Brackney_Dana_2015_Creating_Context_with_prebriefing.pdf

Brydges, R., Carnahan, H., Backstein, D., & Dubrowski, A. (2007). Application of motor learning principles to complex surgical tasks: Searching for the optimal practice schedule. *Journal of Motor Behavior*, 39(1), 40–48. https://doi.org/10.3200/JMBR.39.1.40-48. PMID: 17251170.

Brydges, R., Classen, R., Larmer, J., Xeroulis, G., & Dubrowski, A. (2006). Computer-assisted assessment of one-handed knot tying skills performed within various contexts: A construct validity study. *The American Journal of Surgery*, 192(1), 109–113. https://doi.org/10.1016/j.amjsurg.2005.11.014. PMID: 16769286.

Brydges, R., Dubrowski, A., & Regehr, G. (2010). A new concept of unsupervised learning: Directed self-guided learning in the health professions. *Academic Medicine*, 10 (Suppl), S49–S55. https://doi.org/10.1097/ACM.0b013e3181ed4c96. PMID: 20881703.

Brydges, R., Mallette, C., Pollex, H., Carnahan, H., & Dubrowski, A. (2012). Evaluating the influence of goal setting on intravenous catheterization skill acquisition and transfer in a hybrid simulation training context. *Simulation in Healthcare: The Journal of the Society for Simulation in Healthcare*, 7(4), 236–242. https://doi.org/10.1097/SIH.0b013e31825993f2. PMID: 22722705.

Bucklin, B. A., Asdigian, N. L., Hawkins, J. L., & Klein, U. (2021). Making it stick: Use of active learning strategies in continuing medical education. *BMC Medical Education*, 21(1), 44–44. https://doi.org/10.1186/s12909-020-02447-0

Calvo-Merino, B., Glaser, D. E., Grèzes, J., Passingham, R. E., & Haggard, P. (2005). Action observation and acquired motor skills: An fMRI study with expert dancers. *Cerebral Cortex*, 15(8), 1243–1249. https://doi.org/10.1093/cercor/bhi007

Cepeda, N. J., Pashler, H., Vul, E., Wixted, J. T., & Rohrer, D. (2006). Distributed practice in verbal recall tasks: A review and quantitative synthesis. *Psychological Bulletin*, 132, 354–380.

Cheung, J. J., Koh, J., Brett, C., Bägli, D. J., Kapralos, B., & Dubrowski, A. (2016). Preparation with web-based observational practice improves efficiency of simulation-based mastery learning. *Simulation in Healthcare: Journal of the Society for Simulation in Healthcare*, 11(5), 316–322. https://doi.org/10.1097/SIH.0000000000000171. PMID: 27388862.

Cheung, J. J., Koh, J., Mackinnon, K., Brett, C., Bägli, D., Kapralos, B., & Dubrowski, A. (2013). The use of web-based learning for simulation-based education and training of central venous catheterization in novice learners. *Studies in Health Technology and Informatics*, 184, 71–77. PMID: 23400133.

Chiniara, G., Cole, G., Brisbin, K., Huffman, D., Cragg, B., Lamacchia, M., Norman, D., & Canadian Network for Simulation in Healthcare, Guidelines Working Group (2013). Simulation in healthcare: A taxonomy and a conceptual framework for instructional design and media selection. *Medical Teacher*, 35(8), e1380–e1395. https://doi.org/10.3109/0142159X.2012.733451

Dai, J. C., Lendvay, T. S., & Sorensen, M. D. (2017). Crowdsourcing in surgical skills acquisition: A developing technology in surgical education. *Journal of Graduate Medical Education*, 9(6), 697–705. https://doi.org/10.4300/JGME-D-17-00322.1

Denadai, R., Saad-Hossne, R., Todelo, A. P., Kirylko, L., & Souto, L. R. (2014). Low-fidelity bench models for basic surgical skills training during undergraduate medical education. *Revista do Colégio Brasileiro de Cirurgiões Rev Col Bras Cir*, 41, 137–145.

Donovan, J. J., & Radosevich, D. J. (1999). A meta-analytic review of the distribution of practice effect: Now you see it, now you don't. *Journal of Applied Psychology*, 84, 795–805.

Doody, O., & Condon, M. (2013). Using a simulated environment to support students learning clinical skills. *Nurse Education in Practice*, 13(6), 561–566.

Drews, R., Chiviacowsky, S., & Wulf, G. (2013). Children's motor skill learning is influenced by their conceptions of ability. *Journal of Motor Learning and Development*, 1, 38–44. https://doi.org/10.1123/jmld.1.2.38

Dubrowski, A. (2005). Performance vs. learning curves: What is motor learning and how is it measured? *Surgical Endoscopy*, 19(9), 1290. https://doi.org/10.1007/s00464-004-8261-y

Dubrowski, A., & Backstein, D. (2004). The contributions of kinesiology to surgical education. *The Journal of Bone and Joint Surgery*. American volume, 86(12), 2778–2781. https://doi.org/10.2106/00004623-200412000-00029

Dubrowski, A., Kapralos, B., Peisachovich, E., Da Silva, C., & Torres, A. (2021). A model for an online learning management system for simulation-based acquisition of psychomotor skills in health professions education. *Cureus*, 13(3), e14055. https://doi.org/10.7759/cureus.14055. PMID: 33898139; PMCID: PMC8060984.

Dubrowski, A., & MacRae, H. (2006). Randomised, controlled study investigating the optimal instructor: Student ratios for teaching suturing skills. *Medical Education,* 40(1), 59–63. https://doi.org/10.1111/j.1365-2929.2005.02347.x

Dweck, C. S. (1999). *Self-theories: Their role in motivation, personality, and development.* Psychology Press.

Emmanuel, T., Nicolaides, M., Theodoulou, I., Yoong, W., Lymperopoulos, N., & Sideris, M. (2021). Suturing skills for medical students: A systematic review. *In Vivo,* 35(1), 1–12. https://doi.org/10.21873/invivo.12226

Ende, J. (1983). Feedback in clinical medical education. *The Journal of the American Medical Association,* 250(6), 777–781.

Escher, C., Rystedt, H., Creutzfeldt, J., Meurling, L., Nyström, S., Dahlberg, J., Edelbring, S., Nordahl Amorøe, T., Hult, H., Felländer-Tsai, L., & Abrandt-Dahlgren, M. (2017). Method matters: Impact of in-scenario instruction on simulation-based teamwork training. *Advances in Simulation* (London, England), 2, 25. https://doi.org/10.1186/s41077-017-0059-9

Faulkner, H., Regehr, G., Martin, J., & Reznick, R. (1996). Validation of an objective structured assessment of technical skill for surgical residents. *Academic Medicine: Journal of the Association of American Medical Colleges,* 71(12), 1363–1365. https://doi.org/10.1097/00001888-199612000-00023

Feil, P. H., Guenzel, P. J., Knight, G. W., & Geistfeld, R. (1994). Designing preclinical instruction for psychomotor skills (I)—Theoretical foundations of motor skill performance and their applications to dental education. *Journal of Dental Education,* 58(11–12), 806–812.

Ferrari, M. (1996). Observing the Observer: Self-regulation in the observational learning of motor skills. *Developmental Review,* 16(2), 203–240. https://doi.org/10.1006/drev.1996.0008

Fitts, P. M., & Posner, M. I. (1967). *Human performance.* Brooks/Cole Publishing Company.

Gardner, A. K., Abdelfattah, K., Wiersch, J., Ahmed, R. A., & Willis, R. E. (2015). Embracing errors in simulation-based training: The effect of error training on retention and transfer of central venous catheter skills. *Journal of Surgical Education,* 72(6), e158–e162. https://doi.org/10.1016/j.jsurg.2015.08.002

Gardner, J. (Ed.) (2012). *Assessment and learning.* SAGE Publications Ltd. https://dx.doi.org/10.4135/9781446250808

George, J. H., & Doto, F. X. (2001). A simple five-step method for teaching clinical skills. *Family Medicine,* 33(8), 577–578.

Granados, C., & Wulf, G. (2007). Enhancing motor learning through dyad practice: Contributions of observation and dialogue. *Research Quarterly for Exercise and Sport,* 78(3), 197–203. https://doi.org/10.1080/02701367.2007.10599417

Grantcharov, T. P., & Reznick, R. K. (2008). Teaching procedural skills. *BMJ (Clinical Research Ed.),* 336(7653), 1129–1131. https://doi.org/10.1136/bmj.39517.686956.47

Guadagnoli, M., & Lee, T. D. (2004). Challenge point: A framework for conceptualizing the effects of various practice conditions in motor learning. *Journal of Motor Behavior,* 36, 212–224. http://dx.doi.org/10.3200/JMBR.36.2.212-224

Guadagnoli, M., Morin, M. P., & Dubrowski, A. (2012). The application of the challenge point framework in medical education. *Medical Education,* 46(5), 447–453. https://doi.org/10.1111/j.1365-2923.2011.04210.x

Hadden, C. M. (1998). Concurrent vs. Terminal Augmented Feedback in the Learning of a Discrete Bimanual Coordination Task. https://doi.org/10.31390/gradschool_disstheses.6735

Haji, F. A., Khan, R., Regehr, G., Ng, G., de Ribaupierre, S., Dubrowski, A. (2015). Operationalising elaboration theory for simulation instruction design: A Delphi study. *Medical Education*, 49(6), 576–588. https://doi.org/10.1111/medu.12726. PMID: 25989406.

Issenberg, S. B., McGaghie, W. C., Petrusa, E. R., Lee Gordon, D., & Scalese, R. J. (2005). Features and uses of high-fidelity medical simulations that lead to effective learning: A BEME systematic review. *Medical Education*, 27, 10–28. https://doi.org/10.1080/01421590500046924

Johnson, G. G. R. J., Park, J., Vergis, A., Gillman, L. M., & Rivard, J. D. (2022). Contextual interference for skills development and transfer in laparoscopic surgery: A randomized controlled trial. *Surgical Endoscopy*, 36(9), 6377–6386. https://doi.org/10.1007/s00464-021-08946-5

Jowett, N., LeBlanc, V., Xeroulis, G., MacRae, H., & Dubrowski, A. (2007). Surgical skill acquisition with self-directed practice using computer-based video training. *The American Journal of Surgery*, 193(2), 237–242. https://doi.org/10.1016/j.amjsurg.2006.11.003. PMID: 17236854.

Kantak, S. S., & Winstein, C. J. (2012). Learning-performance distinction and memory processes for motor skills: A focused review and perspective. *Behavioural Brain Research*, 228(1), 219–231. https://doi.org/10.1016/j.bbr.2011.11.028

Kothari, A., McCutcheon, C., & Graham, I. D. (2017). Defining integrated knowledge translation and moving forward: A response to recent commentaries. *International Journal of Health Policy and Management*, 6(5), 299–300. https://doi.org/10.15171/ijhpm.2017.15

Kovacs, G. (1997). Procedural skills in medicine: Linking theory to practice. *Journal of Emergency Medicine*, 15(3), 387–391.

Krishnan, D. G., Keloth, A. V., & Ubedulla, S. (2017). Pros and cons of simulation in medical education: A review. *Education*, 3(6), 84–87.

LeBel, M. E., Haverstock, J., Cristancho, S., van Eimeren, L., & Buckingham, G. (2018). Observational learning during simulation-based training in arthroscopy: Is it useful to novices? *Journal of Surgical Education*, 75(1), 222–230.

Lee, T. D., & Genovese, E. D. (1988). Distribution of practice in motor skill acquisition: Learning and performance effects reconsidered. *Research Quarterly for Exercise and Sport*, 59(4), 277–287. https://doi.org/10.1080/02701367.1988.10609373

Lewthwaite, R., & Wulf, G. (2010a). Grand challenge for movement science and sport psychology: Embracing the social-cognitive-affective-motor nature of motor behavior. *Frontiers in Psychology*, 1 (Article 42), 1–3. https://doi.org/10.3389/fpsyg.2010.00042

Li, Q., Ma, E. L., Liu, J., Fang, L. Q., & Xia, T. (2011). Pre-training evaluation and feedback improve medical students' skills in basic life support. *Medical Teacher*, 33(10), e549–e555. https://doi.org/10.3109/0142159X.2011.600360

MacRae, H., Regehr, G., Leadbetter, W., & Reznick, R. K. (2000). A comprehensive examination for senior surgical residents. *American Journal of Surgery*, 179(3), 190–193. https://doi.org/10.1016/s0002-9610(00)00304-4

Martin, J. A., Regehr, G., Reznick, R., MacRae, H., Murnaghan, J., Hutchison, C., & Brown, M. (1997). Objective structured assessment of technical skill (OSATS) for surgical residents. *The British Journal of Surgery*, 84(2), 273–278. https://doi.org/10.1046/j.1365-2168.1997.02502.x

Maslovat, D., Hayes, S. J., Horn, R., & Hodges, N. J. (2010). *Motor learning through observation: Vision and goal-directed movement: Neurobehavioural perspectives.* Human Kinetics, pp 315–339.

Maxwell, J. P., Masters, R. S., Kerr, E., & Weedon, E. (2001). The implicit benefit of learning without errors. *The Quarterly Journal of Experimental Psychology. A, Human Experimental Psychology*, 54(4), 1049–1068. https://doi.org/10.1080/713756014

McCullagh, P. & Weiss, M. (2001). Modeling: Considerations for motor skill performance and psychological responses. In *Handbook of sport psychology*, vol. 2, Hoboken: Wiley Publishing, pp. 205–238.

Michels, M. E. J., Evans, D. E. & Blok, G. A. (2012) What is a clinical skill? Searching for order in chaos through a modified Delphi process. *Medical Teacher*, 34(8), e573–e581. https://doi.org/10.3109/0142159X.2012.669218

Motola, I., Devine, L. A., Chung, H. S., Sullivan, J. E., & Issenberg, S. B. (2013). Simulation in healthcare education: A best evidence practical guide. AMEE Guide No. 82. *Medical Teacher*, 35(10), e1511–e1530. https://doi.org/10.3109/0142159X.2013.818632

Moulton, C. A., Dubrowski, A., Macrae, H., Graham, B., Grober, E., & Reznick, R. (2006). Teaching surgical skills: What kind of practice makes perfect?: A randomized, controlled trial. *Annals of Surgery*, 244(3), 400–409. https://doi.org/10.1097/01.sla.0000234808.85789.6a. PMID: 16926566; PMCID: PMC1856544.

Nousiainen, M., Brydges, R., Backstein, D., & Dubrowski, A. (2008). Comparison of expert instruction and computer-based video training in teaching fundamental surgical skills to medical students. *Surgery*, 143(4):539–544. https://doi.org/10.1016/j.surg.2007.10.022. PMID: 18374052.

O'Connor, M., Mcgraw, R., Killen, L., & Reich, D. (1998). A computer-based training module for suturing \[1] self-directed basic. *Medical Teacher*, 20(3), 203–206. https://doi.org/10.1080/01421599880922

Oppici, L., Dix, A., & Narciss, S. (2021). When is knowledge of performance (KP) superior to knowledge of results (KR) in promoting motor skill learning? A systematic review. *International Review of Sport and Exercise Psychology*, 14, 1–25.

O'Regan, S., Molloy, E., Watterson, L., & Nestel, D. (2016). Observer roles that optimise learning in healthcare simulation education: A systematic review. *Advances in Simulation*, 1(1), 1–10. https://doi.org/10.1186/s41077-015-0004-8

Palmer, K., Chiviacowsky, S., & Wulf, G. (2016). Enhanced expectancies facilitate golf putting. *Psychology of Sport and Exercise*, 22, 229–232. https://doi.org/10.1016/j.psychsport.2015.08.009

Perry, S., Bridges, S. M., & Burrow, M. F. (2022). A conceptual model for clinical psychomotor skill development in an era of simulated and virtual reality. *European Journal of Dental Education*, 26(2), 263–276. https://doi.org/10.1111/eje.12699

Peyre, S. E, & Ashley, S. W. (2011). Teaching uncommon and highly complex operations: Maximizing the teaching and learning. *Journal of Gastrointestinal Surgery*, 15(10), 1724–1725. https://doi.org/10.1007/s11605-011-1570-2

Price, D. W., Miller, E. K., Rahm, A. K., Brace, N. E., & Larson, R. S. (2010). Assessment of barriers to changing practice as CME outcomes. *The Journal of Continuing Education in the Health Professions*, 30(4), 237–245. https://doi.org/10.1002/chp.20088

Read, E. & Baillie, S. (2013). Using Cognitive Task Analysis to Create a Teaching Protocol for Bovine Dystocia. *Journal of Veterinary Medical Education*, 40(4), 397–401.

Reis, T., Faria, I., Serra, H., & Xavier, M. (2022). Barriers and facilitators to implementing a continuing medical education intervention in a primary health care setting. *BMC Health Services Research*, 22(1), 1–13. https://doi.org/10.1186/s12913-022-08019-w

Reznick, R., Regehr, G., MacRae, H., Martin, J., & McCulloch, W. (1997). Testing technical skill via an innovative "bench station" examination. *American Journal of Surgery*, 173(3), 226–230. https://doi.org/10.1016/s0002-9610(97)89597-9

Rivard, J. D., Vergis, A. S., Unger, B. J., Gillman, L. M., Hardy, K. M., & Park, J. (2015). The effect of blocked versus random task practice schedules on the acquisition and retention of surgical skills. *American Journal of Surgery*, 209(1), 93–100. https://doi.org/10.1016/j.amjsurg.2014.08.038

Rogers, D. A., Regehr, G., & MacDonald, J. (2002). A role for error training in surgical technical skill instruction and evaluation. *American Journal of Surgery*, 183(3), 242–245. https://doi.org/10.1016/s0002-9610(02)00798-5

Rojas, D., Cheung, J. J., Weber, B., Kapralos, B., Carnahan, H., Bägli, D. J., & Dubrowski, A. (2012). An online practice and educational networking system for technical skills: Learning experience in expert facilitated vs. independent learning communities. *Studies in Health Technology and Informatics*, 173, 393–397. PMID: 22357024.

Rojas, D., Kapralos, B., & Dubrowski, A. (2016). The role of game elements in online learning within health professions education. *Studies in Health Technology and Informatics*, 220, 329–334. PMID: 27046600.

Ruch, T. C. (1928). Factors influencing the relative economy of massed and distributed practice in learning. *Psychological Review*, 35(1), 19.

Salmoni, A. W., Schmidt, R. A., & Walter, C. B. (1984). Knowledge of results and motor learning: A review and critical reappraisal. *Psychological Bulletin*, 95(3), 355–386. https://doi.org/10.1037/0033-2909.95.3.355

Sanli, E. A., Patterson, J. T., Bray, S. R., & Lee, T. D. (2013). Understanding self-controlled motor learning protocols through the self-determination theory. *Frontiers in Psychology*, 3, 611. https://doi.org/10.3389/fpsyg.2012.00611

Schmidt, R. A. (1975). A schema theory of discrete motor skill learning. *Psychological Review*, 82(4), 225–260. https://doi.org/10.1037/h0076770

Schmidt, R. A., Zelaznik, H. N., Wulf, G., Winstein, C. J., & Lee, T. D. (2019). *Motor control and learning: A behavioral emphasis*. Human Kinetics.

Schoenherr, J. R., Mahias-Ito, Y., & Li, X. Y. (2024). Collective competence and social learning in the health professions: learning, thinking, and deciding in groups. In Schoenherr, J. R. (ed.), *Fundamentals and Frontiers in Medical Education and Decision-Making: Innovation, Implementation, and Translational Research*. Routledge.

Schoenherr, J. R., Waechter, J., & Lee, C. H. (2024). Quantifying Expertise in the Healthcare Professions: Cognitive Efficiency and Metacognitive Calibration. In Schoenherr, J. R. & McConnell, M. M. (eds.), *Fundamentals and frontiers of medical education and decision-making: Educational theory and psychological practice*. New York: Routledge.

Schoenmaker, J., Houdijk, H., Steenbergen, B., Reinders-Messelink, H. A., & Schoemaker, M. M. (2022). Effectiveness of different extrinsic feedback forms on motor learning in children with cerebral palsy: A systematic review. *Disability and Rehabilitation*, 1–14. https://doi.org/10.1080/09638288.2022.2060333

Scully, D. M., & Newell, K. M. (1985). Observational learning and the acquisition of motor skills: Toward a visual perception perspective. *Journal of Human Movement Studies*, 11, 169–186.

Sharma, D. A., Chevidikunnan, M. F., Khan, F. R., & Gaowgzeh, R. A. (2016). Effectiveness of knowledge of result and knowledge of performance in the learning of a skilled motor activity by healthy young adults. *Journal of Physical Therapy Science*, 28(5), 1482–1486. https://doi.org/10.1589/jpts.28.1482

Shea, C. H., & Kohl, R. M. (1990). Specificity and variability of practice. *Research Quarterly for Exercise and Sport*, 61(2), 169–177. https://doi.org/10.1080/02701 367.1990.10608671

Shea, C. H., Wulf, G., & Whitacre, C. (1999). Enhancing training efficiency and effectiveness through the use of Dyad training. *Journal of Motor Behavior*, 31(2), 119–125. https://doi.org/10.1080/00222899909600983

Shea, J. B., & Morgan, R. L. (1979). Contextual interference effects on the acquisition, retention, and transfer of a motor skill. *Journal of Experimental Psychology: Human Learning and Memory*, 5(2), 179–187. https://doi.org/ 10.1037/0278-7393.5.2.179

Smith, S. M., & Rothkopf, E. Z. (1984). Contextual enrichment and distribution of practice in the classroom. *Cognition and Instruction*, 1(3), 341–358.

Soderstrom, N. C., & Bjork, R. A. (2015). Learning versus performance: An integrative review. *Perspectives on Psychological Science: A Journal of the Association for Psychological Science*, 10(2), 176–199. https://doi.org/10.1177/174569161 5569000

Sullivan, M. E., Yates, K. A., Inaba, K., Lam, L., & Clark, R. E. (2014). The use of cognitive task analysis to reveal the instructional limitations of experts in the teaching of procedural skills. *Academic Medicine: Journal of the Association of American Medical Colleges*, 89(5), 811–816. https://doi.org/10.1097/ACM.00000 00000000224

Taylor, J. A., & Ivry, R. B. (2012). The role of strategies in motor learning. *Annals of the New York Academy of Sciences*, 1251, 1–12. https://doi.org/10.1111/ j.1749-6632.2011.06430.x

Theodoulou, I., Nicolaides, M., Athanasiou, T., Papalois, A., & Sideris, M. (2018). Simulation-based learning strategies to teach undergraduate students basic surgical skills: A systematic review. *Journal of Surgical Education*, 75(5), 1374–1388. https:// doi.org/10.1016/j.jsurg.2018.01.013

Tolsgaard, M. G. (2013). Clinical skills training in undergraduate medical education using a student-centered approach. *Danish Medical Journal*, 60(8), B4690.

Topping, K. J., & Ehly, S. W. (2001). Peer assisted learning: A framework for consultation. *Journal of Educational and Psychological Consultation*, 12(2), 113–132. https://doi. org/10.1207/S1532768XJEPC1202_03

Tyerman, J., Luctkar-Flude, M., Graham, L., Coffey, S., & Olsen-Lynch, E. (2016). Pre-simulation preparation and briefing practices for healthcare professionals and students. *JBI Database of Systematic Reviews and Implementation Reports*, 14(8), 80–89. https://doi.org/10.11124/jbisrir-2016-003055

Verdaasdonk, E. G., Stassen, L. P., van Wijk, R. P., & Dankelman, J. (2007). The influence of different training schedules on the learning of psychomotor skills for endoscopic surgery. *Surgical Endoscopy*, 21, 214–219.

Walker, M., & Peyton, J. W. R. (1998). *Teaching in theatre. Teaching and learning in medical practice*. Rickmansworth, UK: Manticore Europe Limited, 171–180.

Walsh, C. M., Ling, S. C., Wang, C. S., & Carnahan, H. (2009). Concurrent versus terminal feedback: It may be better to wait. *Academic Medicine*, 84(10), S54–S57. doi: https://doi.org/10.1097/ACM.0b013e3181b38daf

Willis, R. E., Curry, E., & Gomez, P. P. (2013). Practice schedules for surgical skills: The role of task characteristics and proactive interference on psychomotor skills acquisition. *Journal of Surgical Education*, 70(6), 789–795. https://doi.org/10.1016/j.jsurg.2013.06.014. Epub 2013 Aug 6. PMID: 24209657.

Wulf, G., Chiviacowsky, S., & Lewthwaite, R. (2012). Altering mindset can enhance motor learning in older adults. *Psychology and Aging*, 27(1), 14–21. https://doi.org/10.1037/a0025718

Xeroulis, G. J., Park, J., Moulton, C. A., Reznick, R. K., Leblanc, V., & Dubrowski, A. (2007). Teaching suturing and knot-tying skills to medical students: A randomized controlled study comparing computer-based video instruction and (concurrent and summary) expert feedback. *Surgery*, 141(4), 442–449. https://doi.org/10.1016/j.surg.2006.09.012

8
QUANTIFYING EXPERTISE IN THE HEALTHCARE PROFESSIONS

Cognitive Efficiency and Metacognitive Calibration

Jordan Richard Schoenherr, Jason Waechter, and Chel Hee Lee

8.1 Introduction

The dynamic environments of healthcare are frequently defined by limited time and information. Achieving effective patient outcomes in these conditions requires quickly narrowing a practitioner's focus of attention to a set of diagnostic cues (e.g., symptoms, history; Krupinski et al., 2006), weighing the evidence to identify the most likely disease model, and responding in an appropriate and timely manner (Norman et al., 2018). As learners transition from novice to expert in an area of practice (Montiero et al., 2024), their ability to recognize and respond to patterns often requires less reflection and deliberation. However, the need for rapid responses makes clinical decision-making susceptible to errors. To ensure effective delivery of care, education and training programs must not only ensure that learners can accurately diagnose and provide treatment recommendations but must also be capable of adapting to limited time.

Despite increased speed in their responses, experienced experts must also recognize when a situation requires more time and attention (Moulton et al., 2007; Moulton et al., 2010). What might initially appear to be a common illness, can turn out to be another, e.g. heart attack for acid reflux, fibrotic breast tissues for breast cancer. Healthcare professionals (HCPs) must also engage in extensive self-directed learning (e.g., Abrham et al., 2011; Lefore et al., 2007; Li et al., 2010; Peine et al., 2016; Yang et al., 2021) which requires reflection on their knowledge and abilities, referred to as metacognition.

Metacognitive strategies are widely regarded as an effective means to reduce biases resulting from automatic responses, by monitoring behavior,

DOI: 10.4324/9781003316091-10

identifying errors, and regulating our responses (e.g., Croskerry, 2000; Croskerry & Norman, 2008; Kosior et al., 2019; Medina et al., 2017; Quirk, 2006; cf. Graber, 2003). Studies have repeated demonstrated that metacognitive assessments of performance are subject to a variety of biases including overconfidence (OC) in prior knowledge (Fischhoff et al., 1977; Moore & Healy, 2008; West & Stanovich, 1997) or believing that they have more knowledge than they do (i.e., overclaiming; Paulhus et al., 2003; Paulhus & Harms, 2004; cf. Hoffman et al., 2022; Ludeke & Makransky, 2016). These biases are not confined to the public but can also be observed in medical decision-making (Baumann et al., 1991; Oskamp, 1965; Naguib et al., 2019; Schoenherr et al., 2018; for a review, see Berner & Graber, 2008) and education (Borracci & Arribalzaga, 2018; Brezis et al., 2019; Massoth et al., 2019; Sanchez & Dunning, 2018). Medical education requires the development of assessment methods that can identify learners' metacognitive accuracy and assess changes over time and between conditions (for complementary approaches, see Gago et al., 2024).

This chapter describes methods of operationalizing HCP expertise along two dimensions: cognitive efficiency and metacognitive calibration. Efficiency is often a poorly defined construct in the healthcare professions, having a dual meaning related to both organizational resources and cognitive resources. Here, we operationalize expertise in terms of an absence of a speed-accuracy trade-off (SAT), such that expertise development requires demonstrating that learners are both faster and more accurate when performing a clinical reasoning task. To demonstrate the utility of an SAT-based approach to expertise, we provide a reanalysis of learner's response accuracy and the speed of their responses in diagnosing an electrocardiogram (ECG) to demonstrate the utility of this method (Waechter et al., 2019).

Alone, efficiency fails to recognize whether clinicians are aware of the limits of their own competencies. In the remainder of the chapter, we present methods for assessing learners' metacognitive abilities. Rather than simply examining a learner's subjective confidence or self-efficacy, we describe calibration indices that capture systematic biases defined by discrepancies between a learner's accuracy and confidence when engaged in professional activities. We argue that, together, the widespread adoption of SAT analyses and calibration indices can ensure a more comprehensive determination of learners' competencies.

8.1.1 The Speed of Thought in Medical Decision-Making

Pattern recognition arguably represents the core of expertise in healthcare (Montiero et al., 2024). Learners must be capable of identifying visual, auditory, haptic, and olfactory patterns that are associated with mental models of a disease (Schoenherr & Le-Bouar, 2024). During the initial stages of learning, the accumulation of evidence requires significant time as novices search people, objects, and environments for diagnostic cues (e.g., Blair et al., 2009). As learners gain more experience, the time taken to complete a task decreases. This process of decreasing effort and response time (RT) is referred to as *automaticity* (Logan, 1988; Schneider & Shiffrin, 1977).

Automaticity is a defining feature of all forms of expertise (e.g., Ericsson, 2007) and features prominently in models of expertise development (e.g., Dreyfus & Dreyfus, 1980; Fitts & Posner, 1967; Abdo et al., 2024). However, rather than increasing the speed of evidence gathering and assessment, reductions in RT can be attributed to the selective processing of evidence (Saling & Philips, 2007). For instance, studies of clinical expertise have found that HCPs focus on diagnostic cues and begin to ignore nondiagnostic information, thereby speeding up their responses (Krupinski et al., 2006).

Rather than assume that later stages of learning are defined by automaticity, models have suggested that reflective cognition occurs in parallel (Norman & Shallice, 1986). Perhaps the most comprehensive model is that provided by Ashby and colleagues (Ashby et al., 1998; Ashby & Valentin, 2017), who assume that explicit verbal systems and implicit nonverbal systems compete during response selection. In this model, effortful processes ('Type 2') such as explicit clinical reasoning dominate the early stages of response selection. Concurrently, comparatively effortless processes ('Type 1')[1] accumulate memory traces of multisensory patterns, creating a basis for clinical intuition. Over time, Type 1 processes begin to become as fast as response selection, leading to a period of high response conflict. Subsequently, Type 1 processes dominate response selection; however, Type 2 processes can monitor the environment for conflicting patterns and regulate behavior if enough conflicting evidence is detected.

Expertise in the healthcare profession is not simply about automaticity. The shift to automaticity can create trade-offs in decision-making. These findings also apply to health professions education. For instance, repeatedly exposing learners to the same task, will not promote generalization from the learning activity to the context of professional practice (Grierson, 2014; see Abdo et al., 2024). Empirical research supports problems with an overreliance on automaticity. Relying exclusively on 'clinical decision-making' (intuition) can often lead to errors in comparison to 'statistical decision-making' (effortful accumulation, weighting, and integration of evidence; Meehl, 1954; for reviews, see Ægisdóttir et al., 2006; Grove et al., 2000). For instance, a meta-analysis of the relationship between 'thinking styles' and performance, found that performance was negatively associated with the use of intuition but positively associated with experience (Philips et al., 2016).

Automaticity trade-offs have also been observed in medical decision-making. During a task that required experienced radiologists to search for the presence of cancer, Drew et al. (2013) found that they frequently overlooked anomalous patterns present in images that were not directly related to their current diagnostic goals (for related examples, see Krupinski et al., 2006; Lum et al., 2005; Potchen, 2006; Williams et al., 2021). Studies have also demonstrated that a clinician's ability to identify a visual pattern can precede clinical diagnostic reasoning (Kelly et al., 2016). Such cognitive factors are frequently associated with diagnostic errors (Graber et al., 2005; Schiff et al., 2009). Given that medical errors can result in a failure to adequately examine and assess symptoms, consider appropriate diagnoses, and consider the availability treatment options (Classen et al., 2011; Kohn et al., 1999; Landrigan et al., 2010; Leape et al., 1993; Makary & Daniel, 2016), metacognitive strategies must be developed to to stop at critical stages of the decision-making process (Croskerry, 2000; Moulton et al., 2007; Moulton et al., 2010).

8.2 Automaticity and Efficiency in Healthcare: Pattern Recognition and Heuristics

Clinical decision-making requires that a clinician can make both fast and accurate decisions. Often, these two criteria are in opposition to one another (Henmon, 1911; MacKay, 1982; Wickelgren, 1977; for a recent review, see Heitz, 2014). Effective diagnosis and treatment can often require an extensive review of considerable information, weighing numerous diagnoses and prognoses, and considering the appropriate courses of treatment given resource limitations, while assessing confidence in their performance. Clinical contexts, such as critical or intensive care, often require that decisions be made rapidly to stabilize a patient or to identify whether one patient requires immediate treatment in a triage situation. Health professions education must develop methods to to assess these facets of clinical competency(Schoenherr, 2020).

Institutional Efficiency. The inherent problem of balancing the demands of accurate diagnosis and expedient healthcare delivery has rarely been considered systematically. For instance, the delivery of care has often been considered in terms of 'efficiency' (e.g., Braddock et al. 2008; Cochrane, 1972; Evans et al., 1991; Milstein & Lee, 2007; Perkins et al., 2012). In healthcare, efficiency has two broad meanings. The first meaning of efficiency relates to the use of the resources of the healthcare system, or *institutional efficiency.* In education, this includes consideration of financial cost (e.g., Salkever et al., 1982) and the number of learners that can be trained within a given task, course, or within the program (e.g., Wulf et al., 2010). In healthcare delivery, this includes the number of practitioners and resources required to treat people within a community. In this sense, efficiency represents a kind of evidence that supports the implementation validity of an educational activity (Schoenherr & Hamstra, 2024).

A recent example of an empirical approach that can be used to inform institutional efficiency was provided by Millington et al. (2017). They examined learners who were provided with extensive training in a lung ultrasound (US) from two institutions. Using a thoracic sonography competency assessment instrument (Assessment of Competency in Thoracic Sonography or ACTS), they were able to demonstrate that learners' performance rapidly increased during early training sessions, but the relative gains in performance leveled off, creating a *performance asymptote*, i.e. ceiling. They suggested that the slope of the response function can be used to inform program evaluation strategies, such that educators provide learners with different tasks once learners are no longer gaining significant benefits from the same educational intervention. This method is also supported by approaches to entrustable professional activities (EPAs; Ma, 2024).

While Millington et al.'s suggestion provides a principled means to inform curriculum development in health professions education programs, an exclusive focus on accuracy assumes that this is the only basis for the assessment of cognitive efficiency. In healthcare delivery settings such as critical/intensive care units and emergency rooms, HCPs must not only be accurate, they must also respond in a timely manner. Consequently, multiple performance dimensions should be considered together.

Cognitive Efficiency. The second formulation of efficiency concerns a clinician's mental resources relative to the decision-making context, or *cognitive efficiency*. For instance, Mauksch et al. (2008) suggested that efficient decisions are those that make 'the best use of available time' (p. 1388). In these cases, the implication is that learners were accurate and that they acted quickly. Such a definition is formally provided by Braddock et al. (2008), noting that efficiency is based on decision quality ('informed decision-making') and the RT.

Formally, cognitive efficiency can be understood in terms of heuristics and biases (Gilovich et al., 2002; Kahneman et al., 1982). For instance, the bounded rationality approach to decision-making assumes that choices occur in environments defined by limited informational, temporal, and cognitive resources (Simon, 1956). In these 'wicked environments', learners typically receive only limited feedback relative to the complex tasks expected of them (Hogarth, 2001). Decision-makers must then use heuristics to respond (Kahneman & Klein, 2009; Gigerenzer & Gaissmaier, 2011).

While the use of general heuristics can lead to systematic errors (i.e., biases), heuristics can facilitate decision-making by accounting for the specific affordances of the situation, i.e., ecological rationality (Gigerenzer & Selten, 2002). The ecological rationality approach assumes that decision-makers must consider the trade-off between performance accuracy and effort, i.e., accuracy-effort trade-off (Gigerenzer & Brighton, 2009).

8.2.1 Speeded Responses, Efficiency, and Performance Trade-Offs

Many studies of perception and decision-making operationalize this problem in terms of a SAT. SATs are defined by situations wherein a decision-maker's accuracy decreases with the speed of their responses (Henmon, 1911; MacKay, 1982; Wickelgren, 1977; Woodworth, 1899). SATs will naturally arise in healthcare settings, as practitioners must make many rapid decisions, often leading to cognitive errors. Cognitive errors have been identified as a major cause of diagnostic errors (Graber et al., 2005) and can occur throughout the course of diagnosis and treatment (Schiff et al., 2009). Consequently, HCPs must develop effective decision-making strategies to address these concerns (Croskerry, 2003; Moulton et al., 2007). However, given that there is evidence that merely increasing the amount of deliberation does not necessarily result in improved performance (Norman et al., 2014), additional research is required to understand the relationship between speed and accuracy. However, studies of health professions education that do consider both speed and accuracy consider them independently rather than conjointly (e.g., Grierson et al., 2013; Waechter et al., 2019).

In that successful performance can be the result of either effortful deliberation or automatic pattern recognition, evidence for automaticity tends to focus on RT. Tasks that are thought to vary in terms of increasing difficulty due to the introduction of more factors should demonstrate increases in RT, leading to a pattern of additivity (e.g., Donders, 1868; Fan et al., 2005: Merkel, 1885; Sanders, 1967). For instance, Donders (1868) assumed that complex tasks were simply the sum of simpler tasks. For instance, diagnosing a patient and providing a prognosis, represents the sum of the time taken to perceive symptoms, retrieve anatomical and physiological knowledge from memory, compare a patient's tissue to patterns retrieved from memory, identify the associated treatment, and execute motor programs for verbal communication and manual treatment.

In contrast to an additive pattern of RT, researchers often find patterns of *overadditivity* and *underadditivity*. Overadditivity is observed when a complicated task takes longer than would be predicted by the sum of the constituent individual tasks. *Underadditive* is observed when a complicated task takes less time than would be predicted by sum of the constituent individual tasks. While overadditivity represents a situation wherein the features of a task affect multiple processes (e.g., conversations in the operating room can affect low-level perceptual identification processes and high-level cognition; Sanders, 1980), underadditivity suggests that a *different* cognitive process is responsible for performing the task, i.e., that performance has become automatic and no longer relies on controlled processes. Violations of additivity have been used to argue for two distinct decision-making and learning systems, i.e. Type 1 and Type 2 processes (Ridderinkhof et al., 1995).

Measures of SAT can be used to understanding the processes and strategies learners use to respond in a decision-making task (Donkin et al., 2014).

Slow and Fast Guessing. In addition to examining whether an overall SAT is evidenced, learners response strategies can also be examined. When clinicians make a choice, they accumulate evidence given a number of possible response (diagnostic) alternatives (e.g., Vickers & Packer, 1982). Trade-offs can be understood in these terms. Adopting this approach, Petrusic (1992) introduced Slow-and-Fast Guessing Theory (SFGT). In addition to overall SATs, Petrusic (1992) additionally assumed that learners adopt response strategies that can be identified by examining the mistakes produced by decision-makers when they attempt to answer a question. For ease of assessment, individual decision-making strategies can be classified as *slow guessing* and *fast guessing* depending on the amount of information they attempt to gather in a situation. Clinicians likely often implicitly consider these strategies throughout the course of their daily practice. SFGT allows for an explicit examination of how they approach clinical decision-making.

In the clinical context, slow and fact guessing strategies have different implications for the delivery of patient care. When slow guessers make an error, they are attempting to accumulate relevant diagnostic information but fail to do so, due to an inability to identify relevant diagnostic cues in the environment. For instance, when presented with an ECG, a clinician might scrutinize it thoroughly to identify any abnormalities that they suspect are present. In contrast, the same clinician might be faced with a triage situation. Due to the self-imposed speeded deadline, they might believe they only have a few moments to spare to inspect the ECG. Consequently, even though abnormalities might be present, they might fail to identify them. Depending on the cases they are presented with, clinicians might shift between these two strategies. Alternatively, they might have a preference due to their own clinical experience. In the following analysis, we consider clinicians' strategies in terms of the SAT.

8.3 SAT as a Multivariate Analysis of Cognitive Efficiency

To understand the overall response strategies of learners and how they change over time, we re-examined an existing dataset that contained extensive training over multiple training modules of the same task (Waechter et al., 2019). In that study, Waechter et al. (2019) limited their analysis to performance increases over the course of learning, how time to respond decreased, and sampled student experiences to inform curriculum development. In the original evaluation of the study, they found that accuracy increased across modules while reaction time decreased across modules.

In this reanalysis, we examined the relationship between these two variables and compared two different measures that reflect trade-offs in performance to identify effective metrics that can be used in medical education and decision-making evaluation (see Appendix for details). First, we consider efficiency. Efficiency is operationalized here as the logarithmic transformation of mean learner accuracy of 14 cases divided by their RT in seconds, reflecting the accuracy per unit of time. This appears to reflect a principled operationalization of how the term is typically used in healthcare professions. The clear benefit of using this measure is that it standardizes learners' performance. For instance, if Learner 1 obtained 60% on a test and took 60 min to complete it whereas Learner 2 obtained a 50% on a test and took 40 min, the efficiency score tells us that Learner 2 (1.25) outperformed Learner 1 (1). This value can then be used to assess whether learners become more efficient over time. Efficiency, however, fails to capture a crucial feature of performance: specific decisions made by learners and decision strategies used by learners.

To examine more specific strategies, we additionally obtained SAT functions and examined micro-SATs. SAT functions can be obtained simply by plotting the speed of the response against the accuracy of the response. Each point on the SAT function represents a given kind of response, i.e., given a particular speed of response, what it provides the expected accuracy. We would expect that with continued learning, both accuracy and speed would increase and that we would observe an increase in efficiency with little to no SAT. In this way, the SAT provides a more specific prediction about how much time is required to achieve a certain level of accuracy within a given task. Unlike efficiency, no transformation is required. Similarly, performance can also be decomposed into correct and incorrect trials to assess learners' response strategies.

8.3.1 Computing Efficiency and Speed-Accuracy Trade-Off

A key feature to identifying an SAT is to consider the relationship between accuracy and RT. Consequently, unlike Waechter et al. (2019), we did not use cumulative module accuracy. Instead, a learner's overall module accuracy and module RT were compared.

Efficiency. Prior to examining an SAT, we first examined the overall trend associated with extensive training to identify when there were noticeable changes in performance. Efficiency was derived using Wickelgren's (1977) formula[2] for speed-accuracy trade-off:

$$d'(t,\lambda,\gamma,\delta) = \lambda\left[1 - e^{-\gamma(1-\delta)}\right]$$

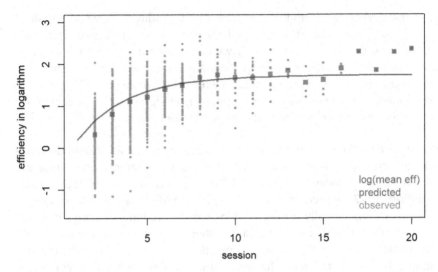

FIGURE 8.1 Changes in efficiency measuring over training modules for observed (gray) and predicted (blue) session performance.

where t is the session (time), λ is the level of efficiency, γ is the increase in efficiency as a function of the session, and δ is the intercept in which efficiency begins to increase. Our measure of efficiency was then plotted against the number of modules completed by the learner (see Figure 8.1).[3] Overall, we observed that relative efficiency reached a performance asymptote at Training Session 4 without any noticeable gains thereafter. Consequently, the remainder of our analyses consider the changes in performance that occur between Training Sessions 1 through 4.

Correlational Analysis. By focusing on only those learners who completed all four of the initial training sessions, the sample population of learners decreased to 156. Prior to conducting a more in-depth analysis of the relationship between a learner's response speed and accuracy, we sought to identify whether there was an overall relationship between these two variables. A correlational analysis revealed that there was a negative correlation between overall module RT and module accuracy, $r(580) = -.227$, $p < .001$. This relationship suggests that learners' time to respond decreased as their accuracy increased. Consequently, there is no evidence for an SAT. Instead, such a pattern reflects automaticity wherein learners become both faster and more accurate.

   In their initial analysis, Waechter et al. (2019) sought to examine whether practice time predicted exam performance. However, to examine the presence of an SAT, we sought to statistically control for exam performance on the grounds that an exam score represents accumulated knowledge. Consequently, the remaining relationship likely reflects a better estimate between decision-making and response strategies. Given that no exam information was available for the three learners, they were excluded from the analysis. After controlling for the effect of exam performance (i.e., overall knowledge), the relationship between speed and accuracy remained, $r(577) = -.221, p < .001$. Consequently, learners' responses appear to be significantly influenced by automatic information retrieval or a response strategy.

Response Functions. A key feature of automaticity is that RT should decrease over the course of learning as information is more rapidly and efficiently retrieved from memory (e.g., Logan, 1988; Saling & Philips, 2007; Schenider & Shiffrin, 1977). Moreover, studies examining SATs have also suggested that participants strategically ignore evidence that is redundant (Donkin et al., 2014). Consequently, the relationship between speed and accuracy should change depending on the amount of practice learners have, i.e., the training module number. To examine changes in responses over time, accuracy scores were grouped into six bins for performance corresponding to accuracy between 50% and 100%. However, given that the program obtained mean responses for each learner, we had to model the overall RT for each session. Consequently, these results can be considered a global measure of both accuracy and speed.

As Figure 8.2 (top) demonstrates, different response patterns were observed for the participants over the course of the four modules. First, module RT decreased over each successive module. With Module 1 RT being the longest ($M_1 = 58.76$ min) and Module 4 RT being the slowest ($M_4 = 31.24$ min). Moreover, Module 1 displayed a curvilinear trend for RTs, with 50% accuracy and 100% accuracy being comparatively faster than intermediate responses. Supporting this, we found that performance was the best fit by a quadratic function (Table 8.1). In contrast, Module 4 demonstrated a linear trend. Due to high accuracy in responses, no 50% confidence category was observed. Intermediate Modules 2 and 3 demonstrated comparable fits across all functions, suggesting that performance was defined by nonlinear non-monotonic responses. However, the low-accuracy responses were slower than high-accuracy responses in both Module 2 ($\Delta M = 5.16$) and Module 3 ($\Delta M = 12.16$). This suggests that learners attempted to provide the correct response but simply failed to do so. This could reflect evidence for a stop-and-think strategy that emerges with experience (e.g., Moulton et al., 2007; Moulton et al., 2010).

In his examination of the relationship between speed and accuracy, Petrusic (1992) reorganized participants' responses to examine correct and error responses to examine macro and micro-SATs. Macro-SATs were evidenced between the high-error and high-correct responses, whereas micro-SATs were evident within each error and correct function. We reorganization our data in

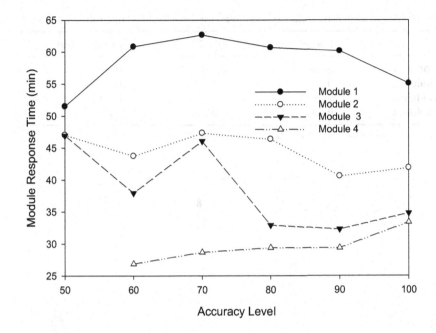

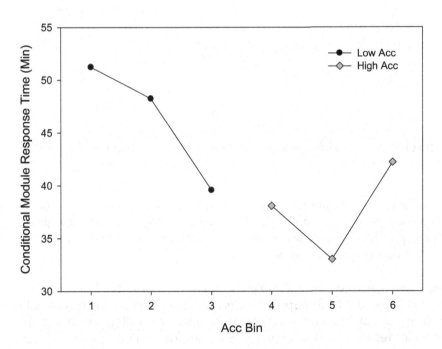

FIGURE 8.2 Speed and accuracy for each module (left). Conditional response times for error and correct responses. Correct responses (unfilled circles) and error responses (filled circles; right).

TABLE 8.1 Proportion of Variance Accounted for Each Best-Fit Function

	Linear	*Exp. Decay*	*Quad. (parab.)*
Module 1	0.03	0.00	**0.90**
Module 2	0.46	0.45	**0.52**
Module 3	0.56	0.57	**0.58**
Module 4	**0.83**	0.00	0.87

Note: Bolded text represents the best fit for each module.

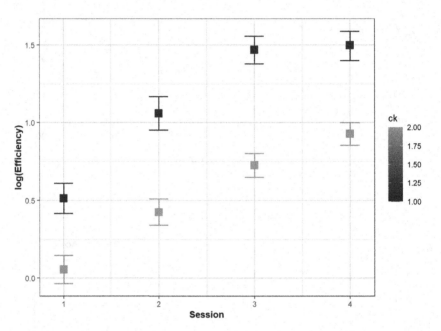

FIGURE 8.3 Slow and fast responders. Error bars reflect standard error of the clusters.

a similar manner (Figure 8.2, right). As Figure 8.2 demonstrates, low-accuracy responses were consistently slower relative to high-accuracy responses. Consequently, the faster learners were to complete the modules, the more likely they were to be accurate.

Slow and Fast Guessing. The foregoing analyses suggest that learners might have developed specific response strategies. Namely, performance in Module 1 suggests that learners were faster to respond when they provided high-accuracy responses or low-accuracy responses. Thus, this could indicate that the retrieval of any answer from memory, if it occurred comparatively rapidly, was used as the basis for the answer. In contrast, Modules 2 and 3 suggest that learners might have adjusted their response strategy. In this case, the strategy reflects a learner-specific approach to learning and decision-making. We used the K-means algorithm to identify different patterns of learning curves characterized by efficiency over four sessions. The optimal number of patterns is found to be two based on the Silhouette measure. We interpreted them as slow- and fast-responder as shown in Figure 8.3.

As Figure 8.3 suggests, slow and fast responders showed very different patterns in their response efficiency. In general, fast responders demonstrated very little trade-off between their speed and accuracy, leading to highly efficient responses over the course of learning. In contrast, slow responders demonstrated considerable SATs, leading to comparatively inefficient performance over time. This might suggest that slow respondents either had difficulties learning or that they did not adjust their response strategy over the course of training. Regardless of the interpretation, the ability to classify learners in this manner can help inform the provision of feedback, allowing educators and learners the ability to identify the source of error and suggest more effective means of problem-solving.

8.4 Measuring Metacognition in Healthcare

Expertise requires more than automatic and efficient processing. Whether novices or experts, HCPs must act autonomously. HCPs must therefore be capable of assessing their own performance by considering any vulnerabilities in the decision-making process (e.g., cognitive biases, limitations in time or attention, team composition), whether they have made any errors, and have had to select treatment options given constraints of the situation (e.g., time, resources, etc.). For instance, if HCPs are aware of an SAT, they might increase or decrease their collection and processing of diagnostic evidence depending on whether there are imminent threats to a patient. These mental processes reflect distinct skills that must be assessed independently of medical knowledge, collectively referred to as metacognition.

To promote autonomous performance, health professions education often focus on developing learner confidence, also referred to as self-efficacy. In its traditionally formulation, self-efficacy represents a person's beliefs about their ability to accomplish a task, i.e., their competency (Bandura, 1977). Self-Efficacy Theory assumes that high self-efficacy will lead learners to increase their efforts when performing a task and remain persistent in the face of failure (Bandura, 1977, 2012; Bandura & Locke, 2003). However, studies of self-efficacy have often found a negative relationship between reported self-efficacy and performance when tasks are ambiguous, suggesting that people are often overly optimistic in their assessment of their abilities (Schmidt & DeShon, 2010; Neal & Yeo, 2003; Vancouver & Kendall, 2006; Vancouver et al., 2001, 2002). To this end, health professions education must

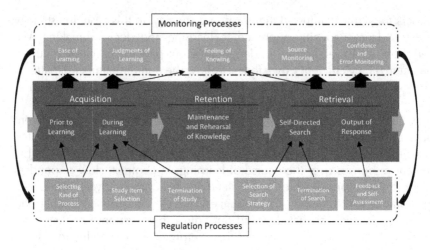

FIGURE 8.4   Monitoring and regulatory metacognitive processes. Healthcare professionals must assess their performance before, during, and after learning, performing a procedure, and consulting. They must also be capable of identifying how to regulate learning and performance. Adapted and extended from Nelson and Narens (1990).

develop self-reflection in learners rather simply confidence in their automatic responses.

Metacognitive processes can be partitioned into two broad kinds: monitoring and control (see Figure 8.4; Nelson & Narens, 1990; Son & Schwartz, 2002). These processes are both functionally and neuroanatomically dissociable (Shimamura, 2008). Monitoring processes use information from the primary decision (e.g., diagnostic cues, lab reports, patient history) as well as situation cues (e.g., time and effort required to choose) to provide an estimate of past, current, or future performance. During the processes of learning, learners might use their general familiarity with a domain to determine how easy it will be to acquire knowledge (ease of learning) or maintain an ongoing estimate of their predicted performance prior to being tested (judgment of learning; Rhodes, 2016). Following their performance on the task, learners might then consider thethe reliability of the source of information and the possibility of error commission.

Learner confidence is believed to play an adaptive role in learning and decision-making. Models of decision-making have suggested that a learner's current level of confidence and their desired level of confidence can be used to determine the effort they will allocate to later learning and decision-making (Chaiken, 1980; Tiedens & Linton, 2001). However, confidence reports are not only determined by evidence collected during the diagnostic process, they additionally rely on how easy it is to learn information that is provided (encoding fluency) or retrieve information from memory (retrieval fluency;

collectively referred to as processing fluency; Alter & Oppenheimer, 2009; Koriat & May'ayan, 2005). Thus, HCPs' automatic and efficient processing might produce high confidence regardless of whether such an assessment is warranted, leading to overconfidence bias.

Measuring Metacognition. The accuracy of subjective assessments of performance has been an ongoing area of study in psychological science. Early introspective methods merely solicited a participant's impression of the task; however, these interpretations demonstrated little correspondence to underlying processes. Much of this work has focused on retrospective confidence reports that are typically obtained by having an individual assign a numeric value, or subjective probability, to the belief that they have provided a correct response (e.g., Henmon, 1911; Pierce & Jastrow, 1884; Sumner, 1898).

Many confidence scales have been used, including lexical scales ('guess', 'certain') and numeric scales (e.g., 50% [guessing] to 100% [certainty][4]). Numeric scales are particularly useful in that they allow a direct comparison between subjective awareness and objective performance. Many of these studies have demonstrated that participants are *overconfident* in perceptual, reasoning, and general knowledge tasks (Kvidera & Koustaal, 2008; Lichtenstein & Fischhoff, 1977; Schoenherr, et al., 2010; Schoenherr & Thomson, 2021; Shynkaruk & Thompson, 2006; West & Stanovich, 1997; for a review, see Hoffrage, 2022). Some studies have attempted to interpret these biases, either in terms of *cognitive penetrability* – an individual's awareness of mental operations – or *task difficulty.* For instance, Ziori and Dienes (2006, 2008) suggested that when confidence and accuracy are correlated, this provides evidence of explicit knowledge, i.e., as learner's knowledge increases, their confidence increases. They additionally argue that when performance is above chance and learners believe they are guessing (i.e., use the 50% category), this suggests the presence of implicit knowledge. They found evidence for both explicit and implicit knowledge. However, despite the intuitive interpretation, by only focusing on guessing responses, their approach ignores *overall* confidence biases. This can lead to erroneous inferences about a learner's awareness. For instance, learners might be underconfident in guessing responses due to regression toward the mean (Dawes & Mulford, 1994). Consequently, overconfidence (OC) bias provides a much better estimate of a learner's awareness and should be used to assess performance (Schoenherr & Lacroix, 2020).

Two measures of biases are typically consider in studies of confidence: subjective calibration and overconfidence bias. The overall degree of correspondence between a participant's mean accuracy when assigning a subjective probability to a response is referred to as *subjective calibration* (Baranski & Petrusic, 1994). Calibration is a general measure of the accuracy of subjective probabilities that can be used to understand the likelihood of events or risk perception. An index of calibration is given by the following:

$$C = \frac{1}{n} \sum_{j=1}^{J} n_j \left(\psi_j - \overline{p(cor)}_j \right)^2$$

Where the squared difference of the jth subjective probability category, ψ_j, and the proportion correct for events, $p(cor)_j$, are calculated (Lichtenstein & Fischhoff, 1977). The product of these responses over the number of trials (n_j) on which they were used is summed across all subjective probability categories (j).

Calibration represents the unsigned difference between objective performance and subjective assessment measured at the level of an individual trial. To be perfectly calibrated, participants' proportion correct (e.g., $p(cor) = 0.70$) should be equivalent to their subjective probabilities (e.g., $mean(conf) = 0.70$), with perfect calibration representing an absence of bias (e.g., $C = 0.00$). Learners are typically only somewhat miscalibrated in perceptual tasks, with biases rarely exceeding $C \leq 0.10$. This suggests that in most perceptual discrimination and judgment tasks, participants exhibit some awareness of their performance, making the use of simple correlation (i.e., Ziori & Dienes, 2006, 2008) problematic. Such results might also explained why clinical reasoning lags behind visual discrimination noted in studies examining clinical reasoning (Kelly et al., 2016).

A measure of OC bias represents the extent to which participants' beliefs overestimate or underestimate their actual performance, provided as the signed difference between the average reported level of confidence within a condition (ψ_j) and the proportion correct $(p(cor)_j)$, given as:

$$OC = \overline{\psi j} - \overline{p(cor)j}$$

In that OC represents a positive or negative value, this information can be used to infer the discrepancies between knowledge and performance for specific tasks or kinds of knowledge. For instance, Lichtenstein and Fischhoff (1977) found that learners tended to overestimate their performance when presented with difficult questions while underestimating their performance for easy questions, referred to as the *Hard-Easy Effect* (Baranski & Petrusic, 1994; Gigerenzer et al., 1991; Griffin & Tversky, 1992; Kvidera & Koustaal, 2008). If questions are hard, learners might not be aware of competing alternative responses or ambiguity in the question, reducing their performance. If questions are easy, learners might be aware of all the possible feature of the question and alternative responses, reducing their uncertainty.

Discrepancies in calibration and OC can be used to understand how learners' subjective awareness of their performance changes over time. Using these methods, studies have found that participants' overconfidence decreases as they gain more experience, referred to as the underconfidence-with-practice (UWP) effect(Finn & Metcalfe, 2007; Koriat et al, 2002; Koriat, 1997; see also Scheck & Nelson, 2005). There are two complementary sources of information that can describe the UWP. First, learners' confidence might remain high. In this case, when = their performance improves, overconfidence decreases. Alternatively, educator or environmental feedback might inform learners that they have overestimated their performance, leading leaners to reduce their confidence. Increased accuracy and decreased confidence can also work together, leading to a need to assess both accuracy and confidence, and how overconfidence changes over time.

8.4.1 Application in the Healthcare Professions

Metacognitive skills must be developed and used in the healthcare professions (Croskerry & Norman, 2008). However, few studies in medical decision-making or education have adopted these psychometric techniques (cf. Mann, 1993). For instance, Meyer et al. (2013) provided clinicians with hard or easy diagnostic vignettes and inferred OC due to aggregate differences in accuracy and confidence. Borracci and Arribalzaga (2018) found both overconfidence and underconfidence in student medical examination performance, with 'better students' demonstrating less OC. In a simulation study, Massoth et al. (2019) found that students who were trained with high-fidelity simulations demonstrated more overconfidence than those trained in low-fidelity simulations, suggesting that confidence was influenced by irrelevant contextual cues (perceived realism).

Similar results have been obtained in self-efficacy reports in medical education. Using self-efficacy ratings of second-year medical students in an OSCE task, Mavis (2001) demonstrated that learners with high self-efficacy (71% correct) outperformed learners with low self-efficacy (51% correct). Critically, despite this general relationship, they failed to obtain a significant correlation between OSCE performance and self-efficacy. Similar results were obtained with examination performance in first-, second-, and third-year students (Khan et al., 2013). Wu et al. (2020) has recently demonstrated that while intrinsic and extrinsic motivations predicted self-efficacy, self-efficacy did not predict performance. Despite these findings, conceptual issues remans concerning how self-efficacy has been defined in medical education, such that these studies must be interpreted with caution (Klassen & Klassen, 2018).

Studies of decision-making and learning within health professions have also replicated more complex patterns observed in the metacognitive literature. During a concurrent training module on cardiac US, Schoenherr et al. (2018) provided learners with a voluntary online test consisting of playable cardiac US videos that were accompanied by diagnostic and treatment questions. Following each set of questions, learners then provided their level of confidence in terms of whether their response was correct.

Schoenherr et al. (2018) replicated both the hard easy effect (HEE) and the UWP (Figure 8.5). When questions were divided into low-, medium-, and high-difficulty categories, they found that learners' overconfidence increased with question difficulty. Overconfidence bias also differed based on the kind of question: learners were more accurate for diagnostic questions, leading to underconfidence, whereas treatment recommendations were associated with greater overconfidence. Moreover, the reported level of prior cardiac US training was also negatively related to the learners' level of overconfidence: learners with more prior training reported less overconfidence than those with little training. However, general US experience was unrelated performance, suggesting that the ability to assess performance is based on domain-specific knowledge.

These techniques can also be adapted for novel diagnostic domains when knowledge about correct diagnoses is limited. Using experts' ratings of learners' performance, Millington et al. (2018) compared expert agreement rather than accuracy to their confidence level. They then used the difference score in an analogous manner to OC bias: the greater the disagreement, the greater the uncertainty in a diagnosis. Replicating patterns of OC bias, the difference scores were all positive, suggesting that confidence was high regardless of the level of expert agreement (Table 8.2). Crucially, replicating the HEE, larger differences between expert agreement and confidence were observed for the relatively complicated diagnostic categories (pneumothorax and atelectasis), and smaller differences between agreement and confidence were observed for relatively simple categories (interstitial syndrome and pleural effusion) and the normal condition where no pathophysiology was present.

Confidence reports must be interpreted with caution. Alone, practitioner or learner confidence does not reflect a robust outcome measure of training and delivery of care as it only reflects the subjective experience. Confidence calibration indices qualify subjective confidence by comparing them to performance. However, the validity of their use depends on certain requirements. Confidence calibration requires trial-by-trial information for both accuracy and confidence. This measure is therefore more precise, but miscalibration does not contain information about the direction of the bias. In contrast, OC bias reflects confidence in a kind of decision but does not reflect performance on any trial. Thus, this measure might obscure meaningful

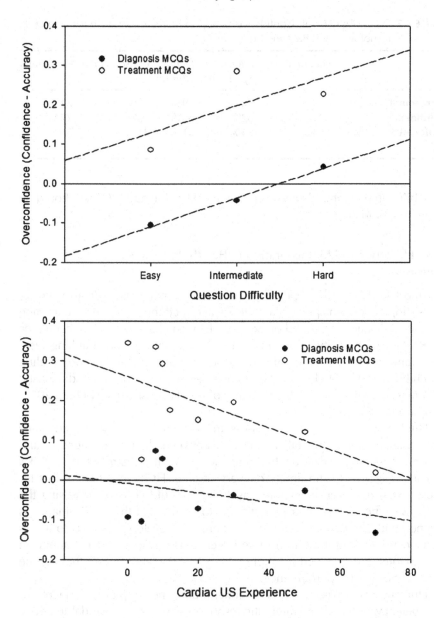

FIGURE 8.5 Increases in overconfidence relative to question difficulty (Hard-Easy Effect) and decreased overconfidence bias associated with experience in US training. Adapted from Schoenherr et al. (2018).

TABLE 8.2 Expert Agreement, Confidence Level, and Difference Score for Five Lung Pathologies and Baseline Condition

	Normal	Pneumothorax	Interstitial Syndrome	Pleural Effusion	Consolidation	Atelectasis
Agreement	60%	31%	58%	59%	47%	21%
Confidence	73%	72%	82%	80%	78%	77%
Difference Score	13%	41%	24%	21%	31%	56%

variability in the data. Ideally, confidence calibration and OC bias should be used in conjunction.

8.5 Efficiency and Metacognition in Health Professions Education

The most fundamental competency that HCPs must master is medical expertise, consisting of domain-specific knowledge acquired through extensive training and specialization. This kind of expertise is often characterized by decreases in RT, or automaticity (Norman et al., 2018). Rather than 'thinking fast', decision-making and problem-solving occur much more efficiently (Saling & Philips, 2007), such that experience results in a focus on diagnostic information and avoiding consideration of nondiagnostic (Drew et al., 2013; Krupinski et al., 2006).

Efficiency requires that we assess the proportion change in accuracy given the amount of time taken to choose between alternative diagnoses and treatment recommendations. In emergency and critical care settings, HCP's efficiency is vital to the timely delivery of care. HCPs might self-select for these roles; however, healthcare institutions should consider assessing the cognitive efficiency of their practitioners to ensure that their performance is aligned with the demands of the environment. Developing means to assess efficiency will contribute to a more effective assessment of competency. In this chapter, we provided a simple means to calculate the SAT that can be used to assess HCP performance.

Efficiency in diagnosis and treatment does not capture all facets of competency. Reliance on automatic responses can result in avoidable errors. HCPs are as susceptible to problem-solving and decision-making biases including overconfidence as any other decision-maker. In many cases, these errors are attributable to cue misidentification, premature closure, and the use of heuristics that are incompatible with the problems being considered. Rather than focusing on learner and HCP confidence as an end, the use of confidence calibration indices allows assessors to determine the condition in which HCPs are miscalibrated and overconfident. This could be used to determine whether learners are prepared to take on entrustable professional activities (EPAs).

Compound measures of competency such as SAT functions and calibration indices provide a principled means to inform competency-based health professions education programs. Both measures can be used to provide learners and practitioners with valuable feedback. Both measures can also be used during the implementation of educational interventions, program development and evaluation. For instance, measures assessing HCPs SAT could be used to evaluate the duration of shifts as well as the length of clinical rotations. Similarly, calibration indices can be used to determine stages of training or areas of practice that are particularly vulnerable to errors. Even if patterns are not immediately clear, data analytics could be used to understand the landscape of education and healthcare delivery in medical schools and hospitals.

Beyond Assessment: Metacognitive Strategies. Effective assessment of efficient decision-making and metacognitive skills presents a first step. HCPs must also be trained to understand the cognitive and situational cues that are associated with decision-making biases and provided with effective debiasing strategies. If diagnostic errors to rapid decision-making, inducing reflective cognition should reduce errors that are attributable to nonanalytic reasoning.

The simplest global strategy is to slow down diagnosis and treatment during the delivery of care. The so-called stop-and-think strategy (Moulton et al., 2007, 2010) requires that HCPs are aware of decision points in a procedure or social cues in the environment that represent vulnerabilities in the individual or collective decision-making process. Similarly, *cognitive forcing strategies* (CFS; Croskerry, 2002, 2003) provide learners with training the describe cognitive biases (*search satisficing* wherein a person stops after identifying an initial diagnosis; *available biases* wherein a person relies on information readily accessible from memory, such as common diagnoses) and provide clinical cases wherein they attempt to identify possible biases. Some evidence shows that these approaches do reduce errors (Sherbino et al., 2011). For instance, in an early review, Lambe et al. (2016) observed that guided reflection and CFS appear to have shown some promise in improving metacognitive ability. However, not all attempts to use CFS have proven effective. For instance, Sherbino et al. (2014) found that CFS training was no better than a control condition in novices (Monteiro et al., 2015). They suggest that learners are not likely to engage in nonanalytic reasoning (Kulatunga-Moruzi et al., 2004), and thus, such training is not aligned with the source of novice errors. Consequently, as in all education interventions, educators must adopt a curriculum perspective, identifying when learners have attained a sufficient level of performance and provide them with training to integrate these separate skills into clinical competency. HCPs must become sensitive to situational cues that are associated with greater risk and uncertainty. When identified – automatically or through controlled processes – HCPs can attempt to consider disconfirming evidence that might suggest an alternative diagnosis or course of treatment. Rather than self-efficacy, health professions education must develop more effective educational interventions to promote accurate self-monitoring.

Appendix

Participants. Three-hundred and eighty-nine first-year medical students from two Canadian institutions (McGill University & University of Calgary) participated in the study (Waechter et al., 2019). To directly compare performance across all sessions, our subsequent analyses were limited to those learners who completed a minimum of four training sessions. This reduced the sample size to 156.

Material. The materials for this study consisted of 14 different ECG diagnostic cases. These cases were selected to correspond to the knowledge required to have acquired competencies in Advanced Cardiac Life Support (ACLS) in order to manage a cardiac arrest.

Procedure. These diagnoses were presented as strip cases on www.teachingm edicine.com/. Three discrete practice modules were created. Completion of the modules was entirely voluntary and self-passed. Consequently, in any given training session, learners we selected were students who had completed 20 modules.

Response accuracy was determined by obtaining the percentage of rhythm strips that were correctly diagnosed by the learner. Correct responses were determined in advance by obtaining unanimous agreement from three expert raters. RT for each practice module was determined by the difference between when learners clicked on the module to start and when they exited the module.

Notes

1   The agnostic terminology of Type 1 and Type 2 corresponds to the evolutionary history of both kinds of processes, assuming that Type 1 is phylogenetically older than Type 2.
2   The original formulation in the study of Wickelgren (1977) describes accuracy as a function of time. In our study, this formulation is differently interpreted. That is, accuracy is replaced by efficiency and reaction time is replaced by session index.
3   For the model fitting process, data from the first 15 sessions are used given that data points between 16 and 20 sessions are very small.

4   These values are used when there are only two alternatives. Guessing will be determined by the number of response alternatives, e.g., 25% when four response alternatives are provided.

References

Abraham, R. R., Fisher, M., Kamath, A., Izzati, T. A., Nabila, S., & Atikah, N. N. (2011). Exploring first-year undergraduate medical students' self-directed learning readiness to physiology. *Advances in Physiology Education*, 35(4), 393–395.

Ægisdóttir, S., White, M. J., Spengler, P. M., Maugherman, A. S., Anderson, L. A., Cook, R. S., ... & Rush, J. D. (2006). The meta-analysis of clinical judgment project: fifty-six years of accumulated research on clinical versus statistical prediction. *The Counseling Psychologist*, 34(3), 341–382.

Alter, A. L., & Oppenheimer, D. M. (2009). Uniting the tribes of fluency to form a metacognitive nation. *Personality and Social Psychology Review*, 13(3), 219–235.

Ashby, F. G., Alfonso-Reese, L. A., & Waldron, E. M. (1998). A neuropsychological theory of multiple systems in category learning. *Psychological Review*, 105(3), 442.

Ashby, F. G., & Valentin, V. V. (2017). Multiple systems of perceptual category learning: Theory and cognitive tests. In *Handbook of Categorization in Cognitive Science* (pp. 157–188). Elsevier.Balakrishnan, J. D., & Ratcliff, R. (1996). Testing models of decision making using confidence ratings in classification. *Journal of Experimental Psychology: Human Perception & Performance*, 22(3), 615–633.

Bandura, A. (1997). *Self-Efficacy: The Exercise of Control*. New York: Freeman.

Bandura, A. (2012). On the functional properties of perceived self-efficacy revisited. *Journal of Management*, 28, 9–44.

Bandura, A., & Jourden, F. J. (1991). Self-regulatory mechanisms governing the impact of social comparison on complex decision-making. *Journal of Personality and Social Psychology*, 60, 941–951.

Bandura, A., & Locke, E. A. (2003). Negative self-efficacy and goal effects revisited. *Journal of Applied Psychology*, 88, 87–99.

Baranski, J. V., & Petrusic, W. M. (1994). The calibration and resolution of confidence in perceptual judgments. *Perception & Psychophysics*, 55(4), 412–428.

Baumann, A. O., Deber, R. B., & Thompson, G. G. (1991). Overconfidence among physicians and nurses: the 'micro-certainty, macro-uncertainty' phenomenon. *Social Science & Medicine*, 32(2), 167–174.

Berner, E. S., & Graber, M. L. (2008). Overconfidence as a cause of diagnostic error in medicine. *The American Journal of Medicine*, 121(5), S2–S23.

Blair, M. R., Watson, M. R., Walshe, R. C., & Maj, F. (2009). Extremely selective attention: eye-tracking studies of the dynamic allocation of attention to stimulus features in categorization. *Journal of Experimental Psychology: Learning, Memory, and Cognition*, 35, 1196–1206.

Borracci, R. A., & Arribalzaga, E. B. (2018). The incidence of overconfidence and underconfidence effects in medical student examinations. *Journal of Surgical Education*, 75(5), 1223–1229.

Braddock III, C., Hudak, P. L., Feldman, J. J., Bereknyei, S., Frankel, R. M., & Levinson, W. (2008). "Surgery is certainly one good option": quality and time-efficiency of informed decision-making in surgery. *The Journal of Bone and Joint Surgery*, 90, 1830.

Brezis, M., Orkin-Bedolach, Y., Fink, D., & Kiderman, A. (2019). Does physician's training induce overconfidence that hampers disclosing errors? *Journal of Patient Safety*, 15(4), 296–298.

Chaiken, S. (1980). Heuristic versus systematic information processing and the use of source versus message cues in persuasion. *Journal of Personality and Social Psychology*, 39(5), 752.

Classen, D., Resar, R., Griffin, F., et al. (2011). Global "trigger tool" shows that adverse events in hospitals may be ten times greater than previously measured. *Health Affairs*, 30, 581–589. https://doi.org/10.1377/hlthaff.2011.0190

Cochrane, A. L. (1972). *Effectiveness and Efficiency: Random Reflection on Health Services*. Nuffield Provincial Hospitals Trust.

Croskerry, P. (2000). The cognitive imperative thinking about how we think. *Academic Emergency Medicine*, 7(11), 1223–1231.

Croskerry, P. (2002). Achieving quality in clinical decision making: Cognitive strategies and detection of bias. *Academic Emergency Medicine*, 9(11), 1184–1204.

Croskerry, P. (2003). The importance of cognitive errors in diagnosis and strategies to minimize them. *Academic Medicine*, 78, 775–780.

Croskerry, P., & Norman, G. (2008). Overconfidence in clinical decision making. *The American Journal of Medicine*, 121(5), S24–S29.

Dawes, R. M. (1980). Confidence in intellectual judgments vs. confidence in perceptual judgments. Lantermann & H. Feger (Eds.), *Similarity and Choice: Papers in Honor of Clyde Coombs*, 327–345.

Dawes, R. M., & Mulford, M. (1996). The false consensus effect and overconfidence: Flaws in judgment or flaws in how we study judgment? *Organizational Behavior and Human Decision Processes*, 65(3), 201–211.

Dijksterhuis, A. (2004). Think different: the merits of unconscious thought in preference development and decision making. *Journal of Personality and Social Psychology*. 87, 586–598.

Dijksterhuis, A., Bos, M. W., Nordgren, L. F., & van Baaren, R. B. (2006). On making the right choice: the deliberation without attention effect. *Science*, 311, 1005–1007.

Dijksterhuis, A., Bos, M. W., van der Leij, A., & van Baaren, R. B. (2009). Predicting soccer matches after unconscious and conscious thought as a function of expertise. *Psychological Science*, 20, 1381–1387.

Dijksterhuis, A., & Nordgren, L. F. (2006). A theory of unconscious thought. *Perspectives in Psychological Science*, 1, 95–109.

Donders, F. C. (1868). On the speed of mental processes. *Arch. Néerland.*, 3, 269–317.

Donkin, C., Little, D. R., & Houpt, J. W. (2014). Assessing the speed-accuracy trade-off effect on the capacity of information processing. *Journal of Experimental Psychology: Human Perception and Performance*, 40, 1183.

Drew, T., Võ, M. L. H., & Wolfe, J. M. (2013). The invisible gorilla strikes again: sustained inattentional blindness in expert observers. *Psychological Science*, 24(9), 1848–1853.

Dreyfus, S. E., & Dreyfus, H. L. (1980). A five-stage model of the mental activities involved in directed skill acquisition. *Operation Research Center Report 80-2*. University of California.

Elliott, D., Hansen, S., Grierson, L. E., Lyons, J., Bennett, S. J., & Hayes, S. J. (2010). Goal-directed aiming: two components but multiple processes. *Psychological Bulletin*, 136, 1023.

Ericsson, K. A. (2007). An expert-performance perspective of research on medical expertise: the study of clinical performance. *Medical Education*, 41, 1124–1130.

Evans, B. J., Stanley, R. O., Mestrovic, R., & Rose, L. (1991). Effects of communication skills training on students' diagnostic efficiency. *Medical Education*, 25, 517–526.

Fan, J., McCandliss, B. D., Fossella, J., Flombaum, J. I., & Posner, M. I. (2005). The activation of attentional networks. *Neuroimage*, 26, 471–479.

Finn, B., & Metcalfe, J. (2007). The role of memory for past test in the underconfidence with practice effect. *Journal of Experimental Psychology: Learning, Memory, and Cognition*, 33(1), 238–244.Fischhoff, B., Slovic, P., & Lichtenstein, S. (1977). Knowing with certainty: The appropriateness of extreme confidence. *Journal of Experimental Psychology: Human Perception and Performance*, 3(4), 552.

Fitts, P. M., & Posner, M. I. (1967). *Human Performance*. Brooke/Cole Publishing Co.

Gago, F., Echagüe, C. L., & Lázaro, M. (2024). Reflection as a core skill in bioethics education: Application to the scientific and healthcare professions. In J. R. Schoenherr & M. M. McConnell (Eds.), *Fundamentals and Frontiers in Medical Education and Decision-Making: Educational Theory and Psychological Practice*. Routledge.

Gigerenzer, G., & Brighton, H. (2009). Homo heuristicus: why biased minds make better inferences. *Topics in Cognitive Science*, 1(1), 107–143.

Gigerenzer, G., & Gaissmaier, W. (2011). Heuristic decision making. *Annual Review of Psychology*, 62, 451–482.

Gigerenzer, G., Hoffrage, U., & Kleinbölting, H. (1991). Probabilistic mental models: a Brunswikian theory of confidence. *Psychological Review*, 98(4), 506-528.Gigerenzer, G., & Selten, R. (Eds.). (2002). *Bounded Rationality: The Adaptive Toolbox*. MIT press.

Gilovich, T., Griffin, D., & Kahneman, D. (Eds.). (2002). *Heuristics and Biases: The Psychology of Intuitive Judgment*. Cambridge University Press.

Graber, M. (2003). Metacognitive training to reduce diagnostic errors: ready for prime time? *Academic Medicine*, 78, 781.

Graber, M. (2005). Diagnostic errors in medicine: a case of neglect. *The Joint Commission Journal on Quality and Patient Safety*, 31(2), 106–113.

Grierson, L. E. (2014). Information processing, specificity of practice, and the transfer of learning: considerations for reconsidering fidelity. *Advances in Health Sciences Education*, 19, 281–289.

Grierson, L. E., Lyons, J. L., & Dubrowski, A. (2013). Gaze-down endoscopic practise leads to better novice performance on gaze-up displays. *Medical Education*, 47, 166–172.

Griffin, D., & Tversky, A. (1992). The weighing of evidence and the determinants of confidence. *Cognitive Psychology*, 24(3), 411-435.Grove, W. M., Zald, D. H., Lebow, B. S., Snitz, B. E., & Nelson, C. (2000). Clinical versus mechanical prediction: a meta-analysis. *Psychological Assessment*, 12(1), 19.

Heitz, R. P. (2014). The speed-accuracy tradeoff: history, physiology, methodology, and behavior. *Frontiers in Neuroscience*, 8, 150.

Henmon, V. A. C. (1911). The relation of the time of a judgment to its accuracy. *Psychological Review*, 18, 186–201. https://doi.org/10.1037/h0074579

Hick, W. E. (1952). On the rate of gain of information. *Quarterly Journal of Experimental Psychology, 4*, 11–26.

Hoffmann, A., Diedenhofen, B., & Müller, S. (2022). The utility of overclaiming questionnaires depends on the fit between test content and application context. *Current Psychology, 42*, 1–11.

Hoffrage, U. (2022). Overconfidence. *Cognitive illusions*, 287–306.Hogarth, R. M. (2001). *Educating Intuition*. University of Chicago Press.

Iregui, M., Ward, S., Sherman, G., Fraser, V. J., & Kollef, M. H. (2002). Clinical importance of delays in the initiation of appropriate antibiotic treatment for ventilator-associated pneumonia. *Chest, 122*, 262–268.

Kahneman, D., & Klein, G. (2009). Conditions for intuitive expertise: a failure to disagree. *American Psychologist, 64*, 515–526.

Kahneman, D., Slovic, P., & Tversky, A. (Eds.). (1982). *Judgment Under Uncertainty: Heuristics and Biases*. Cambridge University Press.Kelly, B. S., Rainford, L. A., Darcy, S. P., Kavanagh, E. C., & Toomey, R. J. (2016). The development of expertise in radiology: in chest radiograph interpretation,"expert" search pattern may predate "expert" levels of diagnostic accuracy for pneumothorax identification. *Radiology, 280*(1), 252–260.

Khan, A. S., Cansever, Z., Avsar, U. Z., & Acemoglu, H. (2013). Perceived self-efficacy and academic performance of medical students at Ataturk University, Turkey. *Journal of the College of Physicians and Surgeons Pakistan, 23*(7), 495–498.

Klassen, R. M., & Klassen, J. R. (2018). Self-efficacy beliefs of medical students: a critical review. *Perspectives on Medical Education, 7*, 76–82.

Klayman, J., Soll, J. B., Gonzalez-Vallejo, C., & Barlas, S. (1999). Overconfidence: it depends on how, what, and whom you ask. *Organizational Behavior and Human Decision Processes, 79*(3), 216–247.

Klein, G. A. (1993). A recognition-primed decision (RPD) model of rapid decision making. In *Decision Making in Action: Models and Methods* (Vol. 5, pp. 138–147). Ablex Publishing.

Klein, G. A. (2017). *Sources of Power: How People Make Decisions*. MIT press.

Kohn, L. T., Corrigan, J. M., & Donaldson, M. S. (1999). *To Err Is Human: Building a Safer Health System*. National Academies Press.Koriat, A. (1997). Monitoring one's own knowledge during study: A cue-utilization approach to judgments of learning. *Journal of Experimental Psychology: General, 126*(4), 349–370.

Koriat, A., & Ma'ayan, H. (2005). The effects of encoding fluency and retrieval fluency on judgments of learning. *Journal of Memory and Language, 52*, 478–492.

Koriat, A., Sheffer, L., & Ma'ayan, H. (2002). Comparing objective and subjective learning curves: judgments of learning exhibit increased underconfidence with practice. *Journal of Experimental Psychology: General, 131*(2), 147–162.Kosior, K., Wall, T., & Ferrero, S. (2019). The role of metacognition in teaching clinical reasoning: theory to practice. *Education in the Health Professions, 2*, 108–114.

Krupinski, E. A., Tillack, A. A., Richter, L., Henderson, J. T., Bhattacharyya, A. K., Scott, K. M., et al. (2006). Eye movement study and human performance using telepathology virtual slides. Implications for medical education and differences with experience. *Human Pathology, 37*, 1543–1556.

Kulatunga-Moruzi, C., Brooks, L. R., & Norman, G. R. (2004). Using comprehensive feature lists to bias medical diagnosis. *Journal of Experimental Psychology: Learning, Memory, and Cognition, 30*(3), 563.

Kvidera, S., & Koutstaal, W. (2008). Confidence and decision type under matched stimulus conditions: Overconfidence in perceptual but not conceptual decisions. *Journal of Behavioral Decision Making*, 21(3), 253–281.Lambe, K. A., O'Reilly, G., Kelly, B. D., & Curristan, S. (2016). Dual-process cognitive interventions to enhance diagnostic reasoning: a systematic review. *BMJ Quality & Safety*, 25, 808–820.

Landrigan, C. P., Parry, G. J., Bones, C. B., Hackbarth, A. D., Goldmannm, D. A., & Sharek, P. J. (2010). Temporal trends in rates of patient harm resulting from medical care. *New England Journal of Medicine*, 363, 2124–2134.

Leape, L. L., Lawthers, A. G., Brennan, T. A., & Johnson, W. G. (1993). Preventing medical injury. *Quality Review Bulletin*, 19, 144–149.

LeFlore, J. L., Anderson, M., Michael, J. L., Engle, W. D., & Anderson, J. (2007). Comparison of self-directed learning versus instructor-modeled learning during a simulated clinical experience. *Simulation in Healthcare*, 2, 170–177.

Li, S. T. T., Paterniti, D. A., & West, D. C. (2010). Successful self-directed lifelong learning in medicine: a conceptual model derived from qualitative analysis of a national survey of pediatric residents. *Academic Medicine*, 85, 1229–1236.

Lichtenstein, S., & Fischhoff, B. (1977). Do those who know more also know more about how much they know?. *Organizational Behavior and Human Performance*, 20(2), 159–183.

Logan, G. D. (1988). Toward an instance theory of automatization. *Psychological Review*, 95(4), 492–527.

Ludeke, S. G., & Makransky, G. (2016). Does the over-claiming questionnaire measure overclaiming? Absent convergent validity in a large community sample. *Psychological Assessment*, 28(6), 765.

Lum, T. E., Fairbanks, R. J., Pennington, E. C., & Zwemer, F. L. (2005). Profiles in patient safety: misplaced femoral line guidewire and multiple failures to detect the foreign body on chest radiography. *Academic Emergency Medicine*, 12(7), 658–662.

MacKay, D. G. (1982). The problems of flexibility, fluency, and speed–accuracy trade-off in skilled behavior. *Psychological Review*, 89, 483–506.

Makary, M. A., & Daniel, M. (2016). Medical error—the third leading cause of death in the US. *British Medical Journal*, 353. https://doi.org/10.1136/bmj.i2139

Mamede, S., Schmidt, H. G., Rikers, R. M., Custers, E. J., Splinter, T. A., & van Saase, J. L. (2010). Conscious thought beats deliberation without attention in diagnostic decision-making: at least when you are an expert. *Psychological Research*, 74, 586–592.

Mann, D. (1993). *The Relationship between Diagnostic Accuracy and Confidence in Medical Students*. Technical Report.

Massoth, C., Röder, H., Ohlenburg, H., Hessler, M., Zarbock, A., Pöpping, D. M., & Wenk, M. (2019). High-fidelity is not superior to low-fidelity simulation but leads to overconfidence in medical students. *BMC Medical Education*, 19(1), 1–8.

Mauksch, L. B., Dugdale, D. C., Dodson, S., & Epstein, R. (2008). Relationship, communication, and efficiency in the medical encounter: creating a clinical model from a literature review. *Archives of Internal Medicine*, 168, 1387–1395. https://doi.org/10.1001/archinte.168.13.1387

Mavis, B. (2001). Self-efficacy and OSCE performance among second year medical students. *Advances in Health Sciences Education*, 6 , 93–102.Medina, M. S., Castleberry, A. N., & Persky, A. M. (2017). Strategies for improving learner metacognition in health professional education. *American Journal of Pharmaceutical Education*, 81(4), 1–14.

Meehl, P. E. (1954). *Clinical versus Statistical Prediction: A Theoretical Analysis and a Review of the Evidence*. University of Minnesota Press.

Merkel, J. (1885). Die zeitlichen verhältnisse der willenstätigkeit. *Philosophical Studies*, 2, 73–127.

Meyer, A. N., Payne, V. L., Meeks, D. W., Rao, R., & Singh, H. (2013). Physicians' diagnostic accuracy, confidence, and resource requests: a vignette study. *JAMA Internal Medicine*, 173(21), 1952–1958.

Millington, S. J., Arntfield, R. T., Guo, R. J., Koenig, S., Kory, P., Noble, V., ... & Schoenherr, J. R. (2018). Expert agreement in the interpretation of lung ultrasound studies performed on mechanically ventilated patients. *Journal of Ultrasound in Medicine*, 37, 2659–2665.

Millington, S. J., Hewak, M., Arntfield, R. T., Beaulieu, Y., Hibbert, B., Koenig, S., ... & Schoenherr, J. R. (2017). Outcomes from extensive training in critical care echocardiography: identifying the optimal number of practice studies required to achieve competency. *Journal of Critical Care*, 40, 99–102.

Milstein, A., & Lee, T. H. (2007). Comparing physicians on efficiency. *New England Journal of Medicine*, 357, 2649–2652.

Monteiro, S. D., Sherbino, J., Patel, A., Mazzetti, I., Norman, G. R., & Howey, E. (2015). Reflecting on diagnostic errors: taking a second look is not enough. *Journal of General Internal Medicine*, 30, 1270–1274.

Moore, D. A., & Healy, P. J. (2008). The trouble with overconfidence. *Psychological Review*, 115(2), 502.

Moulton, C. A., Regehr, G., Lingard, L., Merritt, C., & MacRae, H. (2010). Slowing down to stay out of trouble in the operating room: remaining attentive in automaticity. *Academic Medicine*, 85, 1571–1577.

Moulton, C.A., Regehr, G., Mylopoulos, M., & MacRae, H. M. (2007). Slowing down when you should: a new model of expert judgment. *Academic Medicine*, 82, S109–S116.

Naguib, M., Brull, S. J., Hunter, J. M., Kopman, A. F., Fülesdi, B., Johnson, K. B., & Arkes, H. R. (2019). Anesthesiologists' overconfidence in their perceived knowledge of neuromuscular monitoring and its relevance to all aspects of medical practice: an international survey. *Anesthesia & Analgesia*, 128(6), 1118–1126.

Nallamothu, B., Fox, K. A., Kennelly, B. M., Van de Werf, F., Gore, J. M., Steg, P. G., ... & Eagle, K. A. (2007). Relationship of treatment delays and mortality in patients undergoing fibrinolysis and primary percutaneous coronary intervention. The global registry of acute coronary events. *Heart*, 93, 1552–1555.

Neal, A., & Yeo, G. (2003). Does self-efficacy help or harm performance? An examination of the direction of the relationship between self efficacy and performance at the within person level of analysis. *Australian Journal of Psychology*, 55, 138.

Nelson, T. O., & Narens, L. (1990). Metamemory: A theoretical framework and some new findings. In G. H. Bower (Ed.), *The Psychology of Learning and Motivation* (Vol. 26, pp. 125–173). Academic Press.

Nieuwenstein, M. R., Wierenga, T., Morey, R. D., Wicherts, J. M., Blom, T. N., Wagenmakers, E. J., & van Rijn, H. (2015). On making the right choice: a meta-analysis and large-scale replication attempt of the unconscious thought advantage. *Judgment and Decision Making*, 10(1), 1–17.

Norman, D. A., & Shallice, T. (1986). Attention to action: Willed and automatic control of behavior. In *Consciousness and Self-Regulation: Advances in Research and Theory* (Volume 4; pp. 1–18). Boston, MA: Springer US.

Norman, G. (2017). Generalization and the qualitative–quantitative debate. *Advances in Health Sciences Education*, 22(5), 1051–1055.

Norman, G., Grierson, L. E. M., Sherbino, J., Hamstra, S. J., Schmidt, H. G., & Mamede, S. (2018). Expertise in medicine and surgery. In K. A. Ericsson, R. R. Hoffman, A. Kozbelt, & A. M. Williams (Eds.), *Cambridge Handbooks in Psychology. The Cambridge Handbook of Expertise and Expert Performance* (pp. 331–355). Cambridge University Press.

Norman, G., Sherbino, J., Dore, K., Wood, T., Young, M., Gaissmaier, W., ... & Monteiro, S. (2014). The etiology of diagnostic errors: a controlled trial of system 1 versus system 2 reasoning. *Academic Medicine*, 89, 277–284.

Oskamp, S. (1965). Overconfidence in case-study judgments. *Journal of Consulting Psychology*, 29(3), 261.

Paulhus, D. L., & Harms, P. D. (2004). Measuring cognitive ability with the overclaiming technique. *Intelligence*, 32(3), 297–314.

Paulhus, D. L., Harms, P. D., Bruce, M. N., & Lysy, D. C. (2003). The over-claiming technique: measuring self-enhancement independent of ability. *Journal of Personality and Social Psychology*, 84, 890.

Peine, A., Kabino, K., & Spreckelsen, C. (2016). Self-directed learning can outperform direct instruction in the course of a modern German medical curriculum-results of a mixed methods trial. *BMC Medical Education*, 16, 1–11.

Perkins, G. D., Kimani, P. K., Bullock, I., Clutton-Brock, T., Davies, R. P., Gale, M., ... & Stallard, N. (2012). Improving the efficiency of advanced life support training: a randomized, controlled trial. *Annals of Internal Medicine*, 157, 19–28.

Petrusic, W. M. (1992). Semantic congruity effects and theories of the comparison process. *Journal of Experimental Psychology: Human Perception & Performance*, 18, 962–986.

Phillips, W. J., Fletcher, J. M., Marks, A. D., & Hine, D. W. (2016). Thinking styles and decision making: a meta-analysis. *Psychological Bulletin*, 142(3), 260.

Pierce, C. S., & Jastrow, J. (1884). On small differences in sensation. *Proceedings of the National Academy of Sciences*, 3, 75–83.

Potchen, E. J. (2006). Measuring observer performance in chest radiology: some experiences. *Journal of the American College of Radiology*, 3(6), 423–432.

Proctor, R. W., & Schneider, D. W. (2018). Hick's law for choice reaction time: a review. *Quarterly Journal of Experimental Psychology*, 71(6), 1281–1299.

Proulx, N., Frechette, D., Toye, B., Chan, J., & Kravcik, S. (2005). Delays in the administration of antibiotics are associated with mortality from adult acute bacterial meningitis. *QJM: An International Journal of Medicine*, 98, 291–298.

Quirk, M. (2006). *Intuition and Metacognition in Medical Education: Keys to Developing Expertise*. Springer Publishing Company.

Rhodes, M. G. (2016). Judgments of learning: Methods, data, and theory. In J. Dunlosky & S. K. Tauber (Eds.), *The Oxford Handbook of Metamemory* (pp. 65–80). Oxford University Press.

Ridderinkhof, K. R., van der Molen, M. W., & Bashore, T. R. (1995). Limits on the application of additive factors logic: Violations of stage robustness suggest a dual-process architecture to explain flanker effects on target processing. *Acta Psychologica*, 90(1–3), 29–48.

Saling, L. L., & Philips, J. G. (2007). Automatic behaviour: Efficient not mindless. *Brain Research Bulletin*, 73, 1–20.

Salkever, D. S., Skinner, E. A., Steinwachs, D. M., & Katz, H. (1982). Episode-based efficiency comparisons for physicians and nurse practitioners. *Medical Care*, 143–153.

Sanchez, C., & Dunning, D. (2018). Overconfidence among beginners: is a little learning a dangerous thing?. *Journal of personality and Social Psychology*, 114(1), 10.

Sanders, A. F. (1967). Some aspects of reaction processes, In: A. F. Sanders (Ed.), *Attention and Performance I. Acta Psychologica*, 27, 115–130.

Sanders, A. F. (1980). 20 stage analysis of reaction processes. In *Advances in Psychology* (Vol. 1, pp. 331–354). North-Holland.

Scheck, P., & Nelson, T. O. (2005). Lack of pervasiveness of the underconfidence-with-practice effect: Boundary conditions and an explanation via anchoring. *Journal of Experimental Psychology: General*, 134(1), 124.

Schiff, G. D., Hasan, O., Kim, S., Abrams, R., Cosby, K., Lambert, B. L., ... & Odwazny, R. (2009). Diagnostic error in medicine: analysis of 583 physician-reported errors. *Archives of Internal Medicine*, 169, 1881–1887.

Schmidt, A. M., & DeShon, R. P. (2010). The moderating effects of performance ambiguity on the relationship between self-efficacy and performance. *Journal of Applied Psychology*, 95(3), 572–581.

Schneider, W., & Shiffrin, R. M. (1977). Controlled and automatic human information processing: I. Detection, search, and attention. *Psychological Review*, 84, 1.

Schoenherr, J. R. (2020). Adapting the zone of proximal development to the wicked environments of professional practice. In *International Conference on Human-Computer Interaction* (pp. 394–410). Springer.

Schoenherr, J. R., & Hamstra, S. (2024). Validity in health professions education: From assessment instruments to program innovation and evaluation. In Schoenherr, J. R. & McConnell, M. M. (Eds.), *Fundamentals and Frontiers in Medical Education and Decision-Making: Educational Theory and Psychological Practice*. Routledge.

Schoenherr, J. R., & Lacroix, G. L. (2020). Performance monitoring during categorization with and without prior knowledge: a comparison of confidence calibration indices with the certainty criterion. *Canadian Journal of Experimental Psychology/Revue canadienne de psychologie expérimentale*, 74(4), 302–315.

Schoenherr, J. R., Leth-Steensen, C., & Petrusic, W. M. (2010). Selective attention and subjective confidence calibration. *Attention, Perception, & Psychophysics*, 72(2), 353–368.

Schoenherr, J. R., & Thomson, R. (2021). Persuasive features of scientific explanations: Explanatory schemata of physical and psychosocial phenomena. *Frontiers in Psychology*, 12, 644809.

Schoenherr, J. R., Waechter, J., & Millington, S. J. (2018). Subjective awareness of ultrasound expertise development: individual experience as a determinant of overconfidence. *Advances in Health Sciences Education*, 23, 749–765.

Sherbino, J., Dore, K. L., Siu, E., & Norman, G. R. (2011). The effectiveness of cognitive forcing strategies to decrease diagnostic error: An exploratory study. *Teaching and Learning in Medicine*, 23(1), 78–84.

Sherbino, J., Kulasegaram, K., Howey, E., & Norman, G. (2014). Ineffectiveness of cognitive forcing strategies to reduce biases in diagnostic reasoning: A controlled trial. *Canadian Journal of Emergency Medicine*, 16(1), 34–40.

Shimamura, A. P. (2008). A neurocognitive approach to metacognitive monitoring and control. *Handbook of Metamemory and Memory*, 11, 373–390.

Shynkaruk, J. M., & Thompson, V. A. (2006). Confidence and accuracy in deductive reasoning. *Memory & Cognition*, 34(3), 619–632.

Simon, H. (1956). Rational choice and the structure of the environment. *Psychological Review*, 63(2), 129–138. https://doi.org/10.1037/h0042769

Son, L. K., & Schwartz, B. L. (2002). The relation between metacognitive monitoring and control. In T. J. Perfect & B. L. Schwartz (eds), *Applied Metacognition* (pp. 15–38). Cambridge University Press..

Sumner, F. B. (1898). A statistical study of belief. *Psychological Review*, 5, 616–631.Tiedens, L. Z., & Linton, S. (2001). Judgment under emotional certainty and uncertainty: the effects of specific emotions on information processing. *Journal of Personality and Social Psychology*, 81, 973–988

Usher, M., Russo, Z., Weyers, M., Brauner, R., & Zakay, D. (2011). The impact of the mode of thought in complex decisions: Intuitive decisions are better. *Frontiers in Psychology*, 2, 37.

Vancouver, J. B., & Kendall, L. (2006). When self-efficacy negatively relates to motivation and performance in a learning context. *Journal of Applied Psychology*, 91, 1146 –1153.

Vancouver, J. B., Thompson, C. M., Tischner, E. C., & Putka, D. J. (2002). Two studies examining the negative effect of self-efficacy on performance. *Journal of Applied Psychology*, 87, 506 –516.

Vancouver, J. B., Thompson, C. M., & Williams, A. A. (2001). The changing signs in the relationships among self-efficacy, personal goals, and performance. *Journal of Applied Psychology*, 86, 605–620.

Vickers, D., & Packer, J. (1982). Effects of alternating set for speed or accuracy on response time, accuracy and confidence in a unidimensional discrimination task. *Acta Psychologica*, 50, 179–197.

Waechter, J., Reading, D., Lee, C. H., & Walker, M. (2019). Quantifying the medical student learning curve for ECG rhythm strip interpretation using deliberate practice. *GMS Journal for Medical Education*, 36(4)

West, R. F., & Stanovich, K. E. (1997). The domain specificity and generality of overconfidence: individual differences in performance estimation bias. *Psychonomic Bulletin & Review*, 4(3), 387–392.

Wickelgren, W.A. (1977). Speed-accuracy tradeoff and information processing dynamics. *Acta Psychologica*, 41, 67–85.

Williams, L., Carrigan, A., Auffermann, W., Mills, M., Rich, A., Elmore, J., & Drew, T. (2021). The invisible breast cancer: experience does not protect against inattentional blindness to clinically relevant findings in radiology. *Psychonomic Bulletin & Review*, 28, 503–511.

Woodworth, R. S. (1899). The accuracy of voluntary movement. *Psychological Review*, 3 (Monograph Suppl.), 1–119.

Wu, H., Li, S., Zheng, J., & Guo, J. (2020). Medical students' motivation and academic performance: the mediating roles of self-efficacy and learning engagement. *Medical Education Online*, 25(1), 1742964.

Wulf, G., Shea, C., & Lewthwaite, R. (2010). Motor skill learning and performance: a review of influential factors. *Medical Education*, 44(1), 75–84.

Yang, C., Zhu, Y., Jiang, H., & Qu, B. (2021). Influencing factors of self-directed learning abilities of medical students of mainland China: a cross-sectional study. *BMJ Open*, 11(10), e051590.

Yellott Jr, J. I. (1971). Correction for fast guessing and the speed-accuracy tradeoff in choice reaction time. *Journal of Mathematical Psychology*, 8(2), 159–199.

Ziori, E., & Dienes, Z. (2006). Subjective measures of unconscious knowledge of concepts. *Mind & Society*, 5, 105–122.

Ziori, E., & Dienes, Z. (2008). How does prior knowledge affect implicit and explicit concept learning? *Quarterly Journal of Experimental Psychology*, 61, 601–624.

9

REFLECTION AS A CORE SKILL IN BIOETHICS EDUCATION

Application to the Scientific and Healthcare Professions

Fiorella Gago, Camila López Echagüe, and Marila Lázaro

9.1 Introduction

In recent decades, a series of pedagogical approaches have been consolidated that seek to overcome the classical conception of teaching understood as the transmission of a body of content from the teachers to learners (for accounts of this process, see Ma, 2024; Schoenherr, 2024; Schoenherr & Hamstra, 2024; Schoenherr, Mahias-Ito, & Li, 2024; Schoenherr & McConnell, 2024). Learning also implies developing the capacity to autonomously and reflexively appropriate the knowledge that circulates in the classroom, to link with others in a collaborative process, and to become aware of one's own learning processes, beliefs, and attitudes to critically review them (Freire, 1972; Delors, 1996; Tawil & Cougoureux, 2013).

In the field of science and medical education, the scholarly literature has critiqued traditional models directed toward biologicist and reductionist approaches (Bloom, 1992). These approaches are often criticized for their lack of consideration for social, cultural, and ethical dimensions (Westerhaus et al., 2015). These critiques are validated when considering countries (e.g., Brazil; Venosa et al., 2024) and regions that are defined by medical pluralism (e.g., East Asia; Schoenherr & Beaudoin, 2024). As a result, there is an increasing emphasis on including educational practices that go beyond the mere transmission of content and technical knowledge. Such educational practices include the development of broad competencies like communication, collaboration, and decision-making (e.g., WHO, 2013), critical thinking (Jenicek et al., 2011; Finn, 2011; McConnell, 2024; Monteiro et al., 2024), reflection and metacognition (Schoenherr et al., 2024; Tanner,

DOI: 10.4324/9781003316091-11

2012), while promoting interdisciplinarity and ethical education (Eckles et al., 2005).

In addition to the attitudes and skills deemed essential for expert judgment, several studies have noted the existence of non-analytical resources acquired through experience (Norman & Brooks, 1997), which are part of the professional practice. According to this body of research, in situations where a vast amount of information needs to be processed, expert judgment employs mechanisms such as schemas or pattern recognition to save effort and work more efficiently (Moulton et al., 2007). Nevertheless, although medical practice, for instance, relies on automaticity, we must also acknowledge that the intricate, uncertain, novel, and ethically dilemmatic nature of many emerging issues requires that medical professionals possess the capacity to pause and reflect, deliberate, and make a well-informed judgment (Schoenherr et al., 2024) especially in the domain of ethics.

The dissemination and promotion of medical humanities in educational settings, including Bioethics, try to contribute to more conscientious, responsible, and reflective professionals through interdisciplinary approaches that provide a framework for deliberative decision-making (Evans, 2002; Shapiro et al., 2009). Shapiro et al. (2009) advocate for the adoption of methodologies in medical education that foster reflection and a sense of narrativity that allows students to reconstruct and interpret the situations, cases, and dilemmas they are presented with; identify the complexity and ambiguity in them; and recognize themselves and others as a way to self-awareness and critical reflection (for a discussion of narratives in communication research, see Schoenherr & Le-Bouar, 2024).

In Uruguay, the training of scientists and medical professionals (as well as university students in general) has also been the subject of much discussion, with an emphasis on the importance of introducing changes aimed at providing an interdisciplinary education and promoting other skills and attitudes (Collazo, 2014; Vienni et al., 2015; Martínez Asuaga, 2019; Dapueto et al., 2018; Lázaro et al., 2022). However, it is still necessary to continue advancing in the development of pedagogical and evaluation methodologies. Sharing cases of concrete teaching experiences in undergraduate education can make a significant contribution to this endeavor. For this reason, this chapter aims to share some reflections arising from the experience of a specific university course, "Ethics and Science: Bioethics as a Bridge" course offered by the Faculty of Sciences at the University of the Republic in Uruguay, as well as a formative evaluation tool based on the writing of learning logs.

9.2 Reflection and Metacognition in Bioethics

9.2.1 Bioethics as an Area of Problematization of Practices and Models in the Training of Medical and Science Students

The term medical humanities encompasses a range of disciplines that focus on the study of medical phenomena, including medicine, health, disease, and healthcare, and implies a willingness on the part of medical sciences to engage in interdisciplinary analysis from the perspective of humanities, arts, and social sciences (Bleakley, 2015). Latour (2012) introduced the idea of scientific humanities, which challenges the notion of science and technology as autonomous entities and questions dichotomous distinctions between science and politics, facts and interests (or values), and culture and nature.[1] Both concepts were originally formulated in the context of critiques of the linear model of science and technology and reductionist approaches to knowledge that emerged in the 1960s. They converge in their critique of the idea of evaluative neutrality in science and technology (Gallopin et al., 2001; Ziman, 2000; Wynne, 1991).

Currently, there is significant diversity in how medical and scientific humanities are taught, studied, and understood, with a variety of content, orientation, and pedagogical strategies coexisting in this field (Sánchez González, 2017). The STS (Science, Technology, and Society) approach has generated multiple perspectives on the "extra-scientific" dimensions of science and the importance of incorporating these into teaching and learning processes (Fuller & Collier, 2003). These concepts provide a general framework that justifies and promotes the integration of humanities within medicine and science, particularly in education, that aims to train critical and reflective scientists and medical professionals.

Within the medical humanities, the instruction of ethics has an important role in the training of healthcare practitioners. Bioethics, in particular, as conceived by VR Potter's "Global Bioethics", addresses the imperative of forging a connection between the fields of science and philosophy. Global Bioethics (Potter, 1988) adopts an overtly interdisciplinary approach that expands the notion of community to encompass other living beings, emphasizing the interdependence between humans and the environment.

The interdisciplinary approach proposed by VR Potter has gained recognition as a necessary tool for addressing complex problems at both the local and global levels. Bioethics, as understood through this lens, is not limited to prescribing norms or principles of action but instead provides resources for analysis and interpretation that allow for a deep and reflective consideration of the ethical, political, and social implications of scientific practice. This requires the promotion of certain attitudes related to dialogue and deliberation: respect for others, tolerance, humility in relation to the possibility of fully understanding complex phenomena, accepting the possibility of questioning one's own convictions from the positions and arguments of others, being critical about all types of dogmatism, including scientism (Abel, 1999). As Leon Correa (2008, p. 15) points out, the importance of educational action in Bioethics "is not to get the student to do something, but to want to do something themselves because they find it valuable", as a future doctor or scientist and in general as a person.

To foster ethical deliberation, discussion and reflection on moral dilemmas are fundamental methodological resources for stimulating dialogue and exchange of arguments among students, while avoiding, or at least detecting, prejudices about certain positions or groups of actors. Dilemmas allow for contrasting in which several options and points of view are present to clarify the problem and analyze positions and courses of action (Kohlberg, 1992).

Ultimately, the teaching of Bioethics cannot be conceived solely as the transmission of a set of knowledge, values and conventions, or ethical theories, but as a space for promoting reflective skills, argumentation, metacognition, and critical analysis. Schoenherr and Le-Bouar (2024) refer to "sensemaking" as the process that combines judgment and decision-making, reasoning, and problem-solving strategies to respond to real-world tasks. This can include using beliefs, schemata, social representations, and narratives to reduce uncertainty. The implementation of specific pedagogical strategies aimed at promoting and evaluating these skills can be a complex task, especially without a precise definition of each skill and how to recognize and assess them (Ma, 2024; Schoenherr & Hamstra, 2024). Therefore, some useful models and definitions will be synthesized below to delimit some key concepts that contribute to a more precise understanding of the nature of reflective processes.

9.2.2 Models of Reflection and Metacognition: Practice and Evaluation

Concepts, such as "critical thinking", "reflection", or "metacognition", among others, have been widely praised in the educational framework (Shiau & Chen, 2008; OECD, 2013; Miyamoto et al., 2015; Zhou, 2017). However, there is no clear distinction on how these are defined, making it hard to differentiate among them, especially considering that some of these mental processes are said to rely on others (Wilkinson, 1999; Rogers, 2001).

For instance, when talking about metacognition there are elements of both critical thinking and reflection that will take part of the overall metacognitive process (Ku & Ho, 2010). Metacognition refers to the ability to reflect on and monitor one's own thinking and cognitive processes (Norman et al., 2019; Schoenherr et al., 2024). It involves being aware of one's own knowledge, thinking strategies, and learning processes, as well as being able to regulate and control these processes to improve one's learning and problem-solving abilities (Ku & Ho, 2010). Flavell (1979) was among the first to define metacognition as "knowledge and cognition about cognitive phenomena" (1979, p. 906) and distinguished it from cognition itself, which he defined as "the act or process of knowing". He identified three types of metacognitive knowledge: knowledge of personal variables (knowledge about oneself as a learner), task variables (knowledge about the task to be performed), and strategy variables (knowledge about cognitive strategies and how to use them).

Reflection intuitively seems to be an underlying process that affects the thinking process. Dewey (1910) understood reflection as a process that goes beyond just thinking. He proposed that reflective thought is an "active, persistent, and careful consideration of any belief or supposed form of knowledge in the light of the grounds that support it" (p. 6). Dewey makes a distinction between reflection and critical reflection. Reflection refers to the process of considering an experience or problem in order to gain a better understanding of it by looking back on past experiences, analyzing them, and learning from them. Critical reflection, on the other hand, involves not only looking back on past experiences, but also questioning and challenging assumptions, values, and beliefs that underlie those experiences. Critical reflection involves a deeper level of inquiry and analysis, and it requires an openness to alternative perspectives and ways of thinking. It can lead to transformative learning, where individuals fundamentally change the way they understand themselves and the world. The active aspect of reflection persisted in subsequent discussion on the matter, influencing philosophers, psychologists, and educators such as Schön (1984) and Freire (1972).

While in Dewey's philosophy, reflection is focused on the thinking process, Schön incorporates action as a fundamental element of the reflective process. In contrast, Freire's view challenges this dichotomy by understanding reflection as a process that integrates action. For Freire, the focus is not solely on reflection as a cognitive process but also on its potential as a transformative action.

Schön's work on reflection builds on Dewey's ideas, particularly with respect to the concept of reflection-in-action, focusing mainly on reflection for professional development and for improving the quality of one's professional practice (Schön, 1984). He distinguishes between two types of reflection: reflection *in* action and reflection *on* action. Reflection in action refers to the process of reflecting on one's own actions and adjusting as the situation unfolds. This requires the ability to be flexible and adaptable, and to engage in a continuous process of learning. Reflection on action, on the other hand, involves looking back on one's experiences and analyzing them to gain insight into one's own practice. This type of reflection requires a more deliberate and structured approach, as it involves stepping back from the immediate situation and reflecting on what has happened to identify strengths and weaknesses, and to plan for future action (Schön, 1984).

Freire's influence was mostly seen in Mezirow's transformative learning model which focuses on how individuals can transform their beliefs, values, and assumptions through critical reflection. Mezirow (1981, 1991) assumed that critical reflection is necessary to achieve change and transformation. However, the relationship between the learning and the reflective process is not entirely clear (Denton, 2011).

Hatton and Smith (1995) proposed a model of reflection that would become widely known and among those most used to assess reflection. Based on Schön (1984) and Kolbs' (1984) theories of reflection and learning, Hatton and Smith's (1995) model integrates the importance of attending to self-awareness and exploration of one's own experience critically, and forming new perspectives, all of which can help individuals to learn from their experiences and apply that learning in future situations. The criteria developed by them for recognizing different types of reflective writing consisted in four levels: (1) *descriptive writing*, which consists of reporting events that occurred without any reflections, (2) *descriptive reflection*, where alternative views are recognized and there is superficial attempt to provide justification for events or actions, (3) *dialogic reflection*, which starts by using judgments to explore experiences and actions and alternative explanations, and (4) *critical reflection*, where there is an understanding of multiple historical, and socio-political contexts that influence multiple perspectives.

Another model widely used in education today is the one developed by Moon (1999a, 1999b, 2006). Moon adopts the concept of transformative learning from Mezirow, to propose the stages of her learning model. Part of the utility and diffusion of Moon's model lies in the operationalization of the elements that make up the reflective process. Moon seeks to distinguish critical reflection in the learning process through the analysis of writing. For this, she proposes four progressive levels of reflective writing: (1) descriptive writing; (2) descriptive account with some reflection; (3) reflective writing; (4) reflective writing where description is evidence of a process of reflection (Moon, 1999a, 1999b).

Moon argues that activities such as writing are potentially effective in fostering reflection. Writing is a crucial aspect of the reflective process as it enables individuals to externalize their thoughts and ideas, making them more tangible and easier to analyze (Moon, 1999b). Writing also helps to organize thoughts and ideas and enables them to be subjected to deeper analysis. However, not all writing tasks necessarily induce critical reflection. According to Moon, reflective writing specifically allows for reflective processes to develop. Therefore, resources such as learning logs and diaries are key elements for enhancing, fostering, and analyzing reflective thinking.

9.2.3 Reflective Writing and Learning Logs

Writing is a powerful tool for assessing reflection, as it provides a visible and tangible record of an individual's thoughts, feelings, and experiences. Research in medical education research has demonstrated the efficacy of reflective writing, allowing healthcare professionals to stop, review their mental representations and processes, and consider how their affective state and motivations affect their practice (Charon & Hermann, 2012; Chen & Forbes, 2014; Shapiro et al., 2009; Song & Stewart, 2012; Wald & Reis, 2010; for a review, see Lim et al., 2023). When an individual writes about their reflection, they are forced to organize their thoughts and ideas in a clear and coherent manner. This process requires the individual to critically evaluate their experiences, consider multiple perspectives, and develop a deeper understanding of themselves and their situation (Moon, 1999a).

Furthermore, writing allows for the expression of complex and nuanced ideas that might be difficult to articulate verbally. Writing can help individuals to delve deeper into their thoughts and feelings and explore different perspectives on a particular issue. It can also provide a space for self-expression, allowing individuals to express their emotions and experiences in a safe and non-judgmental way. Overall, writing is an effective means to assess reflection because it allows individuals to reflect deeply, critically evaluate their experiences, and express their thoughts and feelings in a clear and organized manner. It also provides a permanent record of the reflection, which can be reviewed and revisited at a later time for further learning and growth (Francis, 1995; Moon, 1999a; McGuire et al., 2009; Farah, 2012). For these reasons, reflective writing has been used in medical training (Shapiro et al., 2009; Chen & Forbes, 2014; Wald & Reis, 2010).

The interest in recognizing, analyzing, measuring, and fostering reflection has led to an increasing body of research oriented to approach these problems (Mann et al., 2007; Winkel et al., 2017; Triana et al., 2017, Koole et al., 2011). Strategies to foster reflection and summative assessments of the latter go hand-in-hand. When it comes to tackling the development of complex cognitive domains, assessment presents a challenge in and of itself, especially when it comes to assessments that rely on methodologies and tools known as "alternatives", such as the use of rubric-based assessment, especially in a context where quantitative approaches to assessment prevail (Camilloni, 2015). The discussion on the objectivity and reliability of these tools remains under debate (Derakhshan et al., 2011). Embracing the mission of assessing and fostering reflection in university students is, indeed, challenging. But it is still, beyond pedagogical needs, something that needs to be done.

There is a common understanding that imparting subject-specific knowledge falls short in enabling students to effectively tackle complex problems in their professional domains (Schön, 1984). Within ethics education, reflective writing has emerged as a valuable tool in assisting students to identify ethical concerns, comprehend the interplay between theoretical concepts and practical application, and cultivate a sense of commitment when faced with intricate scenarios (McGuire et al., 2009; Moon et al., 2013). The adoption of learning logs presents a promising strategy for advancing reflective writing skills among students and enhancing their metacognitive abilities.

"Learning logs" are logs in which students are encouraged to record their impressions, reflections, and observations throughout the course. They have been widely used to facilitate and enhance learning in medical education (Lim et al., 2023; Niemi, 1997). In addition to serving as a tool for evaluating the skills acquired in a course, the value of learning logs lies in the fact that during the process of creating them, it contributes to strengthening meaningful learning of the topics covered in the classroom and helps students to develop an awareness of their own learning process, fostering active engagement with the subject matter. Learning logs enable students to make sense of their own personal experiences in the context of what they have learned (Boud, 2001; Haigh, 2001). By facilitating the process of revisiting past experiences and reflections, learning logs enable students to reevaluate their previous understanding, become aware of the cognitive processes and emotions present in the recorded experiences, identify the reasoning and beliefs involved, and make the ways in which they are participating in the learning process explicit (Boud, 2001).

Learning logs serve multiple objectives, including the promotion of metacognition, critical and creative thinking, student engagement, expression of personal ideas, and the improvement of professional practice by making it the object of conscious reflection (Moon, 1999a, 2006), and provide a learning space for the interaction between theory and practice (Estrada & Rahmann, 2014). Specifically, they have been used as a tool in the education of scientists (Lázaro et al., 2022) and physicians (Freeman, 2001; Fung et al., 2023; Kelly, 1999).

9.3 Learning Logs Applied in a Bioethics Course

9.3.1 The Case Study: "Ethics and Science: Bioethics as a Bridge"

In Uruguay, there is a heterogeneous offer of courses in Ethics and Bioethics, both in their teaching format, intensity, content covered, and the pedagogical and didactic strategies implemented. Currently, Bioethics courses are provided in both private and public university institutions, societies and associations, and technical institutes. Within public universities, the University of the Republic offers Bioethics courses within the faculties of Medicine, Nursing, Dentistry, Chemistry, Law, and Sciences.

The Faculty of Medicine, for example, has promoted the incorporation of a critical perspective toward the conventional biologicist paradigm by integrating humanities disciplines into medical education (Dapueto et al., 2018). Furthermore, there have been initiatives aimed at enhancing professional practices, albeit their implementation has proven to be challenging (Dapueto et al., 2018). All courses are designed and taught by the Academic Unit of Bioethics, which was consolidated in 2008. During the six years of the degree, Bioethics courses have been incorporated into curricular units that include different subjects. Bioethics content is included during the first, second, third, fifth, and sixth year of the degree in different units. This Faculty is among the three top faculties with the highest enrollment rates of UDELAR. Enrollment rose from 2172 students in 2020, to 2308 in 2021, maintaining this trend in 2023 (Dirección General de Planeamiento, 2021). The high number of students is not usually accompanied by an increase in teaching staff resources, which makes it difficult to maintain face-to-face and workshop teaching modalities. Courses had suffered modifications to adapt to this demand. The use of multiple choice assessments, for instance, is currently the most used form of evaluation to assess Bioethics courses in medical education in this university.

In the Faculty of Sciences, an elective course in Bioethics is provided for students from different disciplines (Biology, Biochemistry, Mathematics, Physics, Geology, Geography, among others) as well as students from other faculties, including those in the Faculty of Medicine. This course is integrated into the Science and Development Unit, established in 1991 to tackle the humanistic and social dimensions of scientific education. More precisely, the unit aims to investigate and teach issues associated with the ethical, social, and political ramifications of scientific practices.

The course's pedagogical objectives are to enable students to identify ethical dilemmas in general (specifically bioethical), analyze them from a global perspective, and justify their positions and possible courses of action. The course design includes open debates among groups, a self-assessment of student performance (integrated into the final grade), as well as an evaluation of the course in those dimensions pre-selected by the students themselves. The course has also implemented various strategies to foster the development of deliberation, interdisciplinarity, metacognition, and critical thinking, such as the use of individual learning logs as a tool to track and evaluate each student's learning process. Within these logs, students are encouraged to engage in an internal dialogue, integrating their own impressions, ideas, doubts, or feelings with the course material and what they have learned (Lázaro et al., 2022).

9.3.2 Examining Reflective Thinking in Learning Logs

In this section, the aim is to present excerpts from learning logs developed by students during the course and their reflections will be analyzed through the lens of various theoretical frameworks. The selected excerpts have been categorized based on the elements deemed noteworthy for reflection analysis. All students participating in this chapter have given their consent. Students have been assigned an ID to keep their privacy. The IDs in this chapter allow the identification of the student's career. BIO: biology, HMB: human biology, BCH: biochemistry, PHY: physics, MED: medicine.

From Description to Inquiry

Most reflective journals tend to focus on descriptive writing. Descriptive writing is an essential part of the reflective process and a steppingstone to developing critical reflection. However, many students do not continue developing and analyzing their ideas. The following excerpt illustrates this point.

> The course began with an exercise about moral assessment, a good warm up. Beyond the specific situations in which we worked, what was interesting was giving the moral discussion a kickstart, that is, trying to justify our moral preferences in general principles. My initial thoughts were outlined toward the above, for example, my anthropocentrism and my idea of minimizing suffering in general were balanced with affirming that it is okay to experiment on animals within reasonable parameters (when it is really necessary) and the overall discussion was like that.
>
> *(PHY1)*

The excerpt above is an example of the use of a learning log as a way of reconstructing situations and as a first step toward reflection. In this case, the student refers to the first workshop held in the course. The student describes their initial thoughts on the matter.

This type of writing is descriptive in the sense that focuses on telling a story, describing situations of feelings and ideas that come naturally to oneself and which are not being "revisited" or analyzed. Moon (1999b) describes that these emotional reactions "are not explored and not related to behavior" and the ideas "are not considered or questioned and the possible impact on behavior or the meaning of events is not mentioned" (Moon, 1999b, p. 161). There is no account of reflection in descriptive writing.

However, descriptive writing can also be a starting point for the development of some kind of inquiry or reflection. During the early stages of learning, before a critical level has been reached, it is common for students to begin to ask questions. As students present the scenario and dilemma through descriptive writing, questions start to emerge to approach these problems. Mezirow (1991) stands on the idea that the presentation of a dilemma elicits strong emotions and prompts a critical examination of the situation. This examination usually starts in the form of a series of questions posted to challenge the assumptions of the dilemma or the opinion and emotions of the student. Moon (1999b) notes that this type of writing elicits some initial level of reflection, although still there is no critical examination.

Throughout the Bioethics course, the dynamic of the debate itself frequently leaves unresolved questions open, to encourage students to continue searching and reflecting beyond the confines of the classroom. The learning log allows for the stimulation of this continued process of reflection and enables to document its outcomes. The following excerpt exemplifies the use of inquiry in writing:

> Now, if all inherently human activity is moral, does that mean that all moral activity is inherently human? This is a question that came up in class and was answered with some examples: some "social" animals exhibit moral or pseudo-moral behaviors. In researching the subject, I have come across several articles and information, mostly from the Dutch primatologist and ethologist Frans de Waal. He shows us his findings, and how he believes that mammals also present moral values. He believes that morality is based on two essential pillars: reciprocity, associated with a sense of justice and fairness; and empathy, associated with compassion. The video shows us several experiments in which we observe these traits: primates that perform favors among themselves unselfishly, elephants that cooperate with each other. Also, primates that feel empathy, from basic expressions such as yawning (which we know is "repeated" in beings with a sense of empathy), to more complex ones, such as animals that comfort others in a similar way to humans. After this presentation, he summarizes by presenting morality as an evolutionary morality, present and continuous in all primates. In Conclusion, I consider this argument a very interesting and very good answer to the question, and I wanted to share it.
>
> *(BIO2)*

In this passage, the student takes a question that emerged during class and continues to investigate it outside of the classroom. The writing goes beyond a simple recollection of events, showcasing an attitude of curiosity, motivation, and a connection to their own field of study. While the inquiry does not lead to a deeper argument or problematization, there is a clear effort to engage with the question and explore it through new avenues.

According to Freire and Faundez ([1985] 2013), posing essential questions is crucial as it triggers new questions that lead to the construction of an argument, where both the answers and the previously posed questions are part of the same discourse. However, in the process of keeping a learning log, students often post questions that are not addressed or analyzed. This behavior is described by Moon (1999b) as a descriptive account with some reflection, a prior level of the process where the problem is still not problematized.

The learning logs allow us to track the development in the process of reflection, as seen in some of the questions posed. These questions serve as a starting point for more complex arguments and discussions. Some of the questions go beyond the surface-level content and identify underlying issues, although they may not explore them fully.

Recognizing and Analyzing Emotions

The interplay between emotions and cognition is still not fully understood but several researchers had hypotheses on the role of emotions in learning, decision-making, perception and most cognitive processes, and vice versa (Lazarus, 1982; Damasio, 1999; Mezirow, 1981, 1991; for a review, see McConnell, 2024). Different theories have linked the ability to recognize emotions and differentiate these emotional responses to the learning potential that can arise from it. Baumeister et al. (2007) state that "automatic affects simply activate approach and avoid tendencies, and conscious emotions stimulate reflection and learning" (p. 170).

When it comes to learning, Mezirow stated that recognizing the emotional aspects in the thinking process is key to fostering a critical approach and to enable reflection, as this allows the person to identify the dynamics that challenge assumptions. However, Mezirow's theory of learning developed a cognitive model of reflection which was mainly a rational conception of a mostly individual process. In 1997, Barnett included an analysis of the "critical being" in his framework of critical reflection, where he included an affective dimension of reflection. Unlike Mezirow's model, Barnett highlighted the positive aspects of the emotions in reflection and integrated a social and community approach to it.

Emotions play a fundamental aspect in developing reflection as they can influence our thoughts and behaviors (Dewey, 1910), potentially leading to making biased decisions. Recognizing and acknowledging emotions can allow us to identify the role of feelings in influencing judgment. To a large extent, the social aspect of reflection, often closer to the concept of reflexivity, lies in an emotional exploration of oneself.

According to Moon (1999a) reflection is enhanced by the emotional dimension that is allowed by journals or logs and encourages exercises that allow writing about experiences and learning from negative events. As an example, consider the excerpt.

I am going home; I cannot tell anyone about my experience. My partner does not want to hear about it because it turns their stomach on everything that has to do with viscera and organs (the fact that it is a mouse is not truly relevant to her). I cannot tell my mother-in-law either because she does not like the subject matter very much. I just sit there, not knowing what to think or what to feel. Nothing happens, no punishment, no reward. Whether I act morally or not in this situation, only matters to me. Then, I understand the reason as to why I am so active with some causes and not with others. I see acts of gender-based violence every day and I know other people are going to be affected and will see me differently based on my stance. That is the big motivator: the sense of justice only leads to guilt and anxiety. Having other people judge me brings me to action. I do not know if this speaks on the importance of collective action and of speaking out (even if no one listens to you), or of the power of inertia in human attitude. But I will definitely continue to process this experience for a long time.

(BCH1)

As the excerpt above shows, many students approach a specific topic (in this case, animal testing) by analyzing their emotions in an everyday scenario and explore their relationships with it. This excerpt also exemplifies the skills that Nussbaum (1997) highlights for "producing people who can function with sensitivity and alertness as citizens of the whole world" (Nussbaum, 1997, p. 8): a critical examination of oneself and the ability to see oneself connected to others.

Being conscious of one's emotional response can serve as a signal that something significant has occurred, indicating the need for attention and reflection. This can be particularly useful for students who experience strong emotional reactions when faced with challenging problems, prompting them to engage in deeper reflection on their thought processes and strategies for problem-solving. Furthermore, emotions can also assist students in regulating their cognitive processes by alerting them to the need for specific cognitive strategies which helps the evaluation of their own learning processes. Through reflection on their emotional responses to various learning situations, students can gain insight into their own strengths and weaknesses as learners, thereby enhancing their metacognitive abilities over time.

Critical Reflection as a Process

Most authors agree that reflective writing should show more than comprehension of the topic, theoretical and empirical sources used as evidence or in support of an argument, the use of questioning, and the recognition of emotions. It should evidence ideas or information that do not come from the situation by itself; it should evidence exploration, analysis, and discussion of the problem and the questions that arise from the process of exploration (Dewey, 1910).

Critical analysis of one's own thought requires skepticism of one's own arguments, challenging unidimensional perspectives, and addition of different viewpoints. Moon (1999b) states that during reflective writing, metacognitive

Fiorella Gago, Camila López Echagüe, and Marila Lázaro

stances can take place and "self-questioning is evident" appearing as internal dialogue.

However, the deep exploration needed to foster a critical point of view cannot be expected to always be reconstructed as a unique and clear moment, or not even as a linear process, but involves continuous revision and re-examination of assumptions and conclusions as new information is acquired or new perspectives are presented. As such, critical reflection is an ongoing process that requires an open and reflective attitude toward constant exploration and analysis of ideas, perspectives, and experiences. In summary, critical reflection is a process that involves a methodical approach and rigorous evaluation of information and requires an attitude of continuous learning and constant questioning.

This requires analyzing the students' writing as a whole. In this sense, analyzing their reflections by brief excerpts imposes difficulties and limitations, as the excerpts only show a small fraction of the students' learning and discussion. Even what can start as a descriptive passage can be highly valuable and potentially turn into a new perspective on a matter. The context of writing and timing offers a platform to let students' own learning process emerge. The following excerpts show the evolution of one student throughout the semester. Each excerpt was extracted from different moments of his learning log. It shows how a specific topic (animal testing) had an impact on himself.

One day I was eating meat and without any apparent reason, I felt strange. I thought about what was in front of me as a corpse, and I lost my appetite. That was the starting point for me to question whether what I had so normalized was wrong. At the beginning of the logbook, I briefly mentioned where my thinking about ethics and morality comes from. There, I made it clear that the mental processes that led me to those conclusions were always very anthropocentric, because the basis for my moral vision was the ability to make agreements with other similar beings. It happens that with animals, it is impossible to make agreements as with those who are similar to oneself, and for this reason, I never had them on my moral radar. Should I change?

(PHY1)

In my personal opinion, there were sincere questioning of certain things, as can be read in previous sections. I mainly highlight the concern that arose for me regarding the morality of eating meat and the feelings that the debate has generated on me; I am even seriously considering reducing my meat consumption, and if it works, I would consider giving it up altogether. For me, all of this is new and therefore I am not in a position to predict what will happen with all of this, but in the immediate future, I would say that it is serious because I have been avoiding meat like never before these days. I emphasize this because these are issues that would not have appeared if it were not for the course of that, I am sure.

(PHY1)

The lesson I take away is not insignificant, I have realized that we are much more irrational beings than I would have been willing to accept at other times in my life. Why do I say this? I always believed that one could justify morality in a rational system that aimed to ensure the well-being of all participants, something like seeking an optimal strategy in the game of life to achieve the Nash equilibrium... When I thought about whether it is moral to kill an animal to eat it, even if there is no real need to do so, I observed that if I am honest with myself the only valid reasons I have to maintain my initial position are: just because, because I like meat, or because I don't care. Without a doubt, they are not entirely rational arguments and this led me to finally understand that most of the time we actually act out of habit or emotion.

(PHY1)

The student's reflection process shows a significant shift in his thinking and understanding regarding the morality of eating meat. He questions his actions and beliefs, leading him to reevaluate his position. These questions were initially sparked by the realization that his moral vision could be anthropocentric, and, if so, it may not consider animals as deserving of moral consideration. This imposes a dilemma as it conflicts with his values. This dilemma leads to an expression of his own concern regarding the moral implications of eating meat. The student reflects on the limitations of rational justifications for morality and the role of habit and emotion in shaping our actions. Overall, the reflection process shows a deep engagement with ethical questions and a willingness to challenge one's own beliefs, leading to self' awareness of the implication of his actions.

Each of these paragraphs was produced over a spaced period of time. Unlike other assessment tools, which reflect the state of knowledge and skills of the student at a given moment (and which are also influenced by factors such as time or pressure), learning logs have the advantage of allowing a glimpse into the phenomenon of reflection and learning as a process. In them, it is possible to detect how students have incorporated different knowledge, skills, and reflective levels over time. Each evolution will be different: there are students who start the course already with high reflective levels, and others who do not. The value does not lie in finding high reflective levels, but in detecting changes, revisions, reconsiderations that imply some kind of evolution or improvement even in those whose writing is predominantly descriptive. It is in this sense that we say that reflective writing allows us to see the "bigger picture".

9.3.3 The Role of the Critical Reflection in the Education of Scientists and Physicians: Mauro's Loop

Despite efforts to consolidate a conception of science that does not elude complexity, historically situated and inseparable from its ethical, political, and cultural dimension, students often have a triumphalist and decontextualized image of science as a neutral activity reflecting the world (Olivé, 2003). In the context of a Bioethics course oriented to scientific and/or medical training, it is important to promote a critical review of this concept. To address any of the problems to be discussed in the course, it is essential to begin by recognizing the value dimension inherent to all scientific practice. It is here that one of the greatest challenges for the course is presented: to promote in students a critical reflection on their deepest beliefs about the nature and meaning of the activity they are studying and to which they intend to dedicate themselves. Many of the reflections in the learning logs reflect this effort to explore issues such as the objectivity-subjectivity dichotomy or the neutrality of science. For example:

> Why do I have the idea that subjectivity is something that is not so good, as something that at a certain point generates problems? Moreover, why do I consider that subjectivity and ethics cannot go hand in hand? I think about it over and over again, and it is like I am in a vicious circle, with no way out, I do not know what the "right" answer is. Why do I see subjectivity so intuitively as a black stain on ethical questions? Now, the fact that I consider that reasons can be given for moral choices, brings with it other considerations: are those reasons fair?, for whom are they fair?, are they fair in any and all backgrounds and times? That is to say, are those justifications for the reason a person does what they do valid and/or accepted in the same way by all of us who are part of the community? Who decides that? Will this problem of objectivity vs. subjectivity with respect to scientific questions be solved by considering the concept of intersubjectivity, raised in class?
>
> (BCH2)

This fragment shows an exercise in self-reflection that aims to critically review one's own ingrained beliefs and attitudes. The student not only applies concepts such as "subjectivity" but from them shows an effort to recognize his own habitual patterns of construction of judgments and reasoning. In this way, he approaches the exercise of metacognitive processes.

During the class, it is common that concerns and discomfort arise around the recognition of one's own subjectivity in the interpretation of the world and the foundation of ethical criteria. The advantage of the learning logs is that they allow taking these concerns and elaborating them, in order to nurture reflection on this value dimension in the light of the topics, concepts, and problems that are being addressed in class. Let us look at an enlightening example. In one of the first classes of one edition of the course, during the initial module in which the course and ethics as a discipline are introduced, a student raised a discomfort that later turned out to be a useful input to stimulate discussion in the group throughout the course. His approach was as follows:

> I find it difficult to climb up the complexity ladder of moral reflection without my personal bias coming out. I think it would be a good thing to minimize bias as much as possible but... I believe it may be impossible and, moreover, considering personal aspects may be beneficial. In this way, I've entered a loop that I can't seem to get out of.
>
> *(BIO3)*

The student's restlessness reveals a common perplexity: they begin to recognize their own biases, beliefs, attitudes permeating their reflections about moral dilemmas or ethical problems in general. Approaching personal bias is essential to critically examine a statement; personal bias has a negative effect in developing critical reflections (Linvill & Mazer, 2012). A common mistake among students is to confuse "ethical reflection" with "personal opinion"; achieving, on the contrary, a critical detachment from one's own beliefs or preferences is one of the main challenges of the course. Some people try, when faced with the recognition of their own subjectivity, to isolate their biases to make impartial, objective judgments; but at the same time, they find this exercise difficult. In the course, the challenge of reflecting on the initial discomfort raised by the aforementioned student was proposed, synthesized under the title "Mauro's loop". We must therefore ask whether it is possible to get out of Mauro's loop. If so, how is this accomplished? Another student reflected on it:

> Regarding this loop, I believe that it is possible to break free from personal bias, at least in certain situations, since the issue sometimes does not only involves overcoming our own bias, but also attempting to completely overcome the bias imposed on us by society, which I consider to be a bit more difficult and convoluted, but is it really possible? Is it something that is accessible to everyone? At the same time, I agree that it can be interesting to take our bias into account, at least if we desire so and if the situation allows it, but this does not mean that we cannot set it aside in another instance.
>
> *(BIO4)*

The previous excerpt shows a common reaction among students at the beginning of the course, where recognition of their own subjectivity provokes rejection, and the strategy to be implemented consists of attempting to "nullify" such subjectivity. While not all students manage to move away from this position, reflections that address this "loop" from the acceptance and integration of personal perspective as an element of analysis usually occur during the semester.

The learning logs are a resource that contributes to complexify and deepen the reflection on the interaction between one's own subjectivity and the elaboration of ethical judgments, since it is a reflection that occurs progressively as students appropriate the analytical and problematizing approach that runs through the course. Thus, toward the end of the semester, it is possible to come across considerations such as the following:

> At the beginning of this module, we started with the analysis of Mauro's loop, which questioned the possibility of human beings setting aside their personal bias when reflecting on our morality. To delve into this discussion, I think it is important to remember the differences between morality and ethics. The former is something inherent to our species, which responds to the question of "what should I do?" based on values and duties that are influenced by our culture and history and are not universal. Ethics, on the other hand, uses morality as its object of study and can be defined as the attempt to analyze and reflect on it, questioning the "why" of that duty raised through critical reflection. Taking into account the above, I believe that the dilemma raised by [B1] is, in essence, the first step towards ethics, as he is precisely questioning and problematizing this morality. Additionally, he is recognizing his own subjectivity, which, in my opinion, is essential when seeking valid arguments and foundations in this reflection. Recognizing this bias is ultimately the first step in questioning our actions and decisions, as if we did not recognize it, we would not even be questioning ourselves. Likewise, I understand that all of this is closely related to what Adela Cortina proposes, mentioning the objective of ethical reflection as "making ourselves intelligible to ourselves".
>
> *(MED1)*

This succession of reflections on the loop serves to illustrate several issues. In the first place, learning logs allow the evaluation of each student's individual process. A student who starts with a descriptive style may, toward the end of the learning log, explore more reflective aspects and even revise their own process. At the same time, learning logs are not just a product of an individual and isolated process of reflection, but there is feedback between the different collective proposals developed throughout the course and the individual process of each student in their learning log. In this case, for example, toward the end of the course, it was proposed to review the best solutions to Mauro's loop, and the last fragment quoted was one of the chosen ones. This shows the necessarily interactive and dialogue-based nature of bioethical reflection. The loop arises from a student's concern, which generates in others a problem to be investigated. The learning logs are individual but result from an internal dialogue whose trigger is the exchange and debate with peers.

This type of teaching and evaluation activities, specifically for the Bioethics course, requires as an indispensable condition, to be based on an exercise of revision, recognition, and critical distance with respect to one's own beliefs, assessments, and conceptions, and that is why it is especially useful in the scientific and medical humanities.

9.4 Conclusion

The field of medical and scientific humanities has emphasized the significance of integrating a holistic perspective into medical education, which encompasses thoughtful consideration of the ethical, political, and cultural ramifications of professional practice. In this context, courses in Bioethics offer an opportune platform for facilitating the cultivation of skills related to critical thinking, introspection, and discourse. Nonetheless, merely addressing the substantive aspects of the discipline does not suffice in realizing this objective; it is imperative to employ pedagogical and evaluative measures that translate this vision into tangible outcomes.

The learning logs produced during the Bioethics courses examined here demonstrate the development of different levels of reflection in the students. It is possible to appreciate the implementation of skills typical of a more descriptive level, such as synthesis, as well as more complex reflection processes. This specific experience of employing learning logs as a learning and assessment strategy in a Bioethics course prompts us to consider the potential of this tool for nurturing reflective and metacognitive aptitudes in medical and scientific professionals. Learning logs offer the benefit of enabling the monitoring and assessment of the individual student's progress throughout the course. However, their implementation may entail certain challenges. The assessment of intricate cognitive processes poses a challenge, particularly given that the prevailing assessment model tends to focus on quantitative tools. An interesting counterpoint that focuses on quantitative methods can be found in the chapter by Schoenherr et al. (2024) in this volume. Moreover, not all students develop deep levels of reflection. The learning log is one of the components of the course, possibly a privileged one in terms of stimulating the individual process in the student. However, other complementary components are needed to stimulate other mental and social processes. For example, collective deliberation or the implementation of more automatable evaluations with rubrics allows self-evaluation exercises, among others.[2]

The increase in the number of university students poses novel challenges for courses aiming to foster critical thinking skills by using instruments that are not automatable for correction. These challenges not only stem from the augmented demand for evaluation time that this tool requires, but also from the ongoing debates concerning its objectivity and reliability. To tackle these challenges, it would be pertinent to continue developing a specific reflection-level protocol for Bioethics courses, which accounts for the distinctive features and objectives of the subject.

In essence, it is imperative to embrace formative evaluation instead of merely relying on summative assessment, which will enhance the learning processes in a comprehensive and interdisciplinary educational setting. The implementation of novel teaching and evaluation methods can indeed prove daunting and intricate. Nevertheless, it is crucial to fortify the training of future professionals who are critical and reflective in their practice.

Notes

1   For instance, Schoenherr and Schoenherr (2024) note how medical education in East Asia has been – and continues to be - influenced by regional belief systems and social institutions, with countries such as North Korea and Vietnam requiring 'political education' in the curriculum for healthcare professionals. See also (Schoenherr, 2024; Venosa et al., 2024).
2   A formative assessment tool to develop ethical thinking skills is currently being designed and validated by our team. The project is being funded by the Comisión Sectorial de Enseñanza (CSE, UDELAR) to whom we express our gratitude for its financial and academic support.

References

Abel, F. (1999). El futuro de la docencia de bioética en España. *Cuadernos de bioética*, 10(37), 11–16.

Barnett, R. (1997). *Higher Education: A Critical Business*. Buckingham: Society for Research into Higher Education and Open University Press.

Baumeister, R. F., Vohs, K. D., Nathan DeWall, C., & Zhang, L (2007). How emotion shapes behavior: Feedback, anticipation, and reflection, rather than direct causation. *Personality and Social Psychology Review*, 11(2), 167–203.

Bleakley, A. (2015). *Medical Humanities and Medical Education: How the Medical Humanities Can Shape Better Doctors*. New York: Routledge.

Bloom, S. W. (1992). Medical education in transition: Paradigm change and organizational status. In: Marston, J. (ed.), *Medical Education in Transition*. Princeton: The Robert-Wood Johnson Foundation.

Boud, D. (2001). Using journal writing to enhance reflective practice. *New Directions for Adult and Continuing Education*, 90, 9–18.

Camilloni, A. (2015). Nudos de debate sobre la evaluación de los aprendizajes en la universidad, necesidades de actualización, profundización e investigación educativa. In: Comisión Sectorial de Enseñanza (ed.), *La evaluación en la educación superior: un escenario de controversia*. Montevideo: Universidad de la República.

Charon, R., & Hermann, M. N. (2012). A sense of story, or why teach reflective writing? *Academic Medicine: Journal of the Association of American Medical Colleges*, 87(1), 5.

Chen, I., & Forbes, C. (2014). Reflective writing and its impact on empathy in medical education: Systematic review. *Journal of Educational Evaluation for Health Professions*, 11, 20.

Collazo, M. (2014). El cambio curricular, una oportunidad para repensar (nos). *InterCambios. Dilemas y transiciones de la Educación Superior*, 1(1), 36–43.

Damasio, A. R. (1999). *The Feeling of What Happens: Body and Emotion in the Making of Consciousness*. New York: Houghton Mifflin Harcourt.

Dapueto, J. J., Viera, M., Samenow, C., Swiggart, W. H., & Steiger, J. (2018). A tale of two countries: Innovation and collaboration aimed at changing the culture of medicine in Uruguay. *Hec forum*, 30, 329–339.

Delors, J. (1996). *Learning: The Treasure Within. Report to UNESCO of the International Commission on Education for the Twenty-First Century*. Paris: UNESCO.

Denton, D. (2011). Reflection and learning: Characteristics, obstacles, and implications. *Educational Philosophy and Theory*, 43(8), 838–852.

Derakhshan, A., Rezaei, S., & Alemi, M. (2011). Alternatives in assessment or alternatives to assessment: A solution or a quandary. *International Journal of English Linguistics*, 1(1), 173–180.

Dewey, J. (1910). *How We Think*. Chicago: D. C. Heath Co. Publishers.

Dirección General de Planeamiento (2021). Ingresos de estudiantes a Carrera 2020. Available online in: https://planeamiento.udelar.edu.uy/publicacion_generica/ingresos-a-carrera-segun-area-y-servicio-por-localizacion-y-sexo-2020/

Eckles, R. E., Meslin, E. M., Gaffney, M., & Helft, P. R. (2005). Medical ethics education: Where are we? Where should we be going? A review. *Academic Medicine*, 80(12), 1143–1152.

Estrada, F. F., & Rahman, M. A. (2014). Reflective journal writing as an approach to enhancing students' learning experience. *Brunei Darussalam Journal of Technology and Commerce*, 8(1), 22–35.

Evans, M. (2002). Medicine, philosophy, and the medical humanities. *The British Journal of General Practice*, 52(479), 447–448.

Farah, M. (2012). Reflective journal writing: An effective technique for the writing process. *An-Najah University Journal for Research (Humanities)*, 30(4), 727–736.

Finn, P. (2011). Critical thinking: Knowledge and skills for evidence-based practice. *Language Speech and Hearing Services in Schools*, 42(1), 69–72.

Flavell, J. H. (1979). Metacognition and cognitive monitoring: A new area of cognitive–developmental inquiry. *American Psychologist*, 34(10), 906–911.

Francis, D. (1995). The reflective journal: A window to preserve teachers' practical knowledge. *Teaching & Teacher Education*, 11(3), 229–241.

Freeman, M. (2001). Reflective logs: An aid to clinical teaching and learning. *International Journal of Language & Communication disorders*, 36(sup1), 411–416.

Freire, P. (1972). *Pedagogía del oprimido*. Buenos Aires: Siglo XXI.

Freire, P., & Faundez, A. ([1985] 2013). *Por una pedagogía de la pregunta. Crítica a una educación basada en respuestas a preguntas inexistentes.* Buenos Aires: Siglo XXI.

Fuller, S., & Collier, J. H. (2003). *Philosophy, Rhetoric, and the End of Knowledge: A New Beginning for Science and Technology Studies.* New York: Routledge.

Fung, O. W., Mulholland, A., Bondy, M., Driedger, M., & Kendall, C. E. (2023). Implementing experiential learning logs addressing social accountability into undergraduate medical clerkship education. *Canadian Medical Education Journal,* 14(2), 146.

Gallopin, G., Funtowicz, S., O'Connor, M., & Ravetz, J. (2001) Science for the twenty-first century: From social contract to the scientific core. *International Social Science Journal,* 168, 220–229.

Haigh, M. J. (2001). Constructing Gaia: Using journals to foster reflective learning. *Journal of Geography in Higher Education,* 25(2), 167–189.

Hatton, N., & Smith, D. (1995). Reflection in teacher education: towards definition and implementation. *Teaching Teacher Education,* 11(1), 33–49.

Jenicek, M., Croskerry, P., & Hitchcock, D. L. (2011). Evidence and its uses in health care and research: The role of critical thinking. *Medical Science Monitor: International Medical Journal of Experimental and Clinical Research,* 17(1), RA12.

Kelly, D. R. (1999). The development and evaluation of a personal learning log for senior house officers. *Medical Education,* 33(4), 260–266.

Kohlberg, L. (1992). *Psicología del desarrollo moral.* Bilbao: Desclée de Brouwer.

Kolb, D. A. (1984). *Experiential Learning: Experience as the Source of Learning and Development.* New Jersey: Prentice-Hall

Koole, S., Dornan, T., Aper, L., Scherpbier, A., Valcke, M., Cohen-Schotanus, J., & Derese, A. (2011). Factors confounding the assessment of reflection: A critical review. *BMC Medical Education,* 11(1), 1–9.

Ku, K. Y. L., & Ho, I. T. (2010). Metacognitive strategies that enhance critical thinking. *Metacognition and Learning,* 5(3), 251–267.

Latour, B. (2012) *Cogitamus: seis cartas sobre las humanidades científicas.* Buenos Aires: Paidós.

Lázaro, M., López Echagüe, C., & Gago, F. (2022). Learning logs: Reflective writing and metacognition in bioethics courses. *Canadian Journal of Bioethics,* 5(4), 68–82.

Lazarus, R. S. (1982). Thoughts on the relations between emotion and cognition. *American Psychologist,* 37(9), 1019–1024.

León Correa, F. J. (2008). Enseñar bioética: cómo trasmitir conocimientos, actitudes y valores. *Acta bioethica,* 14(1), 11–18.

Lim, J. Y., Ong, S. Y. K., Ng, C. Y. H., Chan, K. L. E., Wu, S. Y. E. A., So, W. Z., ... & Krishna, L. K. R. (2023). A systematic scoping review of reflective writing in medical education. *BMC Medical Education,* 23(1), 12.

Linvill, D. L., & Mazer, J. P. (2012). Perceived ideological bias in the college classroom and the role of student reflective thinking: A proposed model. *Journal of the Scholarship of Teaching and Learning,* 11(4), 90–101.

Ma, T. (2024). Considerations for implementation of a competency-based education program for preclerkship courses. In Schoenherr, J. R. & McConnell, M. M. (eds.), *Fundamentals and Frontiers in Medical Education and Decision-Making: Educational Theory and Psychological Practice.* Routledge.

Mann, K., Gordon, J., & MacLeod, A. (2007). Reflection and reflective practice in health professions education: A systematic review. *Advances in Health Sciences Education*, 14(4), 595–621.

Martínez Asuaga, M. (2019). La función de enseñanza de la Facultad de Medicina: desafíos actuales. *Revista Médica del Uruguay*, 35(1), 1–5.

McGuire, L., Lay, K., & Peters, J. (2009). Pedagogy of reflective writing in professional education. *Journal of the Scholarship of Teaching and Learning*, 9(1), 93–107.

Mezirow, J. (1981). A critical theory of adult learning and education. *Adult Education*, 32(1), 3–24.

Mezirow, J. D. (1991). *Transformative Dimensions of Adult Learning*. San Francisco: Jossey-Bass.

Miyamoto, K., Huerta, M. C., & Kubacka, K. (2015). Fostering social and emotional skills for well-being and social progress. *European Journal of Education*, 50, 147–159.

Moon, J. (1999a). *Reflection in Learning and Professional Development*. London: Routledge Falmer.

Moon, J. (1999b). *Learning Journals: A Handbook for Academics, Students and Professional Development*. London: Kogan Page.

Moon, J. (2006). *Learning Journals: A Handbook for Reflective Practice and Professional Development*. London: Routledge Falmer.

Moon, M., Taylor, H., McDonald, E. L., Hughes, M. T., Beach, M. C., & Carrese, J. (2013). Analyzing reflective narratives to assess the ethical reasoning of pediatric residents. *Narrative Inquiry in Bioethics*, 3(2), 165–174.

Moulton, M. P., Carpenter, L. H., & Lubin, B. (2007). Gaia: Using journals to foster reflective learning. *Journal of Geography in Higher Education*, 25(2), 167–189.

Niemi, P. M. (1997). Medical students' professional identity: Self-reflection during the preclinical years. *Medical Education*, 31(6), 408–415.

Norman, E., Pfuhl, G., Sæle, R. G., Svartdal, F., Låg, T., & Dahl, T. I. (2019). Metacognition in psychology. *Review of General Psychology*, 23(4), 403–424.

Norman, G. R., & Brooks, L. R. (1997). The non-analytical basis of clinical reasoning. *Advances in Health Sciences Education*, 2, 173–184.

Nussbaum, M. (1997) *Cultivating Humanity: A Classical Defense of Reform in Liberal Education*. Cambridge: Harvard University Press.

OECD (2013). *OECD Skills Outlook 2013: First Results from the Survey of Adult Skills*. Paris: OECD.

Olivé, L. 2003. La democratización de la ciencia desde la perspectiva de la ética. In: López Cerezo, J. A. (ed.), *La democratización de la ciencia*. San Sebastián: Universidad del País Vasco (UPV/EHU), Colección Poliedro, 159–187

Potter, V. R. (1988). *Global bioethics–Building on the Leopold legacy*. Michigan: Michigan State University Press.

Rogers, R. R. (2001). Reflection in higher education: A concept analysis. *Innovative Higher Education*, 26(1), 37–57.

Sánchez González, M. A. (2017). El humanismo y la enseñanza de las humanidades médicas. *Educación médica*, 18(3), 212–218.

Schoenherr, J. R. (2024). The development and dynamics of Mayan healthcare systems: A socioecological approach. In Schoenherr, J. R. (ed.), *Fundamentals and Frontiers in Medical Education and Decision-Making: Innovation, Implementation, and Translational Research*. Routledge.

Schoenherr, J. R., & Beaudoin, J. (2024). Medical pluralism in East Asian medical education: The evolving landscape of health professions education in East Asia. In Schoenherr, J. R. (ed.), *Fundamentals and Frontiers in Medical Education and Decision-Making: Innovation, Implementation, and Translational Research*. Routledge.

Schoenherr, J. R., & Hamstra, S. J. (2024). Validity in health professions education: From assessment instruments to program innovation and evaluation. In Schoenherr, J. R. & McConnell, M. (eds.), *Fundamentals and Frontiers in Medical Education: Educational Theory and Psychological Practice*. Routledge.

Schoenherr, J. R., Mahias-Ito, Y., & Li, X. Y. (2024). Collective competence and social learning in the health professions: learning, thinking, and deciding in groups. In Schoenherr, J. R. (ed.), *Fundamentals and Frontiers in Medical Education and Decision-Making: Innovation, Implementation, and Translational Research*. Routledge.

Schoenherr, J. R. & McConnell, M. (2024). Human-centered design in health professions education: Informing Competency-Based Education with Psychological Science. In Schoenherr, J. R. & McConnell, M. (eds.), *Fundamentals and Frontiers in Medical Education and Decision-Making: Educational Theory and Psychological Practice*. Routledge.

Schoenherr, J. R., & Le-Bouar, C. (2024). Representing and communicating health information: Fundamentals of persuasive health communication. In Schoenherr, J. R. & McConnell, M. (eds.), *Fundamentals and Frontiers in Medical Education: Educational Theory and Psychological Practice*. Routledge.

Schoenherr, J. R., Waechter, J., & Lee, C. H. (2024). Quantifying expertise in the healthcare professions: Cognitive efficiency and metacognitive calibration. In: Schoenherr, J. R. & McConnell, M. M. (eds.), *Fundamentals and Frontiers of Medical Education and Decision-Making: Educational Theory and Psychological Practice*. Routledge.

Schön, D. (1984). *The Reflective Practitioner: How Professionals Think in Action*. London: Temple Smith.

Shapiro, J., Coulehan, J., Wear, D., & Montello, M. (2009). Medical humanities and their discontents: Definitions, critiques, and implications. *Academic Medicine*, 84(2), 192–198.

Shiau, S.-J., & Chen, C.-H. (2008). Reflection and critical thinking of humanistic care in medical education. *The Kaohsiung Journal of Medical Sciences, 24*(7), 367–372.

Song, P., & Stewart, R. (2012). Reflective writing in medical education. *Medical Teacher, 34*(11), 955–956.

Tanner, K. D. (2012). Promoting student metacognition. *CBE—Life Sciences Education*, 11(2), 113–120.

Tawil, S., & Cougoureux, M. (2013). *Revisiting learning: The Treasure within. Assessing the Impact of the 1996 'Delors Report'*. France: UNESCO Education Research and Foresight Occasional Papers.

Triana, M. J. R., Prieto, L. P., Vozniuk, A., Boroujeni, M. S., Schwendimann, B. A., Holzer, A., & Gillet, D. (2017). Monitoring, awareness and reflection in blended technology enhanced learning: A systematic review. *International Journal of Technology Enhanced Learning, 9*(2/3), 126.

Venosa, A. R., Baroneza, J. E., & Fernandes, R. A. F. (2024). Medical education in Brazil: A history of an evolving pluralistic healthcare system. In Schoenherr,

J. R. (ed.), *Fundamentals and Frontiers in Medical Education and Decision-Making: Innovation, Implementation, and Translational Research*. Routledge.

Vienni-Baptista, B. (2015). Los estudios sobre interdisciplina: Construcción de un ámbito en el campo de la ciencia, tecnología y sociedad. *Redes: Revista de estudios sociales de la ciencia*, 21(41), 141–175.

Wald, H. S., & Reis, S. P. (2010). Beyond the margins: Reflective writing and development of reflective capacity in medical education. *Journal of General Internal Medicine*, 25, 746–749.

Westerhaus, M., Finnegan, A., Haidar, M., Kleinman, A., Mukherjee, J., & Farmer, P. (2015). The necessity of social medicine in medical education. *Academic Medicine*, 90(5), 565–568.

Wilkinson, T. J. (1999). Reflective writing in medical practice: A linguistic perspective. *Text–Interdisciplinary Journal for the Study of Discourse*, 19(3), 331–346.

Winkel, A. F., Yingling, S., Jones, A.-A., & Nicholson, J. (2017). Reflection as a learning tool in graduate medical education: A systematic review. *Journal of Graduate Medical Education*, 9(4), 430–439.

World Health Organization (2013). *Health Education: Theoretical Concepts, Effective Strategies, and Core Competencies*. Cairo: WHO Regional Office for the Eastern Mediterranean.

Wynne, B. (1991). Knowledges in context. *Science, Technology, & Human Values*, 16(1), 111–121.

Zhou, K. (2017). Non-cognitive skills: Potential candidates for global measurement. *European Journal of Education*, 52(4), 487–497. doi:10.1111/ejed.12241

Ziman, J. (2000). *Real Science: What It Is and What It Means*. Cambridge: Cambridge University Press.

10

REPRESENTING AND COMMUNICATING HEALTH INFORMATION

Fundamentals of Persuasive Health Communication

Jordan Richard Schoenherr and Cedric Le-Bouar

10.1 Introduction

We often take our ability to learn and use language for granted. The difficulties in communication become immediately apparent when we examine the professional context of health care. Clinicians and patients might share the same language, but their health literacy, sociocultural background, manner of speech, and roles can create barriers the interfere with the development of a therapeutic alliance. Unlike other approaches to persuasive communication[1], the subject of health communication largely pertains to unobservable phenomena (e.g., 'germs', viruses), delayed consequences (e.g., presentation and spread of disease), and often require conjunctions of factors (e.g., presence of a virus, limited immunity, and access to treatment; Morgan & Miller, 2002; Peltu, 1985).

Beyond everyday practice, the successes and failures of public health communication by public health agencies during the COVID-19 pandemic illustrate the unique requirements of communicating with disparate communities and policymakers. From the announcement of the World Health Organization (WHO) to the subsequent responses of national agencies, stakeholders were inundated with information, misinformation, and disinformation that attempted to explain the causal mechanisms of the virus, the severity of infection, its prevalence in a population, and effective prevention and treatment methodologies. Beyond clarity and consistency of communication, people also questioned the credibility of the message source. The 'infodemic' that paralleled the spread of the virus reinforced the importance of the need to develop effective risk communication strategies within the healthcare community.

DOI: 10.4324/9781003316091-12

Healthcare professionals (HCPs) face additional challenges when working in interprofessional teams when stress, interpersonal discord, or roles and responsibilities are unclear (Schoenherr, Mahias-Ito, & Li, 2024). Whether we consider communication between medical educators and learners, practitioners and patients, or governmental agencies and the public, health communication is an essential competency that all HCPs must master. Failures of communication can have dire consequences. Studies have repeatedly demonstrated that miscommunication leads to negative patient outcomes, including increased mortality (Joint Commission on Accreditation of Healthcare Organizations, 2005; National Patient Safety Goals, 2005; Tiwary et al., 2019). This is especially apparent in acute care settings where time and information are limited (Fagin, 1997; Fisher & Peterson, 1993; Larson, 1999; Tiwary et al., 2019; Zwarenstein & Reeves, 2002). On a larger scale, this was also observed during the COVID-19 pandemic where changes in public health messages created uncertainty, disbelief, and psychological reactance, resulting in divergent information ecosystems that were associated with differences in the adoption of public health measures (for example, in Canada and the United States, see Schoenherr, 2022b; Schoenherr & Thomson, 2020). Given the consequential nature of interpersonal and intergroup communication, HCPs must make efforts to understand how health seekers understand health and illness. This is especially critical in cases of medical pluralism, where health seekers are presented with alternative explanations and therapeutic solutions to their illnesses (Schoenherr, 2024; Schoenherr & Beaudoin, 2024). Theories and methods developed in the social sciences can be used to inform personal practices, professional pedagogy, and public health communication (Glanz & Bishop, 2010).

10.1.1 Health Communication: Motivation, Models, and Methods

In its simplest form, health communication requires that the speaker reduces a listener's *uncertainty*. Traditional approaches frame communication in terms of a 'Code Model' such that the message transmitter (e.g., teacher, clinician, or public health official) encodes their knowledge into symbols such as spoken or written language, and the recipient (e.g., learner, patient, of health information seeker) decodes the message (top, Figure 10.1). Unfortunately, the Code Model ignores the process of interpersonal sensemaking that occurs in both the speaker and listener.

Competent clinicians understand their patients, not simply the diseases that they are treating. Uncertainty reduction requires identifying what information is *relevant* to an audience – it must be novel, timely, and concise. Relevance is ultimately dependent on a listener's health literacy, goals, and direct or indirect experience with illness. These factors will lead to important differences in communication practices depending on whether we consider

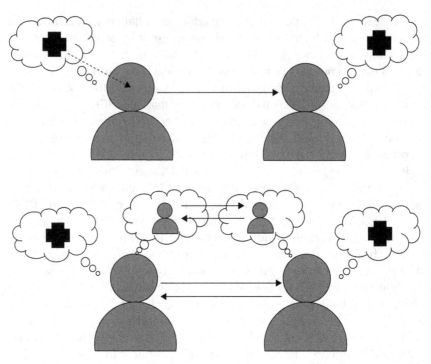

FIGURE 10.1 Two general models of communication. The Code Model of Communication (top) assumes that speakers simply encode a message into language, with listeners decoding the message. The Relevance Model of Communication (bottom) assumes that encoding mental representations into language requires an understanding of the audience (learner) and that linguistic conventions are selected to ensure that a message is relevant to the audience (learner).

interprofessional communication within or between groups of HCPs or extraprofessional communication with stakeholders who have limited literacy and experience in the healthcare domain. Rather than assuming that presenting 'facts' to health seekers conveys knowledge, effective communication requires that we take the perspective of our audience, ensuring that we provide relevant information (bottom, Figure 10.1).

Communication rarely occurs in a single episode. It unfolds over time, requiring the development and maintenance of a relationship between speaker and listener. Relationships that are defined by asymmetries in power can be especially problematic. For intraprofessional and interprofessional communication, psychological safety is a key determinant of whether colleagues will provide information, opinions, and feedback in an unfiltered manner (Grailey et al., 2021; O'Donovan & McAuliffe, 2020a, 2020b). For communication outside of one's profession, the therapeutic alliance developed between health seekers and HCPs will determine whether treatment recommendations are adopted (Elvins & Green, 2008; Kelley et al., 2014; Mao et al., 2021; Martin et al., 2000; Nienhuis et al., 2018; Totura et al., 2018). Rather than framing this as a 'problem of compliance' or a passive process of 'behavioral change', we must see health seekers as partners in making sense of health and illness (Charon, 2008).

Increasingly attention has been directed toward understanding, teaching, and measuring communication skills in the health professions (Berkhof et al., 2011; Cegala & Lenzmeier Broz, 2002; de Sousa et al., 2019; Hamilton et al., 2019; Kyaw et al., 2019; Rehim et al., 2017). Many of these approaches focus on general principles or provide assessment instruments without qualifying the mental processes that cause the observed behavior. In this chapter, we review health communication, focusing on how people represent diseases and illnesses, the features of health messages, and how these factors affect health communication to a large audience.

In Section 1, we review theories and empirical research that describe how people represent health and illness. By understanding the mental models of patients, the public, and professionals (collectively, health seekers), HCPs can more effectively communicate with them. Beyond specific mental models of health and illness, health seekers are also affected by general heuristics and biases. Section 2 reviews research on health communication to identify features of health messages that increase their persuasiveness and adoption of relevant health behaviors. Even if HCPs are only concerned with the treatment of patients, they must also be aware that health seekers are situated in social networks that determine information availability, how it is evaluated, and what channels are relied upon. Section 3 draws together the lessons from our review and provides a brief overview of how information diffuses in social networks, a process referred to as social contagion.

10.2 Representing Health: The Mental Models of Speakers and Listeners

HCPs dedicate years to developing mental representations of illness through lectures, research, direct observations, and indirect experiences through the narratives of their colleagues. As they transition from novice to expert, their knowledge is shaped by formal feedback and informal experience (Abdo et al., 2024; Montiero et al., 2024; e.g., Bing-You et al., 2017; Hatala et al., 2014; Schoenherr, Mahias-Ito, & Li, 2024). Concurrently, patients and the public develop their own representations of illness and disease through education, experiences with family and friends, rumor and gossip, and intuition. This is typically defined in terms of their *health literacy*, how a health information seeker obtains, understands, assesses, and uses health information to make decisions that affect their health. This competency appears to be a critical determinant of health, as low health literacy is associated with lower health outcomes (Berkman et al., 2011; Nutbeam & Lloyd, 2021; Rudd et al., 2023 Sørensen et al., 2012).

Due to disparate experience, the mental models of health seekers are typically defined by folk beliefs that can complement, or conflict, with the biomedical models of HCPs (Schoenherr, 2024). Regardless of their accuracy, HCPs must understand how people represent health beliefs and information. In this section, we review theories that describe and explain the features of these mental models and how they form.

10.2.1 Cognitive and Affective Approaches

Health Belief Model. First developed to understand patients' beliefs about tuberculosis (Rosenstock, 1966), the Health Belief Model (HBM) has subsequently been extended to many other areas of health including promotion of exercise regimens (e.g., Mirotznik et al. 1995), breast cancer self-examination and mammography (e.g., Ronis & Harel, 1989), HIV/AIDS (e.g., Barclay et al., 2007), medication adherence in hemodialysis patients (e.g., Wiebe & Christensen, 1997), and food allergies (e.g., Jones et al., 2015; Hochbaum, 1958; Rosenstock, 1974; Rosenstock, 1960; Kirscht, 1974; for a recent review, see Abraham & Sheeran, 2015).

HBM assumes that mental models of illness are defined by perceived susceptibility and severity, whereas its treatment is defined by the perceived benefits, barriers, and self-efficacy, i.e., the belief that one can perform a behavior (Rosenstock, 1974; Rosenstock et al., 1988). Demographic factors, psychological characteristics, and a patient's general health motivation also contribute to the adoption of health-related behaviors. Reinforcing these mental models, internal (e.g., pain) and external cues to action (e.g., media reminders) can prime mental models, increasing the likelihood of behavior. Due to its simplicity and use of common-sense variables, HBM provides an intuitive model that has generated considerable research (Abraham & Sheeran, 2015; Jones et al., 2015).

Despite its use, HBM has been criticized on several grounds. First, HBM focuses exclusively on cognitive representations of health and illness, leaving affective and emotional responses that can be used as cues for action unaddressed (Ogden, et al., 2019). Second, the factors identified by HBM do not all contribute equally to health decisions. In his meta-analysis of HBM studies, Carpenter (2010) found that treatment factors were the most significant determinants of the HBM with perceived barriers to treatment and benefits of treatment, a result consistent with other meta-analyses (Janz & Becker, 1984; Harrison et al., 1992; Jones et al., 2014; Stretcher et al., 1986). In contrast, factors related to disease models were far less predictive, with disease severity and perceived susceptibility accounting for little variation in behavior. Early reviews attributed these failures to the impact of unhealthy habits, social approval, and environmental influences on individuals' decision-making (Janz & Becker, 1984).

Finally, while HBM provides predictions about the content of mental models, it does not consider how attitudes are formed or changed. This criticism is especially problematic given the widespread use of fear-based messaging in public health campaigns and experimental studies (Leventhal et al., 1967; Ruiter et al., 2014) and the influence of affective and metacognitive systems on responses (e.g., Gago et al., 2024; McConnell, 2024; Schoenherr et al., 2024). Thus, despite the simplicity of the constructs used in HBM (Harrison et al., 1992), the lack of clearly defined variables hinders the predictive utility of HBM (Abraham & Sheeran, 2015).

Protection Motivation Theory. Protection Motivation Theory (PMT) focuses on the efficacy of fear-based appeals (Rogers, 1975). Like HBM, the PMT approach has been used to examine health behaviors including venereal disease prevention (Mewborn & Rogers, 1979), adoption of protective behaviors in pandemics (Bish & Michie, 2010), smoking cessation (Maddux & Rogers, 1983), and physical exercise adherence (Norman et al., 2005).

According to Rogers (1983), the use of fear in communication is effective when (a) an event is perceived to be harmful, (b) the health information seeker will be affected by the event, (c) there is the possibility of avoidance, and (d) the recommendation appears to be an effective strategy. PMT assumes that the experience of fear is a readily accessible cue that initiates the appraisal of the costs and benefits that determine an individual's motivation for action, or protection motivation (Maddux & Rogers, 1983; Mewborn & Rogers, 1979). Protection motivation is a cognitive state that leads to an intent to apply a recommendation by initiating, guiding, and sustaining the individual's response (Rogers, 1975; Maddux & Rogers, 1983; Milne et al., 2000). Individuals' protection motivation is determined by both a threat appraisal process (evaluating severity and probability of an aversive outcome) and a coping appraisal process (evaluation of the coping strategy; Rogers, 1983; Floyd et al., 2000). Self-efficacy is further assumed to be an intervening variable in the coping appraisal process, increasing the likelihood of adopting an adaptive response (Rogers, 1983).

In an early review of literature on pandemics/epidemics (SARS, H5N1, H1N1, and avian flu), perceptions of susceptibility, severity (threat appraisal process), and efficacy of the coping response (coping appraisal process) were all significantly related to health behaviors (Bish & Michie, 2010). Furthermore, two large-scale meta-analyses provided support for the threat and coping appraisal processes of PMT as predictors of health attitudes and behaviors (Floyd et al., 2000; Milne et al., 2000). Finally, these reviews provided significant evidence for the usefulness of self-efficacy as a predictor in PMT due to the strength of its association with attitudes and behaviors (Floyd et al., 2000; Milne et al., 2000).

Health Action Process Approach. Models of attitudes and beliefs, like HBM and PMT, fail to address the fact that attitudes and behaviors are often only weakly related (Glasman & Albarracin, 2006), referred to as the intention-behavior gap (Milne et al., 2000; Norman et al., 2005). The Health Action Process Approach (HAPA) attempts to account for this discrepancy. The key benefit of this approach is that, rather than looking at health behavior at a single point in time, a longitudinal approach allows us to reduce the intention behavior gap (Schwarzer, 2008; Schwarzer et al., 2008). HAPA has been applied to many health issues including smoking cessation, adherence to low-fat diets, and exercise in healthy adults and rehabilitation patients (Schwarzer & Luszczynska, 2008; Schwarzer et al., 2008; Barg et al., 2012).

Building on previous work that identified self-efficacy as a major determinant of health behavior, HAPA distinguishes between three stage-*specific self-efficacy* constructs: action, maintenance, and recovery. Whereas action self-efficacy refers to a person's beliefs in their ability to initiate a behavior, *maintenance self-efficacy* refers to their ability to maintain the behavior. Finally, *recovery self-efficacy* refers to a person's perception of their ability to recover from an illness (Schwarzer, 2008; Schwarzer & Luszczynska, 2008; Schwarzer et al., 2011). Each form of self-efficacy is most relevant during a specific stage (see Figure 10.2).

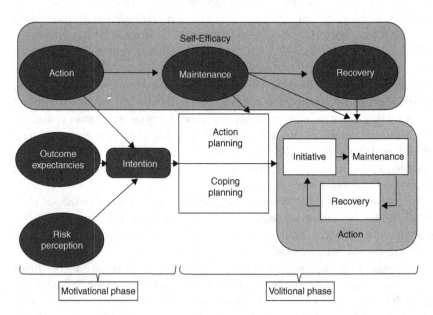

FIGURE 10.2 Health Action Process Approach (HAPA). The model assumes that different kinds of self-efficacy motivation directly and indirectly affect distinct stages of processing from intention formation to action.

Meta-analyses have presented support for many features of HAPA. For instance, Zhang et al. (2019) found that action self-efficacy and outcome expectancies significantly predicted the intentions of health information seekers while intentions, planning, and maintenance self-efficacy predicted their behaviors. However, recovery self-efficacy and risk perception had only minimal influence on health behavior. Collectively, these results support the distinction between the motivational and volitional stages as intentions and behaviors were differentially influenced by each of the stage-specific variables. Zhang et al. additional found that stage-specific self-efficacy constructs affected behavior. However, the variable of risk perception had only minimal influences on behavior, suggesting that health information seekers rely on other types of information and heuristics to make sense of illness. Moreover, despite qualifying the determinants of the intention-behavior gap, HAPA does not consider the influence of others within social networks on an individual's behaviors.

Social Representations Theory. In psychological science, cognitive and affective responses have historically been viewed as individual processes, neglecting the social dimensions of knowledge construction. Social Representation Theory (SRT) instead considers how mental models of illness and disease are created within a social network (Moscovici, 1961, 1988, 2000). While initially used to understand psychoanalysis, SRT has been widely adopted to study a variety of physical diseases and illnesses (e.g., HIV/AIDS; Flick, 1998; Gervais & Jovchelovitch, 1998; Jodelet, 1991; Joffe, 1995).

Moscovici (1961, 2000) assumed that social representations are a means to reduce uncertainty about the physical and social environment by connecting the individual to collective identities consisting of values, ideas, and practices. For instance, an HCP defines themselves by their training, shared knowledge of terminology, practices, and technologies, with the competency to diagnose and treat illnesses and promote health, being a central feature of their identity. Folk medical representation can be understood in similar terms, with a community's representations of health and illness creating common reference points for its members (Schoenherr, 2024; Schoenherr & Beaudoin, 2024).

Social representations are supported by two cognitive processes: anchoring and objectification. Conforming to traditional cognitive approaches, SRT assumes that individuals acquire and retain social categories and schemata in memory. *Anchoring* occurs when novel information is integrated with prior knowledge, such that prior knowledge biases the perception of new information. For instance, the term 'bacteria' is likely to be associated with negativity due to prior experience. When presented with the novel concept of 'probiotic bacteria', a health information seeker might discount any possible benefits of consuming it. The broader meaning of illnesses and diseases creates anchors. Using SRT to study AIDS, Joffe (1995, 1997, 1999) notes that AIDS was understood in terms of epidemics, associating the outbreaks with deviant practices, out-group members (including foreigners). [...] Moreover, marginalized groups often did not challenge these dominant social representations (Herzlich & Pierret, 1984/1987).

Objectification occurs when abstract ideas are physically instantiated, in terms of concrete physical representations (e.g., data are turned into graphs) or verbal representations such as stories (e.g., illness narratives; see below). Thus, communication of health information occurs through multiple mediums. In sharp contrast to other mental models, SRT assumes that the process of production and the availability of public representation are critical features in understanding health beliefs and behavior. Contemporary support for this can be found in social media and internet websites. For instance, websites such as Wikipedia, the Mayo Clinic, or social media act as reference points for learners and other health information seekers.

The biomedical models maintained by Western HCPs also represent social representations held within their community. With home-care general practitioners (GPs) and nurses as their informants, Flick et al. (2002) were able to identify multiple definitions of health maintained by GPs. GPs referenced formal definitions (e.g., WHO), understood health as a relative concept, the patient's ability to adapt to restrictions, used resource analogies, and well-being and mental health. While adopting some similar definitions (e.g., WHO, the relativity of health, prevention), nurses also identified the importance of subjective well-being and autonomy/independence in addition to focusing on the social integration of the patient and a focus on health.

The SRT framework can be used to understand diagnostic rates of disorders. For instance, studies have found regional differences in the prevalence of attentional deficit and hyperactivity disorder (ADHD; e.g., Visser et al., 2014). While such increases might be attributable to environmental changes or changes in diagnostic criteria, evidence suggests that children and adolescents might be over- or underdiagnosed by parents and clinicians (Kazda et al., 2021; Thomas et al., 2015). In one study, Bruchmüller et al. (2012) found that rather than using DSM criteria, prototypical representations of the 'ADHD child' (objectification) biased diagnoses (anchored) of vignettes describing children and symptoms. They found that 16.7% of ambiguous cases were diagnosed as ADHD (false positives) and that vignettes featuring boys were more likely to be diagnosed with ADHD than girls.

10.2.2 Sensemaking Approaches

Mental models are not limited to descriptions. Rather than viewing health and illness beliefs as individual or group-level affective and cognitive representations, we must understand how health seeker's mental models help them make sense of illness.[2] Collectively, we refer to these as sensemaking approaches to illness.

Explanatory Models. Explanatory Models (EMs; Kleinman, 1975) represent the understanding of HCPs and patients about "episodes of sickness and of its treatment that are employed by all of those engaged in the clinical process," (p. 105; Kleinman, 1980). Like other mental representations of health and illness, EMs are created to explain etiology, associated pathophysiology, the timing and mode of the onset of symptoms, course of illness (e.g., severity and sick role [acute, chronic, impairment]), and appropriate treatments. Crucially, Kleinman notes that whereas patient EMs typically only address the most salient features of an illness, HCPs EMs typically attempt to satisfy all five explanatory features: etiology, the onset of symptoms (timing and mode), the disease process (pathophysiology), the course of the illness (sick role, progress, severity, resolution), and treatment (efficacy, function, and side effects). Reviewing ethnographic research, Erickson (2008) identified four general causal mechanisms: (a) the individual's body, (b) the social and economic world, (c) the natural world, and (d) the spiritual world with illness attributed to natural processes, the imbalance between forces, or as punishment (cf. Foster, 1976). Not all EMs address all of these features. For instance, in his study of rural Guatemala, Harris (2007) found that K'iche Maya differentiated between common diseases (*yab'ilal*) that are the normal byproducts of daily activities from curses (*k'oqob'al*) that result from someone else's envy or witchcraft.

Kleinman's approach also prioritizes the use of *metaphors* in reasoning about illness. Analogical reasoning requires that we map features from a familiar domain onto an unfamiliar domain, thereby partially transferring our knowledge of causal relational structures (Harrington, 2012). Analogical reasoning is also quite flexible and can change over time. Studies have demonstrated changes in the use of metaphor throughout the phases of stroke recovery (Boylstein et al., 2007). If metaphors are compatible, this can greatly increase the adoption of healthy attitudes (Landau et al., 2018). However, adopting the wrong metaphor (e.g., 'battling cancer') can negatively affect the perception of the treatment and recovery from illness (Hauser & Schwarz, 2020). Similar observations were made during the COVID-19, such that rather than referring to COVID-19 metaphorically as an 'enemy', defined by a 'tsunami' of cases, a fire metaphor was more productive given that it highlighted urgency and danger, explains the process of contagion, the phases of the pandemic, and the role of healthcare workers, i.e., analogous firefighters (Semino, 2021).

Metaphors are typically culturally embedded (e.g., Chen et al., 2008). For instance, Kleinman (1980) notes that Western metaphors are frequently associated with conflict and war (i.e., one's body is *invaded* by pathogens but can be stopped by our immune *defenses*), whereas Taiwanese metaphors focus on being 'hit'[3] by ghosts intentionally or unintentionally leading to illness while other prominent EMs in East Asian culture focus on imbalances between forces (Schoenherr & Beaudoin, 2024). Depending on the metaphor that is adopted to help understand the disease, health seekers will have different expectations concerning relevant diagnostic features of an illness and the efficacy of treatments. This also highlights the importance of a shared cultural basis for communication in health care.

Narrative Models. Like EMs, *Narrative Models* (NMs) also represent causal explanations of illness (Ezzy, 2000; Frank, 1995; Murray, 2007). Unlike EMs, NMs embed the explanation within a story, often defining multiple causal factors. In this way, narratives are used to *make* meaning. In health professions education, there has been an increased emphasis on the use of narratives to understand and communicate with patients, although this research tends to focus on relationship building, empathy, and perspective-taking rather than understanding the dominance of cross-cultural narratives (e.g., Charon, 2008; Milota et al., 2019; Remein et al., 2020).

Narratives can take multiple forms. Table 10.1 presents common narratives identified in the literature. For instance, Murray (2007) identified four narratives used by injured workers concerning their disability as devastation, a challenge,

TABLE 10.1 Sensemaking Narrative Typology

Narrative Type	Description
Restitutive	An individual minimizes the illness experience, interpreting the event as being a temporary state (interruption) that they must overcome. These linear narratives focus on coping, recovery of impaired (or lost) function, and remoralization that are defined by positive, prospective outcomes.
Chaotic	An individual loses a sense of order in their life and is incapable of developing effective coping strategies. A linear narrative that is disrupted by uncontrollable events. Often associated with experienced violence and shaped by social structure, e.g., comparatively powerless individuals or groups within a society.
Quest	An individual perceives illness as a challenge that must be overcome. Often associated with searching for a cure (e.g., search for alternatives) or an attempt to find meaning. The narratives are often empowering, in that they emphasize agency.
Moral Transgression	An individual views an illness as the consequence of violating a social or universal norm, often perceived as a form of retribution for creating imbalance. The narrative focuses on accepting the transgression and subsequent illness and/or engaging in corrective behavior to restore balance.
Testimony	A story that is explicitly moralized, articulated to 'bear witness' to the illness experience of those suffering. Often associated with extreme or chronic pain. Focusing on the meaning of an illness to an individual or community, such as religion.

an opportunity, or a general phenomenon (see also Gergen & Gergen, 1986). Narrative can typically be understood in terms of *autobiographical memories*, memories of specific consequential events that define the course of an individual's development (Conway & Pleydell-Pearce, 2000), and their relationship with *life scripts*, consisting of culturally proscribed milestones (Munawar et al., 2018). For instance, Bury (1982) frames illness in terms of *biographical disruption* wherein a 'typical' life path is interrupted by an illness. Such narratives have been observed in breast cancer patients, with the diagnosis and treatment representing disruptions to normal life events (Mathieson & Stam, 1995; Yaskowich & Stam, 2003).

Narrative structures can also be found across cultures. In a study by Hatala et al. (2015), they identified narratives of mental illness consisting of 'thinking too much', fright, the date of birth (e.g., fate), and spirit 'attacks'. Other studies have also suggested that narratives underpin the effects of intergenerational trauma, with stories of past events impacting current generations such as those of the First Nations people of Canada (e.g., Crawford, 2014; Hatala et al., 2016; Komanrnisky et al., 2016), holocaust survivors (Adelman, 1995; Békés et al., 2017; Hunter, 2021), Palestinian refugees (Mahamid, 2020; Schirch, 2018; Veronese & Cavazzoni, 2020), slavery in the United States (Gump, 2010; Hicks-Ray, 2004; Leary, 2005), and occupation and war in Asia (Cai & Lee, 2022; Jeong & Vollhardt, 2021; Lee et al., 2019).

More recently, narratives have been used to understand the public's response to COVID-19 (Greenhalgh et al., 2022) and experience of 'long COVID' (Rushforth et al., 2021). The ease with which people can understand narratives can also increase the likelihood that they are shared with others. For instance, Ngai et al. (2020) examined COVID-19 messaging in China using message content analysis. They found that users were more likely to share, comment, and like disease prevention posts that were presented using narratives. In contrast, they found that government information was typically presented in a nonnarrative style. Health seekers are also aware of the efficacy of narratives, with participants recommending brief testimonials as an effective means to support vaccination (Ignacio et al., 2023). Misinformation and disinformation in the form of conspiracy theories can also spread due to their compatibility with existing narratives within a community, a subject we will return to below.

10.3 Health Communication as an Interactive Persuasion Process

Health communication is a form of persuasive communication, either directed toward an individual or an audience. However, health beliefs, are unlikely to remain static. As models like HAPA and SRT suggest, mental models and narratives of illness are continuously constructed and reconstructed as individuals interact within their communities in a *joint* process of sensemaking.

While epidemiology and clinical practices must be informed by evidence, audiences are unlikely to fully understand the accuracy or relevance of this information due to variable health literacy. For instance, health information is typically presented as numerical information (e.g., blood pressure, concentration levels, prevalence of illness in a population) and statistics (e.g., probabilities, percentages, ratios). Such evidence is exceedingly abstract and difficult to understand, leading people (Pennycook et al., 2014) and HCPs to ignore statistical information (Casscells et al., 1978; Offredy, 2002; Smedslund, 1963; cf. Christensen-Szalanski & Bushyhead, 1981). Many health information seekers will instead rely on *heuristics*, simple decision-making rules that focus on a limited number of features that define the health message (Table 10.2). Here, we consider the features of health communication that facilitate changes in attitudes and behaviors by making evidence and arguments more compelling.

10.3.1 Concreteness of Information

For information to be used, it must be recalled. Not all information is equally memorable. Research in psychological science has demonstrated that words that represent abstract concepts (e.g., health, asymptote, threat) are less memorable than words associated with images (e.g., scalpel, syringe, pill; e.g., Dual Coding Theory; Paivio, 1971, 1991; Kounios & Holcomb,

TABLE 10.2 Cues Associated with the Reduced Deliberate Process

Cue Type	Examples
Source	Credibility (reputation), social attractiveness, impartiality, prior experience, group membership
Transmitter	Neutrality, credibility (reputation), past performance of transmitter, social identity
Message Content	Length, number of arguments, sensory properties (e.g., visual design, scent, weight), outcome realism, symbolic content
Communication Context	Crisis, conflict situation, sociocultural context, circumstances of transmission, intergroup communication

Note: Here, we assume that a transmitter can act as a relay for information from a source.

Source: Adapted and modified from Renn (2009).

1994) or scents (Lwin et al., 2010). These effects have been attributed to the 'vividness' of the stimuli. For instance, the Identifiable Victim Effect (IVE) is observed when individuals exhibit more prosocial behaviors toward a single, identifiable victim rather than a group of anonymous, statistical victims (Jenni & Loewenstein, 1997). This effect is typically attributed to an individual's affective responses, i.e., an image is associated with positive or negative affect in memory due to strong prior associations (Erlandsson et al., 2015; Genevsky et al., 2013). Meta-analyses support the IVE's reliability and also suggest that it is most effective when children are presented as suffering (Lee & Feeley, 2016). Thus, health information must be presented in a manner that is as concrete as possible. Moreover, the images that are selected can also frame how the health information seeker perceives the message, provided the audience is aware of the symbols and iconography used in the campaign (e.g., Figure 10.3).

10.3.2 Psychological Distance and the Therapeutic Alliance

Concreteness can also be understood in terms of the relative psychological distance. Psychological distance concerns the temporal (e.g., immediate or delayed rewards/costs; Critchfield & Kollins, 2001; Green et al., 1997; van den Bos & McClure, 2013) and social distance (e.g., self, close other, or distant other; O'Connell et al., 2013) between a decision-maker and the people affected by the outcomes of their choice. For instance, eating now will results in a momentary boost to your energy level (proximal outcome) whereas paying taxes now might support vaccination for someone else at a later date (distant outcome). When psychological distance is great, people tend to discount information and outcomes. This is attributed to failures of affective forecasting, being unaware of how we will feel about our decision in the future (Wilson & Gilbert, 2003). Such failures can be detrimental to effective decision-making, e.g., the outcomes of smoking or failure to wear sunscreen are not observed until later in life.

Psychological distance has been shown to affect health judgments. In her studies of discounting, Chapman (Chapman, 1996; Chapman & Elstein, 1995) presented participants with immediate smaller health outcomes or larger future health outcomes. Participants chose which outcome they valued the most. They observed *less* discounting in the health domain relative to the financial domain: participants were prepared to wait longer for larger future health outcomes than they were for financial outcomes. Using a similar paradigm during COVID-19, Schoenherr (2021) varied the social distance of outcomes (self, close other, or distant other) and temporal distance (now, 3, 6, or 12 months) from participants. He demonstrated that discounting was a function of perceived *familiarity* between the participants and the close and distant others they selected as a comparison standard: the greater the difference in familiarity between close and distant others, the greater the level of discounting.

Psychological distance can also become a concern when there is significant social distance between the status of communicators (e.g., HCPs, patients, and the public), such that health information seekers might adopt a relatively passive role (e.g., Kim et al., 1996, Kim, 1999; Tasaki et al., 1999). To reduce this possibility, HCPs must ensure that they create a sound therapeutic alliance between themselves and their patients that fosters mutual respect and the free exchange of information. HCPs must be aware of the psychological distance between the patients and the outcome and between their relative social distance to the patient to avoid discounting information (see Section 10.3.4).

10.3.3 Framing Effects

Rather than focusing on specific information, health seekers will likely focus on the overall framing of a message. *Framing effects* refer to the different behavioral and attitudinal effects of a message defined by either gains or losses. For instance, vaccination could be framed in terms of the receipt of benefits (e.g., 'stay healthy longer!') or the avoidance of costs (e.g., 'don't get sick!'). Framing effects are believed to work due to loss aversion, such that people would prefer to maintain the status quo rather than the possibility of loss (Tversky & Kahneman, 1981; Rothman & Salovey, 1997).

Message framing has been studied in domains such as breast cancer screening (Meyerowitz & Chaiken, 1987; Consedine et al., 2007), condom use (Garcia-Retamero & Cokely, 2011; Kiene et al., 2005), maternal influenza (Frew et al., 2014), physical activity (Berry & Carson, 2010), dental hygiene (Rothman et al., 1999; Uskul et al., 2009), salt intake reduction (Riet et al., 2010), and vaccination (Penţa & Băban, 2018). Researchers have identified the condition in which gain and loss frames are most effective. In their meta-analysis, Gallagher and Updegraff (2012) found that gain-framed messages were the most successful at promoting adherence to prevention behaviors (e.g., smoking, physical inactivity). Importantly, loss- and gain-framed messages did not significantly affect detection behaviors (e.g., breast self-examination; Gallagher & Opdegraff, 2012). However, other studies have found that loss-framed messages can lead to more behavioral change than gain-framed detection behaviors (Meyerowitz & Chaiken, 1987; Rothman & Salovey, 1997; Rothman et al., 1999).Crucially, exclusively focusing on gain or loss framing ignores many other important factors that are considered by health information seekers, e.g., culture, type of treatment, and threat cues (Gong et al., 2013).

Across the behavioral and social sciences, there is a growing realization that factors associated with culture (e.g., scripts, schemata, conventions), can be critical predictors of behavior. For instance, studies suggest that independent individualists are focused on health consequences to the self, whereas interdependent collectivists are more likely to focus on social consequences (Uskul & Oyserman, 2010). Others have argued that individualists are more likely to adopt a promotion focus whereas collectivists are more likely to adopt a prevention focus, leading to preferences for gain and loss framings, respectively (Aaker & Lee, 2001; Han & Shavitt, 1994; Kreuter et al., 2004; Uskul et al., 2009; Zhang & Gelb, 1996).[4] However, consistent patterns have been observed across cultures. For instance, Yu and Shen (2013) found that Hong Kong and US participants' ratings of perceived message effectiveness, attitude, and behavioral intentions were most influenced by gains for self (e.g., 'Getting a flu shot may benefit you') and by losses to others (e.g., 'Skipping the flu shot may put many at risk'). These results suggest that messaging framing must be compatible with both individual and cultural beliefs.

10.3.4 Roles, Social Categories, and Social Proof

Communication in health care is affected by the degree of trust between both HCPs, the patients, and the public. Health information seekers look for credible sources such as experts and peers (e.g., Jenkins et al., 2020; Kareklas et al., 2015), or technology (Schoenherr, 2022c). Rather than accumulating information about each individual to form a unique impression, people use social categories or stereotypes to inform these judgments. All social categories can be defined in terms of perceived warmth (cooperativeness) and competence (status; Fiske et al., 2002), with high levels of warmth and competence associated with unambivalent in-group categories.

Long-term public opinion surveys provide a useful means to understand the sentiment maintained toward HCPs. Using archival methods, Schoenherr (2022a) found that 'Nurse' and 'Doctor' were both assigned high trust and prestige ratings, reflecting an unambiguous in-group category. In contrast, nurses were rated higher in trust than doctors. Another intriguing finding from this study was the relationship between word frequency and ratings of prestige and trust. Using word frequency corpora (i.e., frequency of word use in movie subtitles, new websites, blog, Twitter frequencies), he found that ratings of prestige (perceived status) were positively associated with word frequency, suggesting a bi-directional relationship: prestige increased references to a social category (i.e., citing credible sources such as doctors), with the additional references increasing the perceived status of the social category (i.e., sources such as doctors appear more credible).

In addition to perceived credibility, social categories also affect whether messages about certain social categories will be relevant. For instance, people tend to devalue the lives and outcomes of outgroup members relative to ingroup members, an extension of psychological distance (Cikara et al., 2010). Consequently, health information seekers and HCPs might be less compelled to act on initiatives directed toward outgroup members, e.g., homeless, mental illness, and 'addicts' (Hansson et al., 2013; Schulze, 2008; see, Section 10.3.2).

BOX 10.1   MULTIMODAL PERSUASIVE MESSAGING IN HEALTH COMMUNICATION

Health and illness are often sensitive topics. Reminders of mortality can result in triggering a fear-based response which is not always an effective means to promote the adoption of the health practices presented in health messages. Clinicians and public HCPs must consider the message content, framing, and imagery used to elicit health-related behaviors. The message must also consider the cognitive limitations of health information seekers in terms of limited attention (main focus) and working memory (total content), variable levels of health literacy (details and information), and motivation.

Consider an effective health message from the 'Share Your Spare' campaign from the Renal Support Network. The brightly colored, laughing cartoon kidneys frame the act of kidney donation as a positive activity. The slogan 'Share your Spare' is simple. The length of the message is below estimates for working memory capacity (i.e., four items; Cowan, 2001) with the similarity in phototactic properties between 'share' and 'spare' facilitating encoding and retention of the message.

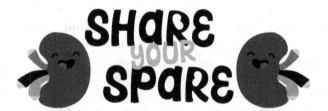

FIGURE 10.3   Image from the share your spare campaign by the Renal Support Network. Image credit and permission obtained from Renal Support Network, RSNhope.org.

The framing of the message is also effective. The term 'spare' implies that an individual can live without a second kidney, reducing the perceived risk of donation of a body part. The term 'share' reduces the complexity and risk associated with surgery required to remove the kidney. The notion of sharing also promotes a communal ethic, such that an individual considers reciprocity with specific others or altruism more generally.

10.3.5 Scripts and Schemata

Rather than treating each situation as novel, social and cultural scripts are often used to guide interpersonal communication. Scripts are routines that individuals follow that define what and when to say and do while interacting (Honeycutt & Bryan, 2011). Like social categories, when scripts contain accurate information, they can facilitate interpersonal interaction. However, if they contain inaccurate information or an inappropriate script is selected, this can lead to confusion and communication traps (Ferrretti et al., 2023).

The Doctor-Nurse Game represents a canonical script in health care (Fagin, 2004). According to Stein (1967; Stein et al., 1990), the script defines the roles, responsibilities, and how information *should* be exchanged between doctors and nurses. In its traditional formulation, 'the game' requires that nurses maintain the appearance of deference and subordination toward the doctor while communicating missed information or misinterpretation made by the clinician and that 'open disagreement between the players must be avoided at all costs… the nurse must communicate her recommendations without appearing to be making a recommendation statement' (p. 699).

Scripts can also be adopted by health seekers, such as the 'sick role', when the patient or family member is subordinate to, and dependent upon, HCPs (Mechanic & Volkart, 1961; Parsons, 1951). This is reinforced in the literature by framing health communication as issues of *compliance* with the recommendations of HCPs. For instance, rather than consulting with a patient, a clinician might simply adhere to a script to communicate information (e.g., contraception; Kelly et al., 2017). Patients likely have scripts related to self-disclosure containing the kind and amount of information sharing (Allen & Arroll, 2015; Farber, 2006). If mental and physical illnesses are associated with stigma and taboo, this can lead to restrictions in terms of what information is offered, or solicited, in interpersonal exchanges (Agne et al., 2000).

10.3.6 Subjective Confidence and Reactance

Confidence in health communication is often framed as an unqualified good, i.e., building confidence in the recommendations of HCPs, the efficacy of treatment, and their self-efficacy in adherence to recommendations (e.g., vaccination, condom use; Askelson et al., 2010; Gilkey et al., 2016; Larson et al., 2011; Larson et al., 2016; Weinstein et al., 2008). Similar assumptions pervade medical education, assuming that a central goal is to build learners' confidence (e.g., Bambini et al., 2009; Eades et al., 2011). Models of judgment and decision-making and persuasive communication assume that people monitor their confidence to determine when greater deliberation is required (Chaiken, 1980; Schoenherr et al., 2024). However, confidence is not good in and of itself. High confidence might lead to premature closure leading to the adoption of diagnoses, treatment recommendations, and behavior that are incorrect (Schoenherr et al., 2018). Similarly, studies of health information seekers have found that objective health literacy and subjective estimates of health literacy are only weakly related, and that objective health literacy was the only significant predictor of healthy behaviors (Schulz et al., 2021). Consequently, HCPs and health seekers might resist information that disconfirms prior beliefs that are associated with high confidence. For instance, changes in messaging regarding masks by public health officials during COVID-19 might have led to greater uncertainty in appropriate behavior or reduced health seekers' confidence in HCP (Zhang et al., 2021).

Message content can also have the opposite of its intended effect. Psychological Reactance Theory considers situations in which attempts at persuasion can lead to a rejection of the message and its intended attitude and behavior change, or a 'boomerang effect' (Brehm, 1966; Brehm & Brehm, 1981; Wicklund, 1974; for reviews, see Rains, 2013; Reynolds-Tylus, 2019). If individuals value their autonomy and freedom to choose, when the ability to choose is threatened, eliminated alternatives become more appealing. When the features of a message threaten an individual's freedom, they experience negative effects and seek to reestablish their freedom. The phenomenon has proven robust including the use of sunscreen, drugs, alcohol, and tobacco (Grandpre et al., 2003; Miller et al., 2007; Quick & Considine, 2008; Quick & Stephenson, 2008; Rains and Turner, 2007).

Psychological reactance, therefore, reflects a variant of a framing effect wherein freedom-threatening language acts as a cue to action. For instance, Dillard and Shen (2005) found that perceived threats to freedom and an individual's proneness to reactance decreased attitudes and behavioral intentions. Unsurprisingly, not all variables are equally likely to produce reactance. In a study conducted by Rains and Turner (2007), argument quality, outcome severity (e.g., strep throat vs. bacterial meningitis), and the magnitude of the freedom-limiting request (e.g., reporting sanitary conditions vs. seeing a doctor immediately upon presentation of symptoms). They found that the main determinant of reactance was the magnitude of the request which affected both the level of self-reported anger as well as negative cognitions.

Despite the general response to freedom-threatening language, cross-cultural differences have been observed. For instance, collectivist societies that place more emphasis on interpersonal accord (harmony) relative to free choice have shown less reactance (Quick & Kim, 2009; for examples, outside of health, see Kim et al., 2017). Response from the public during the COVID-19 pandemic reinforces these results. The requirements to wear masks (and obtain vaccinations) appear to have polarized some individuals within the Western world due to the threats to their autonomy (see Taylor & Asmundson, 2021). However, psychological reactance has also been observed in more collectivist societies (Ye et al., 2023) with evidence suggesting that gain-framed messages were associated with less psychological reactance (Xiang et al., 2023). Thus, social norms and conventions might reduce, but not eliminate, reactance.

10.4 Social Networks, Innovation Diffusion, and Health Communication

HCPs must advocate for the health of their patient's directly to the public or in appeals to policymakers. For instance, in rural areas or disadvantaged communities, the relative inaccessibility of health care might result in community members relying more on folk wisdom and social proof (Schoenherr, 2024). During crisis situations, health communicators must also adapt the basic models described above to social networks where information, misinformation, and disinformation mingle together in information ecosystems that are becoming increasingly segmented and polarized by human and artificial agents. Without understanding the audience of a health message or the channels through which they pass, health messages are unlikely to receive much attention.

Public health communication has long recognized the benefits of understanding the structure and dynamics of social networks (Moorhead et al., 2013; Wright, 2016; Valente, 2010). These networks are defined by agents who are interconnected to varying degrees (e.g., density), with some agents or groups being more connected than others (e.g., centrality), thereby allowing them to receive information from, and transmit information to, a larger audience. In an analogous manner to how epidemiological models are used to understand the spread of disease (Morris, 1993), social contagion models examine how ideas and practices spread within a social network. As social network sites are increasingly used for health communication (Shi et al., 2018), understanding the properties of social networks is critical. Here, we review the basic features of these models.

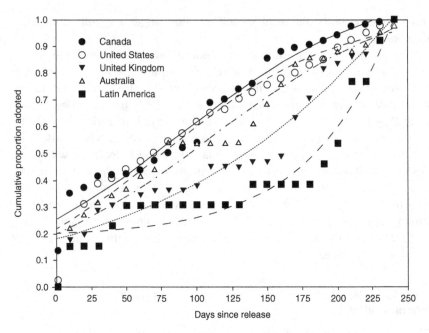

FIGURE 10.4 Adoption behavior of a surgical skills eBook in different social networks. Adapted from Schoenherr et al. (2015).

10.4.1 Social Contagion and Social Network Analysis

Rather than using a passive diffusion metaphor (Katz et al., 1963; Kadushin, 2012; Rogers, 1962/2010; Sultan et al., 1990), social contagion assumes that ideas, conventions, and behaviors actively spread from one individual to another, i.e., an idea is like a virus that replicates within an environment. Qualifying diffusion models, the process of social contagion is affected by multiple factors: social network structure, group identity, and the consequential nature of a topic can affect attitudes and affective responses (e.g., Coviello et al., 2014; Brady et al., 2017). These models require breaking down a social network into agents and understanding how they interact. For instance, in a pedagogical setting, (a) a teacher might provide instructions to a group of learners, with one learner providing information to another learner who was absent during the presentation, this learner can then ask the instructor about the content at a later point; (b) in Web 1.0, health information seekers might only obtain information from a website, without the ability to contribute or correct it, or interact with each other, whereas (c) in Web 2.0, users might interact on a website to varying degrees. By identifying the properties of a health information seekers' social network, HCPs can identify the ways in which patients and the public are influenced through the structure of their interpersonal relationships.

Adoption within Social Network. The efficacy of a public health message will depend on assessing whether information reaches health information seekers in a social network who are at elevated risk. When applied to crisis communication, this requires developing an overall plan (Box 10.2) as well as specifying the unique concerns of the populations that will be targeted with the message. For instance, vulnerable segments of a population can consist of those who are susceptible to a disease, those who have reduced access to specific communication channels (e.g., 'digital divides' such as access to the internet) or health resources (e.g., rural communities), and marginalized communities. For instance, Faife and Kerr (2021) found that fewer Asian (0.9%), Black (1.5%), Latino (1.7%), First Nations (0%), and Middle Eastern (0%) Facebook users were shown Department of Health and Human Service posts during COVID-19 pandemic relative to White users (4.5%). Acceptance of misinformation can also be affected by community membership. Supporting this, studies within the United States have found that medical mistrust and the experience of discrimination (e.g., African Americans) are associated with reduced prevention-seeking behavior and a greater likelihood of endorsing conspiracy beliefs about the origin of diseases including COVID-19 (Bogart et al., 2006; Davis et al., 2018; Hammond et al., 2010; Smith et al., 2022).

Social Contagion and Disinformation. Health communication is increasingly challenged by disinformation (intentional deception) and misinformation (misinterpretation) that can be spread by rumors, gossip, politicians, and media. In crisis situations, the need for rapid responses might lead communicators and audiences to rely more on automatic information processing which can lead to biases. The prevalence of misinformation can be significant. During COVID-19, between 0.2% and 28.8% of COVID-19 posts appear to contain misinformation (Gabarron et al., 2021). Studies have examined the spread of health disinformation and misinformation for many infections and pathologies including the Ebola virus (Fung et al., 2016; Pathak et al., 2015), the Zika virus (Sharma et al., 2017; Sommariva et al., 2018; Wood, 2018), cancer (Chen, B. et al., 2018; Chen, L. et al., 2018; Chua & Banerjee, 2018; Okuhara et al., 2017), cardiology (Chen et al., 2013; Kumar et al., 2014), diabetes (Leong et al., 2017), diet and nutrition (Bessi et al., 2015; Syed-Abdul et al., 2013), naturopathic cancer treatment (Chen et al., 2018b), smoking (Albarracin et al., 2018), and anti-vaccine campaigns (Broniatowski et al., 2018). For instance, in a study of users' online interactions of attitudes toward vaccines, Schmidt et al. (2018) found that most users were only exposed to information that supports *their* prior beliefs about vaccines, creating an echo chamber wherein their opinions are reflected back at them (for a general discussion, see Terren & Borge-Bravo, 2021). The resulting perceived consensus can increase health information seekers' confidence in the accuracy of the information. Thereafter, when individuals have contact with others who hold opposing views, this can lead to group polarization with individuals adopting more extreme views (Iandoli et al., 2021).

BOX 10.2 BASIC STRATEGIES IN CRISIS COMMUNICATION

Crisis communication represents a special case of risk communication in situations wherein there are high-risk threats to individuals, groups, or organizations (e.g., Allen & Caillouet, 1994; Barton, 1993). Threats can consist of imminent direct or indirect physical (e.g., destruction of property or harm), material (e.g., financial loss, loss of information), or social harm (e.g., loss of reputation, or power). For instance, the COVID-19 pandemic presented physical threats (i.e., potential hospitalization or death due to virus), material threats (i.e., lockdowns resulting in job and business loss), and social harms (e.g., mask and vaccine mandates presenting threats to personal autonomy, loss of businesses in communities, representation of dissenters as 'anti-vaxxers' and conspiracy theorists). By failing to carefully craft a health message, it can lead to an audience adopting a contrary position, i.e., psychological reactance. Consequently, numerous best practices have been identified to facilitate the process of crisis communication (e.g., Covello, 2006; Seeger et al., 2003). Health advocacy requires an understanding of the social network, the motivations and knowledge of stakeholders, and logistical considerations (Figure 10.5).

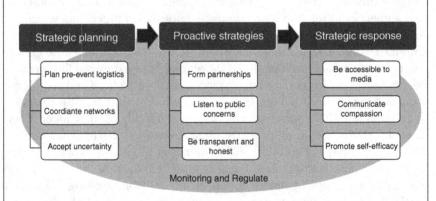

FIGURE 10.5   Best practices in risk and crisis communication. Modified and adapted from Seeger (2006).

This phenomenon was especially apparent in discussions on social media during the COVID-19 pandemic (e.g., Jiang et al., 2021). For instance, Lang et al. (2021) found rhetorical polarization for pro- and anti-maskers in online posts, with the dominant pro-mask groups ignoring the posts from the nondominant anti-mask group. Consequently, political orientation might not *cause* a difference in diffusion rates for mask or vaccine adoption. Instead, people within a social network might share political beliefs, with health-related attitudes and beliefs acting as free riders that are adopted due to imitating the behaviors of other group members who are perceived as peers, i.e., social proof.

Addressing Disinformation. Health communicators must consider how to address disinformation and misinformation. Thankfully, a growing body of literature has begun to address these issues.

The simplest approach is to forewarn an audience of impending dubious messages. Forewarning effects are observed when individuals are cautioned about disinformation and misinformation, or the motivations of a speaker, in advance of being presented with information (Daiku et al., 2020; Dean et al., 1971; Richards & Banas, 2015). Indeed, studies have also found a positive association between the ability to identify disinformation ('fake news'), health literacy, and adoption of health promotion behaviors (Montagni et al., 2021; Schulz et al., 2021). Moreover, when people are forewarned of possible reactance to a freedom-threatening message concerning alcohol consumption, they are less likely to demonstrate reactance (Richards & Banas, 2015; cf. Richards et al., 2017; Richards et al., 2022).

More generally, a meta-analysis by Walter et al. (2020) identified multiple features that predict individuals' ability to successfully identify disinformation. First, correction of disinformation was more difficult when presented by peers relative to news agencies and more effective when delivered by experts relative to non-experts. Second, both simple (rebuttal) and complex (evidence- and logic-based) corrections were equally effective. Taken together, these results reinforce the importance of source credibility and forewarning effects.

10.5 Conclusion

Interpersonal communication is an interactive process, requiring that the speaker and listener actively engage in sensemaking. HCPs face many challenges due to the technical and affectively laden nature of healthcare delivery. Each communication episode can be defined by differences in health literacy, pluralistic representations of disease and illness, how a message is framed, the social scripts that define the roles and responsibilities of communicators, and the structure of social networks.

Health communication must ultimately be *persuasive*. Simply providing a health seeker with diagnoses, prognoses, and treatment recommendations is insufficient. The personal agency of patients and the public requires that analysis and advice are compatible with their beliefs and narratives – about the subject or source – and that they feel empowered to choose. Novel technologies such as artificial intelligence and 'chatbots', despite their opacity, might be preferred by health information seekers, especially in cases where there might be stigma associated with an illness within a community. Healthcare professionals must account for these communication barriers and directly address the limitations of these technologies to health information seekers.

No single approach to health communication can account for every situation. At a macro-level, intraprofessional, interprofessional, and extraprofessional patterns of communication provide distinct challenges. The roles and scripts associated with each one of these relational structures will affect communication. While intraprofessional communication will be facilitated by shared knowledge structures (and language), assumptions of shared knowledge and the potential to self-censor can interfere with communication. In contrast, interprofessional communication might be adversely affected by different power dynamics, such that individuals withhold information due to their role or low perceived psychological safety. Finally, extraprofessional communication between health professionals and health seekers (e.g., doctor-patient communication) will further be hampered by an absence of shared mental models. As health information seekers are presented with alternative sources of health information (e.g., social media, alternative medicine), they might 'shop around' to find individuals who share their beliefs.

HCPs must also understand health communication in terms of social networks. While this is clear when crafting messages for the public, social networks reside behind every interpersonal interaction. The recommendations of a clinician could be discounted if a patient has family, friends, or has a membership in a group that does not share these beliefs. HCPs cannot hope to map out social networks for each patient or health seeker, but they must look for cues and be aware of how they relate to heuristics and biases. Identifying specific health beliefs, explanatory models, and narratives provides a useful starting point. In cases where illnesses might have become politicized, it is important to be aware of, and address, common biases to halt their spread. Periodically surveying information ecosystems for prevalent folk theories, disinformation, and conspiracies will help HCPs to prepare to respond to the concerns of health information seekers and bolster their confidence in the competencies of HCPs.

Notes

1 For example, consumer marketing, political campaigns, cyber hygiene.
2 Some application of SRT can be understood as a sensemaking approach.

3   ch'ung, chhhiong-tioh.
4   This is less likely a product of 'collectivism' than it is about the historical conditions that have led to a collectivist society have emerged, e.g., pathogen prevalence, geographic remoteness, and economic interdependence.

References

Aaker, J. L., & Lee, A. Y. (2001). "I" seek pleasures and "We" avoid pains: The role of self-regulatory goals in information processing and persuasion. *Journal of Consumer Research*, 28(1), 33–49.

Abraham, C., & Sheeran, P. (2015). The health beliefs model. In M. Conner, & P. Norman (Eds.), *Predicting Health Behaviour: Research and Practice with Social Cognition Models* (3. ed., pp. 30–69). Berkshire: Open University Press.

Adelman, A. (1995). Traumatic memory and the intergenerational transmission of Holocaust narratives. The *Psychoanalytic Study of the Child*, 50(1), 343–367.

Agne, R. R., Thompson, T. L., & Cusella, L. P. (2000). Stigma in the line of face: Self-disclosure of patients' HIV status to health care providers. *Journal of Applied Communication Research*, 28, 235–261.

Albarracin, D., Romer, D., Jones, C., Hall Jamieson, K., Jamieson, P. (2018). Misleading claims about tobacco products in YouTube videos: Experimental effects of misinformation on unhealthy attitudes. *Journal of Medical Internet Research*, 20(6), e229.

Alkhateeb, F. M., Khanfar, N. M., & Loudon, D. (2009). Physicians' adoption of pharmaceutical e-detailing: Application of Rogers' innovation-diffusion model. *Services Marketing Quarterly*, 31(1), 116–132.

Allen, E.-C. F., & Arroll, B. (2015). Physician self-disclosure in primary care: A mixed methods study of GPs' attitudes, skills, and behaviour. *The British Journal of General Practice*, 65(638), 601–608.

Allen, M. W., & Caillouet, R. H. (1994). Legitimation endeavors: Impression management strategies used by an organization in crisis. *Communications Monographs*, 61(1), 44–62.

Arroll, B., & Allen, E. C. F. (2015). To self-disclose or not self-disclose? A systematic review of clinical self-disclosure in primary care. *British Journal of General Practice*, 65(638), e609–e616.

Askelson, N. M., Campo, S., Lowem J. B., Smith, S., Dennis, L. K., & Andsager, J. (2010). Using the theory of planned behavior to predict mothers' intentions to vaccinate their daughters against HPV. *The Journal of School Nursing*, 26(3), 194–202.

Bambini, D., Washburn, J., & Perkins, R. (2009). Outcomes of clinical simulation for novice nursing students: Communication, confidence, clinical judgment. *Nursing Education Perspectives*, 30(2), 79–82.

Banon, L. (1993). *Crisis in Organizations: Managing and Communicating in the Heat of Chaos*. College Divisions South-Western.

Barclay, T. R., Hinkin, C. H., Castellon, S. A., Mason, K. I., Reinhard, M. J., Marion, S. D., Levine, A. J., & Durvasula, R. S. (2007). Age-associated predictors of medication adherence in HIV-positive adults: Health beliefs, self-efficacy, and neurocognitive status. *Health Psychology*, 26(2), 40–49.

Barg, C. J., Latimer, A. E., Pomery, E. A., Rivers, S. E., Rench, T. A., Prapavessis, H., & Salovey, P. (2012). Examining predictors of physical activity among inactive middle-aged women: An application of the health action process approach. *Psychology & Health*, 27(7), 829–845.

Békés, V., Perry, J. C., & Starrs, C. J. (2017). Resilience in holocaust survivors: A study of defense mechanisms in holocaust narratives. *Journal of Aggression, Maltreatment & Trauma*, 26(10), 1072–1089.

Berkhof, M., van Rijssen, H. J., Schellart, A. J., Anema, J. R., & van der Beek, A. J. (2011). Effective training strategies for teaching communication skills to physicians: An overview of systematic reviews. *Patient Education and Counseling*, 84(2), 152–162.

Berkman, N. D., Sheridan, S. L., Donahue, K. E., Halpern, D. J., & Crotty, K. (2011). Low health literacy and health outcomes: An updated systematic review. *Annals of Internal Medicine*, 155(2), 97–107.

Berry, T. R., & Carson, V. (2010). Ease of imagination, message framing, and physical activity messages. *British Journal of Health Psychology*, 15(1), 197–211.

Bertrand, J. T. (2004). Diffusion of innovations and HIV/AIDS. *Journal of Health Communication*, 9(S1), 113–121.

Bessi, A., Zollo, F., Vicario, M.D., Scala, A., Caldarelli, G., & Quattrociocchi, W. (2015). Trend of narratives in the age of misinformation. *PLOS One*, 10(8), e0134641.

Bing-You, R., Hayes, V., Varaklis, K., Trowbridge, R., Kemp, H., & McKelvy, D. (2017). Feedback for learners in medical education: What is known? A scoping review. *Academic Medicine*, 92(9), 1346–1354.

Bish, A., & Michie, S. (2010). Demographic and attitudinal determinants of protective behaviours during a pandemic: A review. *British Journal of Health Psychology*, 15(4), 797–824.

Bogart, L. M., & Thorburn, S. (2006). Relationship of African Americans' sociodemographic characteristics to belief in conspiracies about HIV/AIDS and birth control. *Journal of the National Medical Association*, 98(7), 1144–1150.

Boylstein, C., Rittman, M., & Hinojosa, R. (2007). Metaphor shifts in stroke recovery. *Health Communication*, 21(3), 279–287.

Brady, W. J., Wills, J. A., Jost, J. T., Tucker, J. A., & Van Bavel, J. J. (2017). Emotion shapes the diffusion of moralized content in social networks. *Proceedings of the National Academy of Sciences*, 114(28), 7313–7318.

Brehm, J. W. (1966). *A Theory of Psychological Reactance*. New York: Academic Press.

Brehm, S. S., & Brehm, J. W. (1981). *Psychological Reactance: A Theory of Freedom and Control*. New York: Academic Press.

Broniatowski, D. A., Jamison, A. M., Qi, S. H., Alkulaib, L., Chen, T., Benton, A., Quinn, S. C., & Dredze, M. (2018). Weaponized health communication: Twitter bots and Russian trolls amplify the vaccine debate. *Health*, 108(10), 1378–1384.

Bruchmüller, K., Margraf, J., & Schneider, S. (2012). Is ADHD diagnosed in accord with diagnostic criteria? Overdiagnosis and influence of client gender on diagnosis. *Journal of Consulting and Clinical Psychology*, 80(1), 128–138.

Burt, R. S. (1987). A note on missing network data in the general social survey. *Social Networks*, 9(1), 63–73.

Bury, M. (1982). Chronic illness as biographical disruption. *Sociology of Health and Illness*, 4(2), 167–182.

Cai, J., & Lee, R. M. (2022). Intergenerational communication about historical trauma in Asian American families. *Adversity and Resilience Science*, 3(3), 233–245.

Card, K. G. (2022). Collectivism, individualism and COVID-19 prevention: A cross sectional study of personality, culture and behavior among Canadians. *Health Psychology and Behavioral Medicine*, 10(1), 415–438.

Carpenter, C. J. (2010). A meta-analysis of the effectiveness of health belief model variables in predicting behavior. *Health Communication*, 25(8), 661–669.

Casscells, W., Schoenberger, A., & Graboys, T. B. (1978). Interpretation by physicians of clinical laboratory results. *New England Journal of Medicine*, 299, 999–1001.

Cegala, D. J., & Lenzmeier Broz, S. (2002). Physician communication skills training: A review of theoretical backgrounds, objectives and skills. *Medical Education*, 36, 1004–1016.

Chaiken, S. (1980). Heuristic versus systematic information processing and the use of source versus message cues in persuasion. *Journal of Personality and Social Psychology*, 39, 752–766.

Chang, M., Chen, Y. F., Shen, C., & Yu, L. (2009). Dimensions of disease stigma in Taiwan: A multidimensional scaling analysis. *Journal of Psychology in Chinese Societies*, 10, 85–104.

Chapman, B., & Elstein, A. S. (1995). Valuing the future: Temporal discounting of health and money. *Medical Decision Making*, 15, 373–386.

Chapman, G. B. (1996). Temporal discounting and utility for health and money. *Journal of Experimental Psychology: Learning, Memory, and Cognition*, 22, 771–791.

Charon, R. (2008). *Narrative Medicine: Honoring the Stories of Illness*. Oxford University Press.

Chen, B., Shao, J., Liu, K., Cai, G., Jiang, Z., Huang, Y., Gu, H., & Jiang, J. (2018). Does eating chicken feet with pickled peppers cause avian influenza? Observational case study on Chinese social media during the avian influenza A (H7N9) outbreak. *JMIR Public Health and Surveillance*, 4, e32.

Chen, H.-M., Hu, Z.-K., Zheng, X.-L., Yuan, Z.-S., Xu, Z.-B., Yuan, L.-Q., & Liao, X.-B. (2013). Effectiveness of YouTube as a source of medical information on heart transplantation. *Interactive Journal of Medical Research*, 2, e28.

Chen, L., Wang, X., & Peng, T. Q. (2018). Nature and diffusion of gynecologic cancer–related misinformation on social media: Analysis of tweets. *Journal of Medical Internet Research*, 20(10), e11515.

Chen, Z., Mo, L., & Honomichl, R. (2004). Having the memory of an elephant: Long-term retrieval and the use of analogues in problem solving. *Journal of Experimental Psychology: General*, 133(3), 415–433.

Christensen-Szalanski, J. J. J., & Bushyhead, J. B. (1981). Physicians' use of probabilistic information in a real clinical setting. *Journal of Experimental Psychology: Human Perception and Performance*, 7, 928–935.

Chua, A.Y.K., Banerjee, S., 2018. Intentions to trust and share online health rumors: An experiment with medical professionals. *Computers in Human Behavior*, 87, 1–9.

Cikara, M., Farnsworth, R. A., Harris, L. T., & Fiske, S. T. (2010). On the wrong side of the trolley track: Neural correlates of relative social valuation. *Social Cognitive and Affective Neuroscience*, 5, 404–413.

Coleman, J., Katz, E., & Menzel, H. (1957). The diffusion of an innovation among physicians. *Sociometry*, 20, 253–270.

Coleman, J., Katz, E., & Menzel, H. (1966) *Medical Innovation: A Diffusion Study*. Indianapolis: Hobbs-Merrill.

Consedine, N. S., Horton, David., Magai, Carol., & Kukafka, Rita. (2007). Breast screening in response to gain, loss, and empowerment framed messages among diverse, low-income women. *Journal of Health Care for the Poor and Underserved*, 18, 550–566.

Conway, M. A., & Pleydell-Pearce, C. W. (2000). The construction of autobiographical memories in the self-memory system. *Psychological Review*, 107, 261–288.

Covello, V. T. (2006). Risk communication and message mapping: A new tool for communicating effectively in public health emergencies and disasters. *Journal of Emergency Management*, 4(3), 25–40.

Coviello, L., Sohn, Y., Kramer, A. D. I., Marlow, C., Franceschetti, M., Christakis, N. A., & Fowler, J. H. (2014). Detecting emotional contagion in massive social networks. *PLOS One*, 9, e90315.

Cowan, N. (2001). The magical number 4 in short-term memory: A reconsideration of mental storage capacity. *Behavioral and Brain Sciences*, 24(1), 87–114.

Crawford, A. (2014). "The trauma experienced by generations past having an effect in their descendants": Narrative and historical trauma among Inuit in Nunavut, Canada. *Transcultural Psychiatry*, 51(3), 339–369.

Critchfield, T. S., & Kollins, S. H. (2001). Temporal discounting: Basic research and the analysis of socially important behavior. *Journal of Applied Behavior Analysis*, 34(1), 101–122.

Daiku, Y., Kugihara, N., Teraguchi, T., & Watamura, E. (2020). Effective forewarning requires central route processing: Theoretical improvements on the counterargumentation hypothesis and practical implications for scam prevention. *PLOS One*, 15(3), e0229833.

Davis, F. (1989). Perceived usefulness, perceived ease of use, and user acceptance of information technology. *MIS Quarterly*, 13, 319–340.

Davis, J., Wetherell, G., & Henry, P. J. (2018). Social devaluation of African Americans and race-related conspiracy theories. *European Journal of Social Psychology*, 48, 999–1010.

Dean, R. B., Austin, J. A., & Watts, W. A. (1971). Forewarning effects in persuasion: Field and classroom experiments. *Journal of Personality and Social Psychology*, 18(2), 210–221.

de Sousa Mata, A. N., de Azevedo, K. P. M., Braga, L. P., de Medeiros, G. C. B. S., de Oliveira Segundo, V. H., Bezerra, I. N. M., ... & Piuvezam, G. (2019). Training programs in communication skills to improve self-efficacy for health personnel: protocol for a systematic review and meta-analysis. *Medicine*, 98(33), Article e16697, 1–5.

Dillard, J. P., & Shen, L. (2005). On the nature of reactance and its role in persuasive health communication. *Communication Monographs*, 72(2), 144–168.

DiMaggion, P. J., Powell, W. W. (1983). The iron cage revisited: Institutional isomorphism and collective rationality in organizational fields. *American Sociological Review*, 48, 147–160.

Eades, C. E., Ferguson, J. S., & O'Carroll, R. E. (2011). Public health in community pharmacy: A systematic review of pharmacist and consumer views. *BMC Public Health*, 11, 1–13.

Ehrlichman, H., & Halpern, J.N. (1988). Affect and memory: effects of pleasant and unpleasant odors on retrieval of happy and unhappy memories. *Journal of Personality and Social Psychology*, 55, 769–779.

Elvins, R., & Green, J. (2008). The conceptualization and measurement of therapeutic alliance: An empirical review. *Clinical Psychology Review*, 28, 1167–1187.

Erlandsson, A., Björklund, F., & Bäckström, M. (2015). Emotional reactions, perceived impact and perceived responsibility mediate the identifiable victim effect, proportion dominance effect and in-group effect respectively. *Organizational Behavior and Human Decision Processes*, 127, 1–14.

Ezzy, D. (2000). Illness narratives: Time, hope and HIV. *Social Science & Medicine*, 50, 605–617.

Fagin, C. (1997). Collaboration between nurses and physician: No longer a choice. *Academic Medicine*, 5, 295–303.

Fagin, L., & Garelick, A. (2004). The doctor–nurse relationship. *Advances in Psychiatric Treatment*, 10, 277–286.

Faife, C., & Kerr, D. (2021). *Official Information about COVID-19 Is Reaching Fewer Black People on Facebook*. The Markup.

Farber, B. A. (2003). Patient self-disclosure: A review of the research. *Journal of Clinical Psychology*, 59, 589–600.

Farber, B. A. (2006). *Self-Disclosure in Psychotherapy*. New York: Guilford Press.

Fenko, A., & Loock, C. (2014). The influence of ambient scent and music on patients' anxiety in a waiting room of a plastic surgeon. *HERD: Health Environments Research & Design Journal*, 7(3), 38–59.

Ferretti, E., Schoenherr, J. R., Mattiola, A., & Daboval, T. (2023). Vulnerabilities in clinician–parent exchanges and the cascade of communication traps: a review. *Archives of Disease in Childhood*, 108(2), 86–90.

Fisher, B., & Peterson, C. (1993). She won't be dancing anyway: A study of surgeons, surgical nurses, and elder patients. *Qualitative Health Research*, 3, 165–183.

Fiske, S. T., Cuddy, A. J. C., Glick, P., & Xu, J. (2002a). A model of (often mixed) stereotype content: Competence and warmth respectively follow from perceived status and competition. *Journal of Personality and Social Psychology*, 82, 878–902.

Flick, U. (1998). The social construction of individual and public health: Contributions of social representations theory to a social science of health. *Social Science Information*, 37, 639–662.

Flick, U., Fischer, C., Schwartz, F. W., & Walter, U. (2002). Social representations of health held by health professionals: The case of general practitioners and home-care nurses. *Social Science Information*, 41(4), 581–602.

Floyd, D. L., Prentice-Dunn, S., & Rogers, R. W. (2000). A meta-analysis of research on protection motivation theory. *Journal of Applied Social Psychology*, 30, 407–429.

Ford, E. W., Menachemi, N., & Phillips, M. T. (2006). Predicting the adoption of electronic health records by physicians: When will health care be paperless? *Journal of the American Medical Informatics Association*, 13, 106–112.

Foster, G. M. (1976). Disease etiologies in non-western medical systems. *American Anthropologist*, 78, 773–782.

Frank, A. (1995). *The Wounded Storyteller*, Chicago: University of Chicago Press.

Frew, P. M., Saint-Victor, D. S., Owens, L. E., & Omer, S. B. (2014). Socioecological and message framing factors influencing maternal influenza immunization among minority women. *Vaccine*, 32(15), 1736–1744.

Fung, I. C. H., Fu, K. W., Chan, C. H., Chan, B. S. B., Cheung, C. N., Abraham, T., & Tse, Z. T. H. (2016). Social media's initial reaction to information and misinformation on Ebola, August 2014: Facts and rumors. *Public Health Reports*, 131, 461–473.

Gabarron, E., Oyeyemi, S. O., & Wynn, R. (2021). COVID-19-related misinformation on social media: a systematic review. *Bulletin of the World Health Organization*, 99, 455–463.

Gago, F., Echagüe, C. L., & Lázaro, M. (2024). Reflection as a core skill in bioethics education: Application to the scientific and healthcare professions. In Schoenherr, J. R. & McConnell, M. M. (Eds.), *Fundamentals and Frontiers in Medical Education and Decision-Making: Educational Theory and Psychological Practice.* New York: Routledge.

Gallagher, K. M., & Updegraff, J. A. (2012). Health message framing effects on attitudes, intentions, and behavior: A meta-analytic review. *Annals of Behavioral Medicine, 43,* 101–116.

Garcia-Retamero, R., & Cokely, E. T. (2011). Effective communication of risks to young adults: Using message framing and visual aids to increase condom use and STD screening. *Journal of Experimental Psychology: Applied, 17,* 270–287.

Garvar, A., & Schmelkin, L. P. (1989). A multidimensional scaling study of administrators' and teachers' perceptions of disabilities. *The Journal of Special Education, 22,* 463–478.

Gelfand, M. J., Jackson, J. C., Pan, X., Nau, D., Pieper, D., Denison, E., ... & Wang, M. (2021). The relationship between cultural tightness–looseness and COVID-19 cases and deaths: a global analysis. *The Lancet Planetary Health, 5*(3), e135–e144.

Gelfand, M. J., Nishii, L. H., & Raver, J. L. (2006). On the nature and importance of cultural tightness-looseness. *Journal of Applied Psychology, 91*(6), 1225–1244.

Gelfand, M. J., Raver, J. L., Nishii, L., Leslie, L. M., Lun, J., Lim, B. C., ... & Yamaguchi, S. (2011). Differences between tight and loose cultures: A 33-nation study. *Science, 332*(6033), 1100–1104.

Genevsky, A., Västfjäll, D., Slovic, P., & Knutson, B. (2013). Neural underpinnings of the identifiable victim effect: Affect shifts preferences for giving. *Journal of Neuroscience, 33,* 17188–17196.

Gergen, K. J., & Gergen, M. M. (1986). Narrative form and the construction of psychological science. In T. R. Sarbin (Ed.), *Narrative Psychology: The Storied Nature of Human Conduct* (pp. 22–44). Westport, CT: Praeger Publishers/ Greenwood Publishing Group.

Gervais, M. C. & Jovchelovitch, S. (1998). Health and identity: The case of the Chinese community in England. *Social Science Information, 37,* 709–730.

Gilkey, M. B., Calo, W. A., Moss, J. L., Shah, P. D., Marciniak, M. W., & Brewer, N. T. (2016). Provider communication and HPV vaccination: The impact of recommendation quality. *Vaccine, 34,* 1187–1192.

Gilliam, A., Schwartz, D. B., Godoy, R., Boduroglu, A., & Gutchess, A. (2022). Does state tightness-looseness predict behavior and attitudes early in the COVID-19 pandemic in the USA?. *Journal of Cross-Cultural Psychology, 53*(5), 522–542.

Glanz, K., & Bishop, D. B. (2010). The role of behavioral science theory in development and implementation of public health interventions. *Annual Review of Public Health, 31,* 399–418.

Glasman, L. R., & Albarracín, D. (2006). Forming attitudes that predict future behavior: A meta-analysis of the attitude-behavior relation. *Psychological Bulletin, 132*(5), 778–822.

Gong, J., Zhang, Y., Yang, Z., Huang, Y., Feng, J., & Zhang, W. (2013). The framing effect in medical decision-making: A review of the literature. *Psychology, Health & Medicine, 18*(6), 645–653.

Grailey, K. E., Murray, E., Reader, T., & Brett, S. J. (2021). The presence and potential impact of psychological safety in the healthcare setting: An evidence synthesis. *BMC Health Services Research, 21,* 1–15.

Grandpre, J., Alvaro, E. M., Burgoon, M., Miller, C. H., & Hall, J. R. (2003). Adolescent reactance and anti-smoking campaigns: A theoretical approach. *Health Communication*, 15, 349–366.

Green, L., Myerson, J., & McFadden, E. (1997). Rate of temporal discounting decreases with amount of reward. *Memory & Cognition*, 25, 715–723.

Greenhalgh, T., Ozbilgin, M., & Tomlinson, D. (2022). How COVID-19 spreads: Narratives, counter narratives, and social dramas. *British Medical Journal*, 378, Article e069940, 1–9.

Gump, J. P. (2010). Reality matters: The shadow of trauma on African American subjectivity. *Psychoanalytic Psychology*, 27(1), 42.

Haider, M., & Kreps, G. L. (2004). Forty years of diffusion of innovations: Utility and value in public health. *Journal of Health Communication*, 9(S1), 3–11.

Hamilton, A. L., Kerins, J., MacCrossan, M. A., & Tallentire, V. R. (2019). Medical students' non-technical skills (Medi-StuNTS): Preliminary work developing a behavioural marker system for the non-technical skills of medical students in acute care. *BMJ Simulation & Technology Enhanced Learning*, 5(3), 130–139.

Hammond, W. P., Matthews, D., Mohottige, D., Agyemang, A., & Corbie-Smith, G. (2010). Masculinity, medical mistrust, and preventive health services delays among community-dwelling African-American men. *Journal of General Internal Medicine*, 25, 1300–1308.

Han, S., & Shavitt, S. (1994). Persuasion and culture: Advertising appeals in individualistic and collectivistic societies. *Journal of Experimental Social Psychology*, 30(4), 326–350.

Hannan, T. H., & McDowell, J. M. (1987). Rival precedence and the dynamics of technology adoption: An empirical analysis. *Economica*, 54(214), 155–171.

Hansson, L., Jormfeldt, H., Svedberg, P., & Svensson, B. (2013). Mental health professionals' attitudes towards people with mental illness: Do they differ from attitudes held by people with mental illness?. *International Journal of Social Psychiatry*, 59(1), 48–54.

Harrington, K. J. (2012). The use of metaphor in discourse about cancer: A review of the literature. *Clinical Journal of Oncology Nursing*, 16(4), 408–412.

Harris, J. (2007). "Someone is making you sick": Conceptions of disease in Santa Catarina Ixtahuacán. In Adams, W. R., & Hawkins, J. P. (Eds.), *Health Care in Maya Guatemala: Confronting Medical Pluralism in a Developing Country*. (pp. 179–193). Norman, OK: University of Oklahoma Press.

Harrison, J. A., Mullen, P. D., & Green, L. W. (1992). A meta-analysis of studies of the health belief model with adults. *Health Education Research*, 7(1), 107–116.

Hatala, A. R., Desjardins, M., & Bombay, A. (2016). Reframing narratives of Aboriginal health inequity: Exploring Cree elder resilience and well-being in contexts of historical trauma. *Qualitative Health Research*, 26(14), 1911–1927.

Hatala, A. R., Waldram, J. B., & Caal, T. (2015). Narrative structures of Maya mental disorders. *Culture, Medicine, and Psychiatry*, 39, 449–486.

Hatala, R., Cook, D. A., Zendejas, B., Hamstra, S. J., & Brydges, R. (2014). Feedback for simulation-based procedural skills training: A meta-analysis and critical narrative synthesis. *Advances in Health Sciences Education*, 19, 251–272.

Hauser, D. J., & Schwarz, N. (2020). The war on prevention II: Battle metaphors undermine cancer treatment and prevention and do not increase vigilance. *Health Communication*, 35(13), 1698–1704.

Herzlich, C., & Pierret, J. (1984). *Malades d'hier, malades d'aujourd'hui: De la mort collective au devoir de guérison*. Paris: Payot.

Herzlich, C. & Pierret, J. (1984/1987) *Illness and Self in Society*. Baltimore: Johns Hopkins University Press.

Hicks-Ray, D. (2004). The pain didn't start here: Trauma and violence in the African American community. Atlanta, GA: TSA Communications.

Hochbaum, G. M. (1958). Public participation in medical screening programs: A sociopsychological study. *Public Health Service Publication*, 572, 1–23.

Homer, J. B. (1987). A diffusion model with application to evolving medical technologies. *Technological Forecasting and Social Change*, 31(3), 197–218.

Honeycutt, J. M., & Bryan, S. P. (2011). *Scripts and Communication for Relationships*. New York: Peter Lang.

Hunter, A. C. (2021). 'To tell the story': Cultural trauma and holocaust metanarrative. In *Trauma & Memory* (pp. 14-30). Routledge.

Iandoli, L., Primario, S., & Zollo, G. (2021). The impact of group polarization on the quality of online debate in social media: A systematic literature review. *Technological Forecasting and Social Change*, 170, 120924.

Ignacio, M., Oesterle, S., Mercado, M., Carver, A., Lopez, G., Wolfersteig, W., ... & Doubeni, C. (2023). Narratives from African American/Black, American Indian/ Alaska Native, and Hispanic/Latinx community members in Arizona to enhance COVID-19 vaccine and vaccination uptake. *Journal of Behavioral Medicine*, 46(1–2), 140–152.

Janz, N. K., & Becker, M. H. (1984). The health belief model: A decade later. *Health Education Quarterly*, 11(1), 1–47.

Jenkins, E. L., Ilicic, J., Barklamb, A. M., & McCaffrey, T. A. (2020). Assessing the credibility and authenticity of social media content for applications in health communication: Scoping review. *Journal of Medical Internet Research*, 22(7), e17296.

Jenni, K., & Loewenstein, G. (1997). Explaining the identifiable victim effect. *Journal of Risk and Uncertainty*, 14, 235–257.

Jeong, H. Y., & Vollhardt, J. R. (2021). Koreans' collective victim beliefs about Japanese colonization. *Peace and Conflict: Journal of Peace Psychology*, 27(4), 629.

Jiang, J., Ren, X., & Ferrara, E. (2021). Social media polarization and echo chambers in the context of COVID-19: Case study. *JMIRx Med*, 2(3), e29570.

Jodelet, D. (1991). *Madness and Social Representations*. Hemel Hempstead: Harvester/ Wheatsheaf.

Joffe, H. (1995) Social Representations of AIDS: Towards encompassing issues of power. *Papers on Social Representations*, 4(1), 29–40.

Joffe, H. (1997). Juxtaposing positivist and non-positivist approaches to social scientific AIDS research: Reply to Fife-Schaw's commentary. *British Journal of Medical Psychology*, 70(1), 75–83.

Joffe, H. (1999). *Risk and 'the Other'*. Cambridge University Press.

Joint Commission on Accreditation of Healthcare Organizations (2005). National Patient Safety Goals.

Jones, C. J., Llewellyn, C. D., Frew, A. J., Du Toit, G., Mukhopadhyay, S., & Smith, H. (2015). Factors associated with good adherence to self-care behaviours amongst adolescents with food allergy. *Pediatric Allergy and Immunology*, 26(2), 111–118.

Jones, C. J., Smith, H., & Llewellyn, C. (2014). Evaluating the effectiveness of health belief model interventions in improving adherence: A systematic review. *Health Psychology Review*, 8(3), 253–269.

Jones, C. L., Jensen, J. D., Scherr, C. L., Brown, N. R., Christy, K., & Weaver, J. (2015). The health belief model as an explanatory framework in communication research: Exploring parallel, serial, and moderated mediation. *Health Communication*, 30, 566–576.

Kadushin, C. (2012). *Understanding Social Networks: Theories, Concepts, and Findings*. New York: Oxford University Press.

Kareklas, I., Muehling, D. D., & Weber, T. J. (2015). Reexamining health messages in the digital age: A fresh look at source credibility effects. *Journal of Advertising*, 44, 88–104.

Katz, E., Levin, M. L., Hamilton, H. (1963). Traditions of research on the diffusion of innovation. *American Sociological Review*, 28, 237–252.

Kazda, L., Bell, K., Thomas, R., McGeechan, K., Sims, R., & Barratt, A. (2021). Overdiagnosis of attention-deficit/hyperactivity disorder in children and adolescents: A systematic scoping review. *JAMA Network Open*, 4(4), e215335–e215335.

Kelley, J. M., Kraft-Todd, G., Schapira, L., Kossowsky, J., & Riess, H. (2014). The influence of the patient-clinician relationship on healthcare outcomes: A systematic review and meta-analysis of randomized controlled trials. *PLOS One*, 9, e94207.

Kelly, L., Runge, J., & Spencer, C. (2015). Predictors of compassion fatigue and compassion satisfaction in acute care nurses: Compassion fatigue. *Journal of Nursing Scholarship*, 47(6), 522–528.

Kelly, M., Inoue, K., Black, K. I., Barratt, A., Bateson, D., Rutherford, A., ... & Richters, J. (2017). Doctors' experience of the contraceptive consultation: A qualitative study in Australia. *Journal of Family Planning and Reproductive Health Care*, 43(2), 119–125.

Kiene, S. M., Barta, W. D., Zelenski, J. M., & Cothran, D. L. (2005). Why are you bringing up condoms now? The effect of message content on framing effects of condom use messages. *Health Psychology*, 24(3), 321–326.

Kim, M. S. (1999). Cross-cultural perspectives on motivations of verbal communication: Review, critique, and a theoretical framework. In M. Roloff (Ed.), *Communication Yearbook 22* (pp. 51–89). Thousand Oaks: Sage.

Kim, M. S., Hunter, J. E., Miyahara, A., Horvath, A. M., Bresnahan, M., & Yoon, H. J. (1996). Individual-vs. culture-level dimensions of individualism and collectivism: Effects on preferred conversational styles. *Communications Monographs*, 63(1), 29–49.

Kim, Y., Baek, T. H., Yoon, S., Oh, S., & Choi, Y. K. (2017). Assertive environmental advertising and reactance: Differences between South Koreans and Americans. *Journal of Advertising*, 46(4), 550–564.

Kirscht, J. P., (1974). The health belief model and illness behavior. *Health Education Monographs*, 2(4). 387–408.

Kleinman, A. (1975). Explanatory models in health care relationships. *Health of the Family* (pp. 159–172). Washington, DC: National Council for International Health.

Kleinman, A. (1978). Concepts and a model for the comparison of medical systems as cultural systems. *Social Science & Medicine. Part B: Medical Anthropology*, 12, 85–93.

Kleinman, A. (1980). *Patients and Healers in the Context of Culture: An Exploration of the Borderland between Anthropology, Medicine, and Psychiatry*. Los Angeles: University of California Press.

Komarnisky, S., Hackett, P., Abonyi, S., Heffernan, C., & Long, R. (2016). "Years ago": reconciliation and First Nations narratives of tuberculosis in the Canadian Prairie Provinces. *Critical Public Health*, 26(4), 381–393.

Kounios, J., & Holcomb, P. J. (1994). Concreteness effects in semantic processing: ERP evidence supporting dual-coding theory. *Journal of Experimental Psychology: Learning, Memory, and Cognition*, 20, 804–823.

Kreuter, M. W., & McClure, S. M. (2004). The role of culture in health communication. *Annual Review of Public Health*, 25, 439–455.

Kumar, N., Pandey, A., Venkatraman, A., Garg, N., 2014. Are video sharing Web sites a useful source of information on hypertension? *Journal of the American Society of Hypertension*, 8, 481–490.

Kyaw, B. M., Posadzki, P., Paddock, S., Car, J., Campbell, J., & Tudor Car, L. (2019). Effectiveness of digital education on communication skills among medical students: Systematic review and meta-analysis by the digital health education collaboration. *Journal of Medical Internet Research*, 21, e12967.

Landau, M. J., Arndt, J., & Cameron, L. D. (2018). Do metaphors in health messages work? Exploring emotional and cognitive factors. *Journal of Experimental Social Psychology*, 74, 135–149.

Lang, J., Erickson, W. W., & Jing-Schmidt, Z. (2021). #MaskOn! #MaskOff! Digital polarization of mask-wearing in the United States during COVID-19. *PLOS One*, 16(4), e0250817.

Larson, E. (1999). The impact of physician-nurse interaction on patient care. *Holistic Nurse Practice*, 13, 38–47.

Larson, H. J., Cooper, L. Z., Eskola, J., Katz, S. L., & Ratzan, S. (2011). Addressing the vaccine confidence gap. *The Lancet*, 378(9790), 526–535.

Larson, H. J., de Figueiredo, A., Xiahong, Z., Schulz, W. S., Verger, P., Johnston, I. G., Cook, A. R., & Jones, N. S. (2016). The state of vaccine confidence 2016: Global insights through a 67-country survey. *EBioMedicine*, 12, 295–301.

Leary, J. D. (2005). *Post traumatic Slave Syndrome: America's Legacy of Enduring Injury and Healing*. Milwaukie, OR: Uptone Press

Lee, J., Kwak, Y. S., Kim, Y. J., Kim, E. J., Park, E. J., Shin, Y., ... & Lee, S. I. (2019). Transgenerational transmission of trauma: Psychiatric evaluation of offspring of former "comfort women," survivors of the Japanese military sexual slavery during World War II. *Psychiatry Investigation*, 16(3), 249.

Lee, S., & Feeley, T. H. (2016). The identifiable victim effect: A meta-analytic review. *Social Influence*, 11(3), 199–215.

Leong, A.Y., Sanghera, R., Jhajj, J., Desai, N., Jammu, B.S., Makowsky, M.J., 2017. Is YouTube useful as a source of health information for adults with type 2 diabetes? A South Asian perspective. *Canadian Journal of Diabetes*, 42(4), 495–403.

Leventhal, H., Watts, J. C., & Pagano, F. (1967). Effects of fear and instructions on how to cope with danger. *Journal of Personality and Social Psychology*, 6(3), 313–321.

Lien, A. S. Y., & Jiang, Y. D. (2017). Integration of diffusion of innovation theory into diabetes care. *Journal of diabetes investigation*, 8(3), 259–260.

Lu, J. G., Jin, P., & English, A. S. (2021). Collectivism predicts mask use during COVID-19. *Proceedings of the National Academy of Sciences*, 118(23), e2021793118.

Lwin, M. O., Morrin, M., & Krishna, A. (2010). Exploring the superadditive effects of scent and pictures on verbal recall: An extension of dual coding theory. *Journal of Consumer Psychology*, 20(3), 317–326.

Maaravi, Y., Levy, A., Gur, T., Confino, D., & Segal, S. (2021). "The tragedy of the commons": How individualism and collectivism affected the spread of the COVID-19 pandemic. *Frontiers in Public Health*, 9, 627559.

Maddux, J. E., & Rogers, R. W. (1983). Protection motivation and self-efficacy: A revised theory of fear appeals and attitude change. *Journal of Experimental Social Psychology*, 19(5), 469–479.

Mahamid, F. A. (2020). Collective trauma, quality of life and resilience in narratives of third generation Palestinian refugee children. *Child Indicators Research*, 13(6), 2181–2204.

Mao, Y., Ning, W., Zhang, N., Xie, T., Liu, J., Lu, Y., & Zhu, B. (2021). The therapeutic relationship in China: A systematic review and meta-analysis. *International Journal of Environmental Research and Public Health*, 18, 3460.

Martin, D. J., Garske, J. P., & Davis, M. K. (2000). Relation of the therapeutic alliance with outcome and other variables: A meta-analytic review. *Journal of Consulting and Clinical Psychology*, 68(3), 438–450.

Mathieson, C. M., & Stam, H. J. (1995). Renegotiating identity: Cancer narratives. *Sociology of Health & Illness*, 17, 283–306.

McConnell, M. (2024). Emotion and clinical decision-making. In Schoenherr, J. R. & McConnell, M. M. (eds.), *Fundamentals and Frontiers in Medical Education and Decision-Making: Educational Theory and Psychological Practice*. New York: Routledge.

Mechanic, D., & Volkart, E. H. (1961). Stress, illness behavior, and the sick role. *American Sociological Review*, 51–58.

Mewborn, C. R., & Rogers, R. W. (1979). Effects of threatening and reassuring components of fear appeals on physiological and verbal measures of emotion and attitudes. *Journal of Experimental Social Psychology*, 15(3), 242–253.

Meyerowitz, B. E., & Chaiken, S. (1987). The effect of message framing on breast self-examination attitudes, intentions, and behavior. *Journal of Personality and Social Psychology*, 52(3), 500–510.

Miller, C. H., Lane, L. T., Deatrick, L. M., Young, A. M., & Potts, K. A. (2007). Psychological reactance and promotional health messages: The effects of controlling language, lexical concreteness, and the restoration of freedom. *Human Communication Research*, 33, 219–240.

Milne, S., Sheeran, P., & Orbell, S. (2000). Prediction and intervention in health-related behavior: A meta-analytic review of protection motivation theory. *Journal of Applied Social Psychology*, 30, 106–143.

Milota, M. M., van Thiel, G. J., & van Delden, J. J. (2019). Narrative medicine as a medical education tool: A systematic review. *Medical Teacher*, 41, 802–810.

Mirotznik, J., Feldman, L., & Stein, R. (1995). The health belief model and adherence with a community center-based, supervised coronary heart disease exercise program. *Journal of Community Health*, 20(3), 233–247.

Montagni, I., Ouazzani-Touhami, K., Mebarki, A., Texier, N., Schück, S., Tzourio, C., & Confins Group. (2021). Acceptance of a Covid-19 vaccine is associated with ability to detect fake news and health literacy. *Journal of Public Health*, 43, 695–702.

Moorhead, S. A., Hazlett, D. E., Harrison, L., Carroll, J. K., Irwin, A., & Hoving, C. (2013). A new dimension of health care: Systematic review of the uses, benefits, and limitations of social media for health communication. *Journal of Medical Internet Research*, 15(4), e85.

Morgan, S. E., & Miller, J. K. (2002). Beyond the organ donor card: The effect of knowledge, attitudes, and values on willingness to communicate about organ donation to family members. *Health Communication*, 14, 121–134.

Morris, M. (1993). Epidemiology and social networks. *Sociological Methods and Research*, 22(1), 99–126.

Moscovici, S. (1961) *La Psychanalyse, Son Image et Son Public*. Paris: Presses Universitaires de France.

Moscovici, S. (1988). Notes towards a description of social representations. *European Journal of Social Psychology*, 18(3), 211–250.

Moscovici, S. (2000). *Social Representations: Explorations in Social Psychology*. Cambridge: Polity.

Munawar, K., Kuhn, S. K., & Haque, S. (2018). Understanding the reminiscence bump: A systematic review. *PLOS One*, 13(12), e0208595.

Murray, M. (2007). "It's in the blood and you're not going to change it": Fish harvesters' narrative accounts of injuries and disability. *Work*, 28(2), 165–174.

Ngai, C. S. B., Singh, R. G., Lu, W., & Koon, A. C. (2020). Grappling with the COVID-19 health crisis: Content analysis of communication strategies and their effects on public engagement on social media. *Journal of Medical Internet Research*, 22(8), e21360.

Nienhuis, J. B., Owen, J., Valentine, J. C., Winkeljohn Black, S., Halford, T. C., Parazak, S. E., … & Hilsenroth, M. (2018). Therapeutic alliance, empathy, and genuineness in individual adult psychotherapy: A meta-analytic review. *Psychotherapy Research*, 28, 593–605.

Nisbett, R. E., & Ross, L. (1980). *Human Inference: Strategies and Shortcomings of Social Judgment*. Englewood Cliffs: Prentice-Hall.

Norman, P., Henk, B., Seydel, E. S. (2005) Protection motivation theory. In M. Conner, & P. Norman (Eds.), *Predicting Health Behaviour: Research and Practice with Social Cognition Models* (2. ed., pp. 81–126). Open University Press.

Nutbeam, D., & Lloyd, J. E. (2021). Understanding and responding to health literacy as a social determinant of health. *Annual Review of Public Health*, 42(1), 159–73.

O'Connell, G., Christakou, A., Haffey, A. T., & Chakrabarti, B. (2013). The role of empathy in choosing rewards from another's perspective. *Frontiers in Human Neuroscience*, 7, Article 174, 1–5.

O'Donovan, R., & McAuliffe, E. (2020a). A systematic review of factors that enable psychological safety in healthcare teams. *International Journal for Quality in Health Care*, 32(4), 240–250.

O'Donovan, R., & McAuliffe, E. (2020b). A systematic review exploring the content and outcomes of interventions to improve psychological safety, speaking up and voice behaviour. *BMC Health Services Research*, 20, Article 101.

Offredy, M. (2002). Decision-making in primary care: Outcomes from a study using patient scenarios. *Journal of Advanced Nursing*, 40(5), 532–541.

Ogden, J. (2019). *Health Psychology* (6. ed.). McGraw-Hill.

Okuhara, T., Ishikawa, H., Okada, M., Kato, M., Kiuchi, T., 2017. Assertions of Japanese websites for and against cancer screening: A text mining analysis. *Asian Pacific Journal of Cancer Prevention*, 18 (4), 1069–1075.

Paivio, A. (1971). Imagery and language. In S. J. Segal (Ed.), *Imagery: Current Cognitive Approaches*. New York: Academic Press.

Paivio, A. (1991). Dual coding theory: Retrospect and current status. *Canadian Journal of Psychology/Revue canadienne de psychologie*, 45(3), 255–287.

Parsons, T. (1951). *The Social System*. The Free Press.

Pathak, R., Poudel, D.R., Karmacharya, P., Pathak, A., Aryal, M.R., Mahmood, M., Donato, A.A., 2015. YouTube as a source of information on Ebola virus disease. *North American Journal of Medicine & Science*, 7 (7), 306–309

Peltu, M. (1985). The role of communications media. In H. Otway & M. Peltu (Eds.), *Regulating Industrial Risks* (pp. 128–148). Oxford: Butterworth-Heinemann Ltd.

Pennycook, G., Trippas, D., Handley, S. J., & Thompson, V. A. (2014). Base rates: Both neglected and intuitive. *Journal of Experimental Psychology: Learning, Memory, and Cognition*, 40(2), 544–554.

Penţa, M. A., & Băban, A. (2018). Message framing in vaccine communication: A systematic review of published literature. *Health Communication*, 33(3), 299–314.

Polgar, S. (1962). Health and human behavior: Areas of interest common to the social and medical sciences. *Current Anthropology*, 3(2), 159–205.

Quick, B. L., & Considine, J. R. (2008). Examining the use of forceful language when designing exercise persuasive messages for adults: A test of conceptualizing reactance arousal as a two-step process. *Health Communication*, 23, 483–491.

Quick, B. L., & Kim, D. K. (2009). Examining reactance and reactance restoration with South Korean adolescents: A test of psychological reactance within a collectivist culture. *Communication Research*, 36(5), 765–782.

Quick, B. L., & Stephenson, M. T. (2007). Further evidence that psychological reactance can be modeled as a combination of anger and negative cognitions. *Communication Research*, 34, 255–276.

Rains, S. A. (2013). The nature of psychological reactance revisited: A meta-analytic review. *Human Communication Research*, 39, 47–73.

Rains, S. A., & Turner, M. M. (2007). Psychological reactance and persuasive health communication: A test and extension of the intertwined model. *Human Communication Research*, 33(2), 241-269.

Rehim, S. A., DeMoor, S., Olmsted, R., Dent, D. L., & Parker-Raley, J. (2017). Tools for assessment of communication skills of hospital action teams: A systematic review. *Journal of Surgical Education*, 74(2), 341–351.

Remein, C. D., Childs, E., Pasco, J. C., Trinquart, L., Flynn, D. B., Wingerter, S. L., … & Benjamin, E. J. (2020). Content and outcomes of narrative medicine programmes: A systematic review of the literature through 2019. *BMJ Open*, 10(1), e031568.

Renn, O. (2020). Risk communication: Insights and requirements for designing successful communication programs on health and environmental hazards. In *Handbook of Risk and Crisis Communication* (pp. 80–98). Routledge.

Reynolds-Tylus, T. (2019). Psychological reactance and persuasive health communication: A review of the literature. *Frontiers in Communication*, 4, Article 56.

Richards, A. S., & Banas, J. A. (2015). Inoculating against reactance to persuasive health messages. *Health Communication*, 30, 451–460.

Richards, A. S., Banas, J. A., & Magid, Y. (2017). More on inoculating against reactance to persuasive health messages: The paradox of threat. *Health Communication*, 32, 890–902.

Richards, A. S., Bessarabova, E., Banas, J. A., & Bernard, D. R. (2022). Reducing psychological reactance to health promotion messages: Comparing preemptive and postscript mitigation strategies. *Health Communication*, 37, 366–374.

Riet, J. V. 'T, Ruiter, R. A. C., Smerecnik, C., & Vries, H. D. (2010). Examining the influence of self-efficacy on message-framing effects: Reducing salt consumption in the general population. *Basic and Applied Social Psychology*, 32(2), 165–172.

Rogers. E. M. (1962/2010). *Diffusion of Innovation*. New York: New York Free Press.

Rogers, E. M. (2004). A prospective and retrospective look at the diffusion model. *Journal of Health Communication*, 9(S1), 13–19.

Rogers, R. W. (1975). A protection motivation theory of fear appeals and attitude change. *The Journal of Psychology*, 91(1), 93–114.

Rogers, R. W. (1983). Cognitive and physiological processes in fear appeals and attitude change: A revised theory of protection motivation. In J. T. Cacioppo & R. E. Petty (Eds.), *Social Psychophysiology* (pp. 153–174). New York: The Gilford Press.

Ronis, D. L., & Harel, Y. (1989). Health beliefs and breast examination behaviors: Analyses of linear structural relations. *Psychology & Health*, 3(4), 259–285.

Rosenstock, I. M. (1960). What research in motivation suggests for public health. *American Journal of Public Health*, 50(3), 295–302.

Rosenstock, I. M. (1966). Why people use health services. *The Milbank Memorial Fund Quarterly*, 44(3), 94–127.

Rosenstock, I. M. (1974). Historical origins of the health belief model. *Health Education Monographs*, 2(4), 328–325.

Rosenstock, I. M., Strecher, V. J., & Becker, M. H. (1988). Social learning theory and the health belief model. *Health Education Quarterly*, 15(2), 175–183.

Rothman, A. J., Martino, S. C., Bedell, B. T., Detweiler, J. B., & Salovey, P. (1999). The systematic influence of gain-and loss-framed messages on interest in and use of different types of health behavior. *Personality and Social Psychology Bulletin*, 25(11), 1355–1369.

Rothman, A. J., & Salovey, P. (1997). Shaping perceptions to motivate healthy behavior: The role of message framing. *Psychological Bulletin*, 121, 3–19.

Rounds, J. B., & Zevon, M. A. (1993). Cancer stereotypes: A multidimensional scaling analysis. *Journal of Behavioral Medicine*, 16(5), 485–496.

Rudd, R. E., Anderson, J. E., Oppenheimer, S., & Nath, C. (2023). Health literacy: An update of medical and public health literature. In *Review of Adult Learning and Literacy*, Volume 7 (pp. 175–204). New York: Routledge.

Ruiter, R. A. C., Kessels, L. T. E., Peters, G. Y., & Kok, G. (2014). Sixty years of fear appeal research: Current state of the evidence. *International Journal of Psychology*, 49(2), 63–70.

Rushforth, A., Ladds, E., Wieringa, S., Taylor, S., Husain, L., & Greenhalgh, T. (2021). Long covid–the illness narratives. *Social Science & Medicine*, 286, 114326.

Schirch, L. (2018). Trauma triggers and narratives on Israel and Palestine. *Journal of Peacebuilding & Development*, 13(3), 108–114.

Schmelkin, L. P. (1982). Perceptions of disabilities: A multidimensional scaling approach. *The Journal of Special Education*, 16(2), 161–177.

Schmidt, A. L., Zollo, F., Scala, A., Betsch, C., & Quattrociocchi, W. (2018). Polarization of the vaccination debate on Facebook. *Vaccine*, 36(25), 3606–3612.

Schoenherr, J. R. (2021). Social categories in/of cyberspace: Frequency effects and trust in Media. In *2022 IEEE International Symposium on Technology and Society (ISTAS)*, (pp. 1–7). IEEE.

Schoenherr, J. R. (2022a). Social categories in/of cyberspace: Frequency effects and trust in media. In *2022 IEEE International Symposium on Technology and Society (ISTAS)* (pp. 1–7). New York: IEEE.

Schoenherr, J. R. (2022b). Vaccination, values, and health information search behaviour in the New Folk medicine. In *2022 IEEE International Symposium on Technology and Society (ISTAS)*, pp. 1–10. New York: IEEE.

Schoenherr, J. R. (2022c). Folkmedical Technologies and the sociotechnical systems of healthcare. *IEEE Technology and Society Magazine*, 41(3), 38–49.

Schoenherr, J. R. (2024). The development and dynamics of Mayan healthcare systems: A socioecological approach. In Schoenherr, J. R. (ed.), *Fundamentals and Frontiers in Medical Education and Decision-Making: Innovation, Implementation, and Translational Research*. Routledge.

Schoenherr, J. R., & Beaudoin, J. (2024). Medical pluralism in East Asian medical education: The evolving landscape of health professions education in East Asia. In Schoenherr, J. R. & McConnell, M. M. (Eds.), *Fundamentals and Frontiers in Medical Education and Decision-Making: Innovation, Implementation, and Translational Research*. New York: Routledge.

Schoenherr, J. R., & Thomson, R. (2020). Health information seeking behaviour, risk communication, and mobility during COVID-19. In *2020 IEEE International Symposium on Technology and Society (ISTAS)* (pp. 283–289). New York: IEEE.

Schoenherr, J. R., & Thomson, R. (2021). Persuasive features of scientific explanations: Explanatory schemata of physical and psychosocial phenomena. *Frontiers in Psychology*, 12, 644809.

Schoenherr, J. R., Waechter, J., & Lee, C. H. (2024). Quantifying expertise in the healthcare professions: Cognitive efficiency and metacognitive calibration. In Schoenherr, J. R. & McConnell, M. M. (Eds.), *Fundamentals and Frontiers in Medical Education: Educational Theory and Psychological Practice*. New York: Routledge,.

Schoenherr, J. R., Mahias-Ito, Y., & Li, X. Y. (2024). Collective competence and social learning in the health professions: learning, thinking, and deciding in groups. In Schoenherr, J. R. (ed.), *Fundamentals and Frontiers in Medical Education and Decision-Making: Innovation, Implementation, and Translational Research*. Routledge.

Schulz, P. J., Pessina, A., Hartung, U., & Petrocchi, S. (2021). Effects of objective and subjective health literacy on patients' accurate judgment of health information and decision-making ability: Survey study. *Journal of Medical Internet Research*, 23(1), e20457.

Schulze, B. (2008). Evaluating programmatic needs concerning the stigma of mental illness. In Arboleda-Florez, J. and Sartorius, N. (eds.), *Understanding the Stigma of Mental Illness: Theory and Interventions*, 85–124.

Schwarzer, R. (2001). Social-cognitive factors in changing health-related behaviors. *Current Directions in Psychological Science*, 10, 47–51.

Schwarzer, R. (2008). Modeling health behavior change: How to predict and modify the adoption and maintenance of health behaviors. *Applied Psychology*, 57, 1–29.

Schwarzer, R., Lippke, S., & Luszczynska, A. (2011). Mechanisms of health behavior change in persons with chronic illness or disability: The Health Action Process Approach (HAPA). *Rehabilitation Psychology*, 56(3), 161–170.

Schwarzer, R., & Luszczynska, A. (2008). How to overcome health-compromising behaviors: The health action process approach. *European Psychologist*, 13(2), 141–151.

Schwarzer, R., Luszczynska, A., Ziegelmann, J. P., Scholz, U., & Lippke, S. (2008). Social-cognitive predictors of physical exercise adherence: Three longitudinal studies in rehabilitation. *Health Psychology*, 27(1, Suppl), S54–S63.

Seeger, M. W., Sellnow, T. L., & Ulmer, R. R. (2003). *Communication and Organizational Crisis* (p. 144). Westport, CT: Praeger.

Semino, E. (2021). "Not soldiers but fire-fighters"–metaphors and Covid-19. *Health Communication*, 36(1), 50–58.

Sexton J. (2002). Error, stress, and teamwork in medicine and aviation: Cross sectional surveys. *British Medical Journal*, 320, 745–749.

Sharma, M., Yadav, K., Yadav, N., Ferdinand, K.C., 2017. Zika virus pandemic-analysis of Facebook as a social media health information platform. *American Journal of Infection Control*, 45, 301–302.

Shi, J., Poorisat, T., & Salmon, C. T. (2018). The use of social networking sites (SNSs) in health communication campaigns: Review and recommendations. *Health Communication*, 33, 49–56.

Smedslund, J. (1963). The concept of correlation in adults. *Scandinavian Journal of Psychology*, 4(1), 165–173.

Smith, A. C., Woerner, J., Perera, R., Haeny, A. M., & Cox, J. M. (2022). An investigation of associations between race, ethnicity, and past experiences of discrimination with medical mistrust and COVID-19 protective strategies. *Journal of Racial and Ethnic Health Disparities*, 9, 1430–1442.

Sommariva, S., Vamos, C., Mantzarlis, A., Đào, L.U.-L., Tyson, D.M., 2018. Spreading the (fake) news: Exploring health messages on social media and the implications for health professionals using a case study. *American Journal of Health Education*, 49, 246–255.

Sørensen, K., Van den Broucke, S., Fullam, J., Doyle, G., Pelikan, J., Slonska, Z., & Brand, H. (2012). Health literacy and public health: A systematic review and integration of definitions and models. *BMC Public Health*, 12(1), 1–13.

Stein, L. (1967). The doctor-nurse game. *Archives of General Psychiatry*, 16(6), 699–703.

Stein, L., Watts, D. T., & Howell, T. (1990). The doctor-nurse game revisited. *Nursing Outlook*, 322(8), 264–8

Strecher, V. J., McEvoy DeVellis, B., Becker, M. H., & Rosenstock, I. M. (1986). The role of self-efficacy in achieving health behavior change. *Health Education Quarterly*, 13(1), 73–91.

Sultan, F., Farley, J. U., Lehmann, D. R. (1990). A meta-analysis of applications of diffusion models. *Journal of Marketing Research*, 27(1), 70–77.

Syed-Abdul, S., Fernandez-Luque, L., Jian, W.-S., Li, Y.-C., Crain, S., Hsu, M.-H., Wang, Y.-C., Khandregzen, D., Chuluunbaatar, E., Nguyen, P. A., & Liou, D.-M. (2013). Misleading health-related information promoted through video-based social media: Anorexia on YouTube. *Journal of Medical Internet Research*, 15(2), e30.

Tasaki, K., Kim, M. S., & Miller, M. D. (1999). The effects of social status on cognitive elaboration and post-message attitude: Focusing on self-construals. *Communication Quarterly*, 47(2), 196–214.

Taylor, S., & Asmundson, G. J. G. (2021). Negative attitudes about facemasks during the COVID-19 pandemic: The dual importance of perceived ineffectiveness and psychological reactance. *PLOS One*, 16(2), e0246317.

Terren, L., & Borge-Bravo, R. (2021). Echo chambers on social media: A systematic review of the literature. *Review of Communication Research*, 9, 99–118.

Thomas, R., Sanders, S., Doust, J., Beller, E., & Glasziou, P. (2015). Prevalence of attention-deficit/hyperactivity disorder: A systematic review and meta-analysis. *Pediatrics*, 135(4), e994–e1001.

Tiwary, A., Rimal, A., Paudyal, B., Sigdel, K. R., & Basnyat, B. (2019). Poor communication by health care professionals may lead to life-threatening complications: Examples from two case reports. *Wellcome Open Research*, 4:7.

Totura, C. M. W., Fields, S. A., & Karver, M. S. (2018). The role of the therapeutic relationship in psychopharmacological treatment outcomes: A meta-analytic review. *Psychiatric Services*, 69(1), 41–47.

Tversky, A., & Kahneman, D. (1981). The framing of decisions and the psychology of choice. *Science*, 211(4481), 453–458.

Uskul, A. K., & Oyserman, D. (2010). When message-frame fits salient cultural-frame, messages feel more persuasive. *Psychology & Health*, 25(3), 321–337.

Uskul, A. K., Sherman, D. K., & Fitzgibbon, J. (2009). The cultural congruency effect: Culture, regulatory focus, and the effectiveness of gain–vs. loss-framed health messages. *Journal of Experimental Social Psychology*, 45(3), 535–541.

Valente, T. W. (2010). *Social Networks and Health: Models, Methods, and Applications*. New York: Oxford University Press.

van den Bos, W., & McClure, S. M. (2013). Towards a general model of temporal discounting. *Journal of the Experimental Analysis of Behavior*, 99(1), 58–73.

Van den Bulte, C., & Lilien, G. L. (2001). Medical innovation revisited: Social contagion versus marketing effort. *American Journal of Sociology*, 106(5), 1409–1435.

Veronese, G., & Cavazzoni, F. (2020). "I hope I will be able to go back to my home city": Narratives of suffering and survival of children in Palestine. *Psychological Studies*, 65(1), 51–63.

Visser, S. N., Danielson, M. L., Bitsko, R. H., Holbrook, J. R., Kogan, M. D., Ghandour, R. M., … & Blumberg, S. J. (2014). Trends in the parent-report of health care provider-diagnosed and medicated attention-deficit/hyperactivity disorder: United States, 2003–2011. *Journal of the American Academy of Child & Adolescent Psychiatry*, 53(1), 34–46.

Walter, N., & Tukachinsky, R. (2020). A meta-analytic examination of the continued influence of misinformation in the face of correction: How powerful is it, why does it happen, and how to stop it? *Communication Research*, 47(2), 155–177.

Weinstein, R. B., Walsh, J. L., & Ward, L. M. (2008). Testing a new measure of sexual health knowledge and its connections to students' sex education, communication, confidence, and condom use. *International Journal of Sexual Health*, 20(3), 212–221.

Wicklund, R. A. (1974). *Freedom and Reactance*. Potomac: Lawrence Erlbaum Associates, Inc.

Wiebe, J. S., & Christensen, A. J. (1997). Health beliefs, personality, and adherence in hemodialysis patients: An interactional perspective. *Annals of Behavioral Medicine*, 19(1), 30–35.

Wilson, T. D., & Gilbert, D. T. (2003). Affective forecasting. *Advances in Experimental Social Psychology*, 35(35), 345–411.

Wood, M. J. (2018). Propagating and debunking conspiracy theories on Twitter during the 2015–2016 Zika virus outbreak. *Cyberpsychology, Behavior, and Social Networking*, 21(8), 485–490.

Wright, K. (2016). Social networks, interpersonal social support, and health outcomes: A health communication perspective. *Frontiers in Communication*, 1, Article 10.

Xiang, H., Li, Y., & Guo, Y. (2023). Promoting COVID-19 booster vaccines in Macao: A psychological reactance perspective. *Social Science & Medicine*, 332, 116128.

Yaskowich, K. M., & Stam, H. J. (2003). Cancer narratives and the cancer support group. *Journal of Health Psychology*, 8(6), 720–737.

Ye, X., Lee, H. H., Hui, K. H., Xin, M., & Mo, P. K. (2023). Effects of Negative Attitudes towards Vaccination in General and Trust in Government on Uptake of a Booster Dose of COVID-19 Vaccine and the Moderating Role of Psychological Reactance: An Observational Prospective Cohort Study in Hong Kong. *Vaccines*, 11(2), 393.

Yu, N., & Shen, F. (2013). Benefits for me or risks for others: A cross-culture investigation of the effects of message frames and cultural appeals. *Health Communication*, 28(2), 133–145.

Zhang, C.-Q., Zhang, R., Schwarzer, R., & Hagger, M. S. (2019). A meta-analysis of the health action process approach. *Health Psychology*, 38(7), 623–637.

Zhang, Y., & Gelb, B. D. (1996). Matching advertising appeals to culture: The influence of products' use conditions. *Journal of Advertising*, 25(3), 29–46.

Zhang, Y. S. D., Young Leslie, H., Sharafaddin-Zadeh, Y., Noels, K., & Lou, N. M. (2021). Public health messages about face masks early in the COVID-19 pandemic: Perceptions of and impacts on Canadians. *Journal of Community Health*, 46(5), 903–912.

Zolnierek, K. B. H., & DiMatteo, M. R. (2009). Physician communication and patient adherence to treatment: A meta-analysis. *Medical Care*, 47(8), 826–834.

Zwarenstein, M., & Reeves, S. (2002). Working together but apart: Barriers and routes to nurse-physician collaboration. *Joint Commission Journal on Quality Improvement*, 28, 242–247.

INDEX

institutional efficiency 216–17; metacognition 232–3
emotion 6, 21, 22, 75, 254, 259, 274; affect 6, 21, 274; appraisal 141, 143–4; attention 144–6, 180; clinical decision-making 153–7; decision-making and reasoning 139–40, 148–53; definition 140–3; expression 251; memory 146–8; mood 140–1, 148–52, 155–8; reflection 256–7; theory 143–4, 256
entrustable professional activities (EPA) 4, 10, 18, 48–9, 87, 95, 111–12, 116–17, 233
equity, diversity, and inclusion (EDI) 39, 115
errors 188, 193, 195, 211, 214, 215, 225, 232; biases 217; clinical 151, 215; cognitive 151, 218; diagnostic 137, 151, 155, 218, 233; fixation errors 156; medical 7, 21, 153, 216; memory 148; psychomotor 187; reasoning 152
ethics 123; bioethics 247–8, 252–3, 255; education (*see* validity (values and social consequences))
expertise 6, 12, 14, 15, 18, 22, 64, 176, 180, 203, 204, 214–15, 225–7, 255; competencies 9; development of 19–22, 187; educational design and implementation 94–5; efficiency 232–3; folk theories 7; intuition 8; levels of 188; medical 8, 9, 82, 169; metacognition assessment 227–9; metacognitive strategies 233–4
explanatory models *see* illness models

familiarity *see* heuristics
feedback 13, 15, 20, 22, 23, 45, 58, 60, 63, 85, 96, 126, 129, 188, 190; assessment 45, 47, 54, 56, 113–14, 116; communication 272; false-positive 191; interpretation of 83; learning 18, 19, 55, 59, 63, 116, 187, 197, 273; metacognition 229, 262; narrative 125; practice-based feedback 128; programmatic 128; quality 118, 122; teaching 116; timing and quantity 191, 192, 194, 201–4, 217, 224
fidelity *see* simulation
formative assessment *see* assessment
functional task alignment 85

health communication *see* communication
health professions education *see* medical education
help-seeking 155
heuristics and biases *see* cognition
human-centred design *see* design

Identifiable Victim Effect 283
illness models 214; explanatory models 279–80; narrative models 280–1; social representations 277–8
implementation: implementation validity (*see* validity)
individualism-collectivism *see* collectivism
incivility 155
indigenous 6
innovation 5, 83, 84, 88–9, 91, 92, 99, 101; adoption and implementation 96, 128, 290; dependency 94–6; learning analytics 127–8; role of leadership 93
intensive care unit *see* critical care unit

large language model (LLM) *see* AI
learning: analytics (*see* data analytics); associative 18, 24, 187; educational models of 203, 204, 215, 225, 245; learning engineering 6, 14, 17, 18, 22, 24, 63; learning logs 22, 246, 250–3, 256; science of 63; self-paced learning 114; transfer of (transfer appropriate processing) 186, 188–90, 198, 202, 279; *see also* cognition and competence

machine learning *see* AI
medical education: continuing professional development 17, 23, 111–12, 114, 118; graduate 9, 37; post-graduate 111–12, 116–18, 127; undergraduate 111–12, 115–16; *see also* health professions education
medical pluralism 20, 245
metacognition 21, 148, 172, 177–8, 180, 213, 232, 233, 245; quantitative measurement of 225–9; qualitative assessment of 248–9, 252
models of learning: apprenticeship model (*see* competence); competency-based medical education (*see* competence); *see also* learning

Printed in the United States
by Baker & Taylor Publisher Services

Printed in the United States
by Baker & Taylor Publisher Services